NEUROANATOMY
P R I M E R

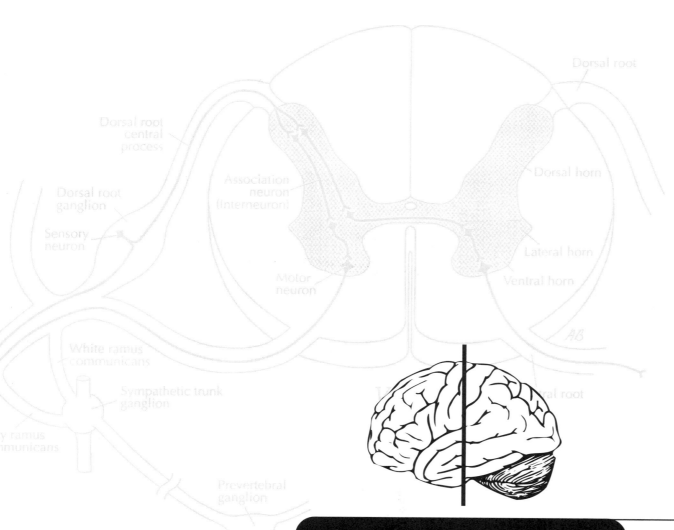

Dorsal root

Dorsal root
central
process

Association
neuron
(Interneuron)

Dorsal horn

Dorsal root
ganglion

Sensory
neuron

Lateral horn

Motor
neuron

Ventral horn

White ramus
communicans

Sympathetic trunk
ganglion

ral root

Gray ramus
communicans

Prevertebral
ganglion

COLOR TO LEARN

NEUROANATOMY
P R I M E R

M. Evelyn McNeill, Ph.D.
Department of Anatomy and Cell Biology
East Carolina University School of Medicine
Greenville, North Carolina

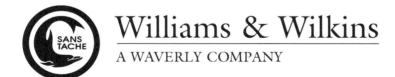

Williams & Wilkins
A WAVERLY COMPANY

BALTIMORE • PHILADELPHIA • LONDON • PARIS • BANGKOK
HONG KONG • MUNICH • SYDNEY • TOKYO • WROCLAW

COLOR TO LEARN

Editor: Jane Velker
Managing Editor: Crystal Taylor
Production Coordinator: Danielle Hagan
Book Project Editor: Robert D. Magee
Designer: Nancy Hagan Abbott
Cover Designer: Nancy Hagan Abbott
Typesetter: Peirce Graphic Services, Inc.
Printer: Edwards Brothers Incorporated
Binder: Edwards Brothers Incorporated

351 West Camden Street
Baltimore, Maryland 21201-2436 USA

Rose Tree Corporate Center
1400 North Providence Road
Building II, Suite 5025
Media, Pennsylvania 19063-2043 USA

Accurate indications, adverse reactions and dosage schedules for drugs are provided in this book, but it is possible that they may change. The reader is urged to review the package information data of the manufacturers of the medications mentioned.

Printed in the United States of America

First Edition

Library of Congress Cataloging-in-Publication Data

McNeill, M. Evelyn.
   Neuroanatomy primer : color to learn / M. Evelyn McNeill.—1st ed.
       p.   cm.
   Includes index.
   ISBN 0-683-30067-9
   1. Neuroanatomy—Atlases.   2. Neuroanatomy—Problems, exercises, etc.   3. Neuroanatomy—Examinations, questions, etc.   4. Coloring books.   I. Title.
   [DNLM: 1.   Central   Nervous   System—anatomy & history—atlases.
2.   Central   Nervous   System—anatomy & histology—examination   questions.
3. Magnetic Resonance Imaging—atlases.   4. Magnetic Resonance Imaging—examination questions.   WL   17   M478n   1997]
QM451.M37   1997
611′.8—dc21
DNLM/DLC
for Library of Congress   96-46125
                                                                                          CIP

The publishers have made every effort to trace the copyright holders for borrowed material. If they have inadvertently overlooked any, they will be pleased to make the necessary arrangements at the first opportunity.

To purchase additional copies of this book, call our customer service department at **(800) 638-0672** or fax orders to **(800) 447-8438.** For other book services, including chapter reprints and large quantity sales, ask for the Special Sales department. Canadian customers should call **(800) 268-4178,** or fax **(905) 470-6780.** For all other calls originating outside of the United States, please call **(410) 528-4223** or fax us at **(410) 528-8550.**

Visit Williams & Wilkins on the Internet: **http://www.wwilkins.com** or contact our customer service department at **custserv@wwilkins.com.** Williams & Wilkins customer service representatives are available from 8:30 am to 6:00 pm, EST, Monday through Friday, for telephone access.

97 98 99
1 2 3 4 5 6 7 8 9 10

Dedication

To Mary Lee Watson McNeill

1901-1995

As a white candle in a holy place, so is the beauty of an aged face. — Joseph Campbell

Preface

Midway into the "Decade of the Brain," exciting and novel technology continues to expand our knowledge of the human nervous system and to create an enormous focus on the neurosciences. Recent discoveries are so intriguing, it is tempting to favor functional studies and bypass basic neuroanatomy. There is, however, a "core" knowledge of vocabulary, concepts, and topographical relationships of the nervous system that is essential for understanding the most complex system of the body. Difficulties encountered by students beginning to unravel the mysteries of the brain include the:

1. Inability to visualize spatial relationships

2. Frustration of deciding which facts are significant, and

3. Interconnectivity of the nervous system, making it difficult to understand until a considerable volume of the material is mastered

My priorities in creating *Neuroanatomy Primer: Color to Learn* have been accuracy, visual clarity, and clinical relevance. The purpose of the visual format is to present the basics of a difficult subject as clearly as possible, to counter the problems listed above, and to whet student interest in a fascinating subject! Brevity and quick access to vital information are of paramount importance to students.

"[T]here appear to be two modes of thinking, verbal and nonverbal, represented rather separately in left and right hemispheres, respectively, and that our educational system, as well as science in general, tends to neglect the nonverbal form of intellect. What it comes down to is that modern society discriminates against the right hemisphere."

—Nobel Laureate Roger W. Sperry

Most learning programs deal first with verbal information, which is supported by visual complements. The aim of this book, which is formatted into double-page spreads of corresponding text and art pages, is to equalize the right-left hemisphere involvement to help students in their study of neuroanatomy. Holistic or gestalt perception is attributed to the right hemisphere.

Neuroanatomy Primer: Color to Learn includes professional line drawings, which are linked to the "Color to Learn" feature, magnetic resonance images (MRIs), and dissection photographs. The interactivity of "Color to Learn" and the way in which the illustrations are labeled encourage students to test themselves in recalling names, spelling, spatial relationships, and connectivity of the nervous system. The MRIs include sagittal, coronal, and axial planes. The coronal MRIs are especially helpful in showing the ventricular system and negating the need for actual dissections in that plane. Among the dissection visuals in this book are eight dissections prepared by the Klingler method and reprinted with permission from Ludwig and Klingler's *Atlas Cerebri Humani,* which is out of print. In particular, the dissections from the medial and lateral surfaces help one appreciate fiber connections through the core of the diencephalon and telencephalon. It is my hope that appreciating the beauty of the brain will lessen the significant challenge of understanding it.

Neuroanatomy Primer: Color to Learn, created to serve as a visual companion to an in-depth text, also includes study questions with answers and explanations at the end of each chapter. Composite summaries in the two-page spreads form a particularly valuable tool to aid students in their initial study of the central nervous system and for the United States Medical Licensing Examination (USMLE) or other paramedical licensing examinations. Basic "Clinical Correlations" are visually set apart as an important feature to facilitate licensure preparation.

coronal – crown, ~~bisect~~

sagittal – bisects

Acknowledgments

Alan E. Branigan of the Center for Health Sciences Communication (CHSC) at East Carolina University School of Medicine (ECU-SOM) has painstakingly produced superbly simple, aesthetic drawings of complex concepts. As Artwork Director, Alan called forth his artistic talent, knowledge of neuroanatomy, and computer technology. In addition to overseeing all of the art, he is responsible for the artwork in Chapters 2, 3, and 5. The delicacy of Alan's pen work invites one to explore his drawings. I acknowledge Alan's perfectionist skill with deep appreciation.

Laurels go to three additional artists: Charlotte A. Bauer, largely responsible for the drawings in Chapter 1; Wayne C. Williams, who provided drawings for Chapter 4; and Juan Garcia, who created most of the blood supply drawings in Chapter 6.

I gratefully acknowledge Dr. Michael D. Weaver's intellectual and technical assistance in creating the magnetic resonance images (MRIs) in Chapter 7 and an angiogram and computed tomogram (CT) in Chapter 6.

I am particularly grateful to Ms. Debbie H. Nichols for typing the manuscript.

Neuroanatomy Primer: Color to Learn evolved through innumerable suggestions from medical, graduate, and undergraduate students since 1986. My heartfelt thanks go to every student whose input has played a valuable role in creating this learning tool. I especially wish to thank Drs. Charles D. Finley and Robin M. Moherek who, as students, assisted me on this project one summer.

Numerous colleagues have contributed to this endeavor. Dr. Robert L. Timmons deserves special recognition for the spirit in which he instigated and coordinated the clinical lectures on the nervous system at East Carolina University School of Medicine. Dr. Jacqueline F. McGinty made helpful suggestions relative to the illustrations of the hypothalamus and limbic system. Drs. Jack E. Brinn and Irvin E. Lawrence, Jr. have provided encouragement through their interest, advice, and support. I am indebted to Dr. Ervin Powell for introducing me to the dissection method of Dr. Klingler.

I also wish to thank my colleagues who reviewed the manuscript. Drs. Hubert W. Burden and Gary M. Peterson carefully critiqued the cranial nerves, and Dr. David M. Terrian reviewed the section on the cerebellum. Professor Emeritus, Isabel Lockard, Ph.D., author of *Desk Reference for Neuroscience,* graciously critiqued the manuscript. Dr. Lennart Heimer, author of *The Human Brain and Spinal Cord,* offered valuable comments regarding olfactory connections. Dr. Duane E. Haines, author of *Neuroanatomy: An Atlas of Structures, Sections, and Systems,* provided a thorough review of the entire book. Drs. Stuart K. Lee and Griffith J. Steel offered valuable critiques on Chapter 6, as did Joe Coleman, Bryan Edwards, David Lutz, Ness Kahn, and Julie Nelson.

I am particularly indebted to my colleague Dr. Ronald W. Dudek, who read the entire manuscript while it was in progress. I greatly appreciate his ability to immediately perceive problem areas and his manner of making suggestions without dogma. Criticisms are easy to accept when they are attended so promptly and so nonassertively.

Finally, I wish to express my appreciation to the staff at Williams and Wilkins who found solutions to whatever problems were encountered. In particular I thank Debra Dreger, Jane Velker, Crystal Taylor, and Danielle Hagan for bringing this project to fruition.

M. Evelyn McNeill
Greenville, North Carolina

Introduction

In the experience of the author, color coding motor and sensory pathways and the seven different functional components of spinal and cranial nerves has proven immensely beneficial to students. The proprioceptive act and mental concentration involved keep one motivated and help to commit information to memory. However, this needs to be kept as simple as possible.

A set of colored pencils has been provided with this book; they are preferable to felt-tipped pens, as pencils do not bleed through the page. Generally, the structures of the central nervous system (brain and spinal cord) are bilaterally symmetrical (identical left and right sides). For visual simplicity, it seems to work best to study a pathway and to color one side only.

Descending pathways that end in motor nuclei are described as efferent; color these red. The motor component or final common pathway of spinal nerves may end on striated skeletal muscle or in autonomic ganglia for relay to visceral structures, e.g., smooth muscle. Consequently, they are classified, respectively, as general somatic efferent (GSE) and general visceral efferent (GVE). Ascending pathways are described as afferent, or sensory; color these blue. The functional components of spinal and cranial nerves will be explained in the text. These components may be colored as follows:

General somatic afferent (GSA): blue
General somatic efferent (GSE): red
General visceral afferent (GVA): purple

General visceral efferent (GVE): orange
Special somatic afferent (SSA): yellow
Special visceral afferent (SVA): brown
Special visceral efferent (SVE): green

For many students, the "Color to Learn" method seems to be an effective way to commit to memory the functions of the various cranial nerves. Understanding cranial nerve functions is crucial to doing a physical examination. The combined presentation of the peripheral course of cranial nerves and the brain stem location of the nuclei in dorsal, midsagittal, and transverse planes is particularly beneficial.

Study guides, board review books with questions, and advice from professionals who have cleared the hurdle of licensure examinations are helpful. Nonetheless, these measures pale in comparison with the value of creating your own review source. Whether you are qualifying to practice medicine, nursing, physical, occupational, or speech therapy, or to become a psychology counselor, using the "Color to Learn" feature along with compiling your personal notes in this book is worthy of the effort. This will enable you to maximize your review time, and, just perhaps, to enjoy it!

Contents

Chapter One: Gross Brain

Descriptive Terms 2, 3
Development of the Mature Brain From the Brain Vesicles 4, 5
Sutures and Fontanels in the Skull of a Neonate 6, 7
Ventricles, Lateral View 8, 9
Ventricles, Superior View 10, 11
Venous Sinuses of Dura Mater 12, 13
Cranial Fossae, Dural Venous Sinuses, Tentorium Cerebelli 14, 15
Tentorium Cerebelli, Descending Herniations 16, 17
Lobes of the Cerebral Hemisphere 18, 19
Sulci of the Cerebral Hemisphere 20, 21
Gyri of the Lateral Surface 22, 23
Gyri of the Medial Surface 24, 25
Gyri and Other Structures of the Inferior Surface: Cerebellum and
    Brain Stem Removed 26, 27
Selected Brodmann's Areas, Lateral Surface 28, 29
Selected Brodmann's Areas, Medial Surface 30, 31
Fibers of the Cerebral Hemispheres 32, 33
A Superior View of the Cerebrum 34, 35
Medial Surface of the Brain with Blood Vessels Removed Showing Sulci,
    Gyri, and Median Features 36, 37
Lateral Surface of the Left Cerebral Hemisphere Showing Sulci and Gyri 38, 39
Dissection of the Left Hemisphere from the Lateral Surface 40, 41
Chapter One Study Questions 42, 44
Answers and Explanations for Chapter One Study Questions 43, 45

Chapter Two: The Spinal Cord

The Relation of the Spinal Cord and Spinal Nerves to the Meninges
    and Vertebral Column 46, 47
Transverse Section of the Spinal Cord Showing a Somatic Reflex Arc 48, 49
Spinal Cord at Lumbosacral Enlargement (S1) 50, 51
Spinal Cord at High Lumbar level (L2) 52, 53
Spinal Cord at High Thoracic Level (T2) 54, 55
Spinal Cord at Cervical Enlargement (C7) 56, 57
Spinal Cord Summary Including Blood Supply 58, 59
Chapter Two Study Questions 60
Answers and Explanations for Chapter Two Study Questions 61

Chapter Three: The Brain Stem, Cranial Nerves and Cerebellum

Medial View of Brain Stem Nuclei Excluding Cranial Nerve Nuclei 62, 63
Cross-Sectional Levels 64, 65
Caudal Medulla at Level of Pyramidal (Motor) Decussation 66, 67
Medulla at Level of Decussation of Medial Lemniscus (Sensory Decussation) 68, 69
"Open" Medulla at Level of Inferior Olivary Nucleus 70, 71
Rostral Medulla at Level of Dorsal Cochlear Nucleus 72, 73
Oblique Section Through Caudal Pons Medullopontine Junction 74, 75
Pons at Level of Trapezoid Body and Facial Colliculus 76, 77
Rostral Pons at Level of Locus Ceruleus 78, 79
Pons at Level of Isthmus 80, 81
Mesencephalon at Level of Inferior Colliculus 82, 83
Mesencephalon at Level of Superior Colliculus 84, 85
Cranial Nerve Summary 86
Cranial Nerve Nuclei and Components 87
Cranial Nerve I, Olfactory 88, 89
Cranial Nerve II, Optic 90, 91
Cranial Nerve III, Oculomotor 92, 93
Cranial Nerve IV, Trochlear 94, 95
Cranial Nerve V, Trigeminal 96, 97
Cranial Nerve VI, Abducens 98, 99
Cranial Nerve VII, Facial 100, 101
Cranial Nerve VIII, Vestibulocochlear 102, 103
Cranial Nerve IX, Glossopharyngeal 104, 105
Cranial Nerve X, Vagus 106, 107
Cranial Nerve XI, (Spinal) Accessory 108, 109
Cranial Nerve XII, Hypoglossal 110, 111
Intramedullary Course of the Cranial Nerves 112, 113
Basal View of the Diencephalon, Brain Stem and Cerebellum 114, 115
Base of Skull, Calvaria Removed, Internal Aspect 116. 117
Median Section Through the Skull, Internal Aspect of the Left Basal Portion 118, 119
Dorsal and Ventral Spinocerebellar and Cuneocerebellar Tracts:
    Proprioceptive Input 120, 121
Brain Stem Lesions and Syndromes 122, 123
Chapter Three Study Questions 124
Answers and Explanations for Chapter Three Study Questions 125

Chapter Four: Pathways

Lateral View of Major Pathways in the Brain Stem 126, 127
Ventrolateral System: Pain, Temperature and Nondiscriminative Touch 128, 129
Trigeminal System: Pain, Temperature, Touch, Pressure and Proprioception 130, 131
Dorsal Column—Medial Lemniscal System: Proprioception, Vibration, Pressure
    and Discriminative Touch 132, 133
Spinal Cord Ascending Pathways: Somatosensory Pathways (Limbs and Trunk) 134
Spinal Cord Ascending Pathways 135
Lateral and Ventral Corticospinal Tracts: Volitional Control of Limbs and Trunk . . 136, 137
Descending Pathways Converge on Motor Neurons 138, 139
Corticobulbar Tract: Volitional Control of the Face and Head 140, 141
Corticobulbar and Corticospinal Summary 142, 143
Sympathetic (Thoracolumbar) Division of the Autonomic Nervous System 144, 145
Parasympathetic (Craniosacral) Division of the Autonomic Nervous System 146, 147
Dissection of the Left Hemisphere and Brain Stem From the Lateral Surface 148, 149
Dissection of the Left Hemisphere from the Medial Surface with Brain Stem and
    Cerebellum Cut Midsagittally 150, 151
Chapter Four Study Questions 152
Answers and Explanations for Chapter Four Study Questions 153

Chapter Five: The Forebrain

Forebrain at the Level of the Striatum and Nucleus Accumbens 154, 155
Forebrain at the Level of the Anterior Nucleus of the Thalamus 156, 157
Forebrain at the Level of the Midthalamus 158, 159
Thalamic Nuclei 160, 161
Hypothalamic Nuclei 162
Medial View of the Hypothalamus and Coronal Section 163
A Horizontal Section of the Brain through the Basal Ganglia, Thalamus
    and Internal Capsule 164, 165
Limbic System Structures: Dissection of the Right Hemisphere
    from the Medial Surface, Thalamic Radiations Exposed 166, 167
Limbic System Connections 168, 169
Dissection of the Right Hemisphere from the Lateral Surface, Putamen
    and Hippocampus Exposed 170, 171
Dissection of the Right Hemisphere from the Lateral Surface, Internal Capsule and
    Optic Radiations Exposed 172, 173
Dissection of the Right Hemisphere from the Medial Surface, Caudate Nucleus and
    Limbic Structures Exposed 174, 175
Chapter Five Study Questions 176, 178
Answers and Explanations for Chapter Five Study Questions 177, 179

Chapter Six: Blood Supply of the Forebrain

Circle of Willis 180, 181
General Blood Supply of the Brain 182, 183
Blood Supply of the Basal Ganglia, Thalamus and Internal Capsule 184, 185
Blood Supply of the Brain, Lateral View 186, 187
Blood Supply of the Brain, Medial View 188, 189
Blood Supply of the Visual System 190, 191
Regional Blood Supply of the Main Cerebral Arteries 192, 193
Computed Tomography Demonstration of Intracranial Hemorrhage 194, 195
Angiography, Aneurysms and an Angiogram of an Internal Carotid Aneurysm 196
Angiogram of an Internal Carotid Aneurysm 197
Chapter Six Study Questions 198
Answers and Explanations for Chapter Six Study Questions 199

Chapter Seven: T1 Magnetic Resonance Images (MRI)

Midline Sagittal T1 MRI Through the Cerebral Aqueduct 200, 201
Sagittal T1 MRI Through the Cerebral Peduncle 202, 203
Sagittal T1 MRI Through the Lateral Ventricle, Inferior Horn 204, 205
Coronal T1 MRI Through the Lateral Ventricle, Anterior Horn 206, 207
Coronal T1 MRI Through the Caudate Nucleus, Head 208, 209
Coronal T1 MRI Through the Internal Capsule, Posterior Limb 210, 211
Coronal T1 MRI Through the Lateral Ventricle, Posterior Horn 212, 213
Axial T1 MRI Through the Diencephalon 214, 215
Axial T1 MRI Through the Midbrain 216, 217
Axial T1 MRI Through the Pons 218, 219
Axial T1 MRI Through the "Open" Medulla 220, 221
Chapter Seven Study Questions 222
Answers and Explanations for Chapter Seven Study Questions 223

Index 224

Chapter One **Gross Brain**	Chapter Two **The Spinal Cord**	Chapter Three **Brain Stem, Cranial Nerves and Cerebellum**	Chapter Four **Pathways**	Chapter Five **The Forebrain**	Chapter Six **Blood Supply of the Forebrain**	Chapter Seven **T1 Magnetic Resonance Images (MRI)**
2	**46**	**62**	**126**	**154**	**180**	**200**

CHAPTER 1 Descriptive Terms

The **sagittal (median) plane,** named after the cranial suture, divides the brain vertically into right and left halves.

Coronal (frontal) planes, named after the coronal suture, are vertical planes at right angles to the median plane.

Horizontal (axial) planes are those which traverse the brain at right angles to both the median and coronal planes.

Rostral indicates that a particular entity is nearer the rostrum (beak or nose) and is therefore anterior. **Caudal** refers to the tail or posterior position.

Proximal and **distal** refer to positions nearer to or farther from, respectively, the median plane or any designated starting point.

Self-explanatory combined terms are used for intermediate positional arrangements. An example is **anterolateral.**

In anatomy, **unilateral** refers to entities or functions located on or affecting only one side, whereas **bilateral** describes those affecting both sides of the body or central nervous system (CNS).

Ipsilateral refers to structures or events situated on or affecting the same side of the body, e.g., cerebral cortex, whereas **contralateral** means occurring on or acting in conjunction with similar parts on the opposite side.

Supratentorial and **infratentorial** refer to structures above or below the tentorium cerebelli, which anatomically separates the brain stem and cerebellum from the cerebral hemispheres (see pages 15 and 17).

The **telencephalon** is the most anterior subdivision of the embryonic brain; the cerebral hemispheres develop from it. The telencephalon is derived from the prosencephalon (forebrain).

The **gray matter** consists of cell bodies of neurons that are specialized for communication. They aggregate on the surface in layers and in subcortical masses of various shapes. Gray matter describes cellular regions.

The **white matter** consists of nerve fibers and their myelin sheaths, which are white in freshly cut sections.

Cerebral cortex (bark) is the outer region covering each hemisphere. It is composed of nerve cells arranged in 3 to 6 horizontal layers and identified by Roman numerals I–VI, from the surface to the underlying white matter, respectively.

The **diencephalon** is the most medial gray subdivision of the prosencephalon. It consists of the **epithalamus,** the **thalamus,** the **subthalamus,** and **the hypothalamus.**

Basal ganglia are subcortical masses of gray matter of the telencephalon, classically comprising the **caudate nucleus, putamen, globus pallidus, amygdala,** and **claustrum.** Most often this term is limited to the **corpus striatum,** i.e., the **caudate nucleus, putamen,** and **globus pallidus,** which is important in the control of movement.

The **thalamus** is the part of the diencephalon located on either side of the third ventricle just above the hypothalamic sulcus. It is bounded laterally by the internal capsule and is considered to be the "gateway" to the cortex.

The **internal capsule** is a mass of nerve fibers (white matter) located between the caudate and thalamic nuclei medially and the **lenticular nucleus** (i.e., putamen and globus pallidus) laterally. It connects the cerebral cortex with various subcortical centers.

The **cerebral hemisphere** comprises the cerebral cortex, the medullary center (white matter), the olfactory system, and the corpus striatum.

 Color the cortex blue in the coronal and horizontal views of the telencephalon (bottom row). Color the thalamus blue. Color the caudate, putamen, and lenticular nuclei red.

Descriptive Terms

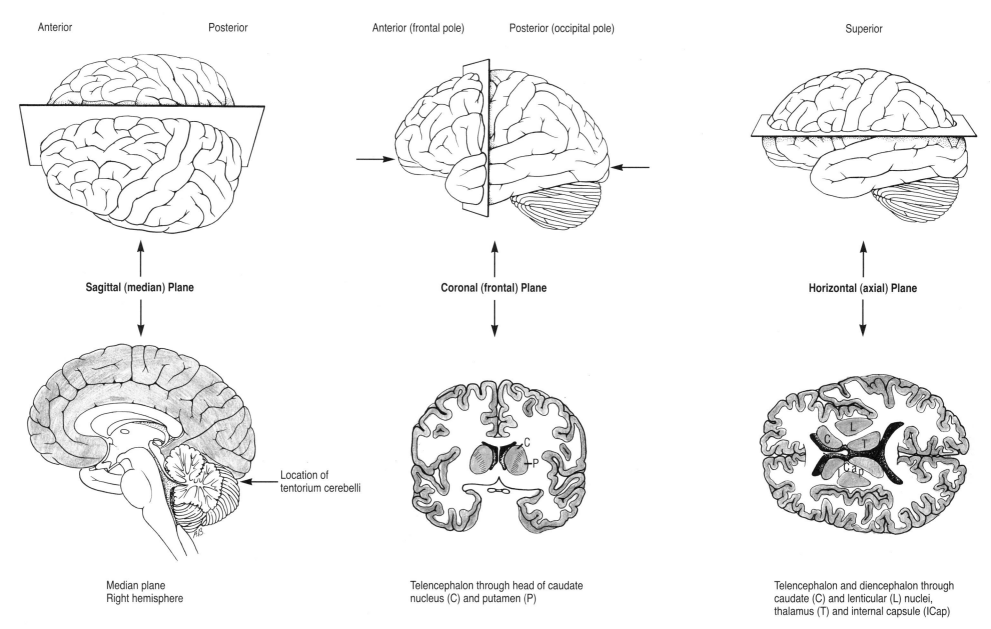

Anterior   Posterior

Anterior (frontal pole)   Posterior (occipital pole)

Superior

Sagittal (median) Plane

Coronal (frontal) Plane

Horizontal (axial) Plane

Location of
tentorium cerebelli

Median plane
Right hemisphere

Telencephalon through head of caudate
nucleus (C) and putamen (P)

Telencephalon and diencephalon through
caudate (C) and lenticular (L) nuclei,
thalamus (T) and internal capsule (ICap)

Development of the Mature Brain from the Brain Subdivisions

The brain and spinal cord are derived from the ectoderm of the embryo. The **neural plate,** whose formation is induced by the developing notochord, invaginates on day 18 and forms a longitudinal median groove with **neural folds** on either side. By the end of week 3, the neural folds move together to form the **neural tube,** which has openings at either end called the **rostral** and **caudal neuropores.** The brain and spinal cord make up the CNS whereas the cranial and spinal nerves and all their branches, together with the autonomic and sensory ganglia, make up the peripheral nervous system (PNS). The **neural crest,** which lies on either wide of the neural tube, forms most elements of the PNS (see page 48).

Neurulation describes the processes involved in the formation of the neural plate, neural folds, and neural tube. The neural folds at the rostal end become prominent at the first sign of brain development. Neurulation is completed when the cranial and caudal neuropores close during week 4. Failure of the neural tube to close normally results in congenital malformations of the CNS (Clinical Correlations).

At week 4, the major divisions of the CNS are present such that the neural tube consists of three subdivisions: the **prosencephalon (forebrain), mesencephalon (midbrain),** and **rhombencephalon (hindbrain).** By the end of week 5 there are five subdivisions. The prosencephalon differentiates into the **telencephalon** and **diencephalon;** the configuration of the **mesencephalon** remains unchanged, and the rhombencephalon differentiates into the **metencephalon** and **myelencephalon.**

The lumen of the neural tube is the forerunner of the ependyma-lined ventricular cavities in the core of the brain. The lateral ventricles are bilateral cavities away from the midline that extend into the frontal, parietal, temporal, and occipital lobes of the telencephalon. The **third** and **fourth ventricles** are single cavities connected by the narrow **cerebral aqueduct** (CA) of the midbrain (also called the aqueduct of Sylvius). The **third ventricle** is in the midline in the **diencephalon** and the **fourth ventricle** is dorsal to the **pons** and **rostral** (open) **medulla** and ventral to the **cerebellum.** The **caudal** (closed) **medulla** contains a small cavity that is continuous with the central canal of the spinal cord.

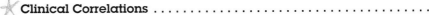

Clinical Correlations

Anencephaly occurs when the cerebral hemispheres (and frequently the diencephalon) fail to develop due to lack of fusion of the neural folds at the rostral end of the developing neural tube. It is the most serious malformation seen in stillbirths and is incompatible with life, but occurs in approximately 1 of every 1000 live births. The neural tube defects show marked epidemiologic variations, which suggests environmental influences. **Spina bifida cystica** occurs when there is incomplete fusion at the caudal neuropore and there is herniation of the meninges (**meningocele**) or of the spinal cord and the meninges (**meningomyelocele**) through a vertebral defect. In **spina bifida occulta** there is defective closure of one or more vertebrae; however, the dura and skin remain intact. The skin overlying the defect is often marked by a tuft of hair; usually, there are no symptoms. However, the bony defect may predispose an individual to injury such as trauma sustained in a fall or in an automobile accident.

Cerebrospinal fluid that fills the ventricles is clear and colorless. Nonetheless, color the cavities light blue to facilitate imprinting the important fact that only the lateral ventricles are bilateral and are therefore away from the midline. The primary goal at this point is to learn terminology and spelling. The secondary goal is to associate the ventricles with their location in the neuraxis. The tertiary goal is to relate the mature structures to one of the five subdivisions of the brain.

Development of the Mature Brain from the Brain Subdivisions

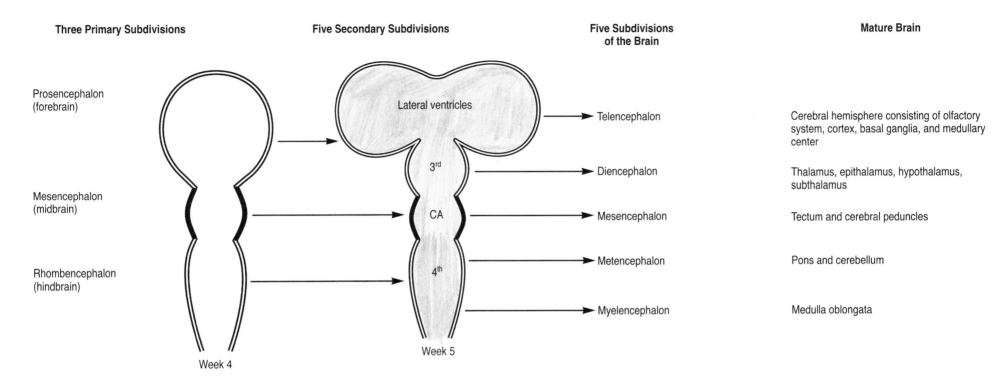

Three Primary Subdivisions	Five Secondary Subdivisions	Five Subdivisions of the Brain	Mature Brain

Prosencephalon (forebrain)

Mesencephalon (midbrain)

Rhombencephalon (hindbrain)

Lateral ventricles

3rd

CA

4th

Week 4

Week 5

→ Telencephalon → Cerebral hemisphere consisting of olfactory system, cortex, basal ganglia, and medullary center

→ Diencephalon → Thalamus, epithalamus, hypothalamus, subthalamus

→ Mesencephalon → Tectum and cerebral peduncles

→ Metencephalon → Pons and cerebellum

→ Myelencephalon → Medulla oblongata

Sutures and Fontanels in the Skull of a Neonate

Definitions

Bregma is the point on the skull where the coronal and sagittal sutures meet, at the juncture of the frontal bones with the two parietal bones.

Lambda is the point of juncture of the occipital bone and the two parietal bones of the skull where the lambdoid and sagittal sutures meet in the form of a lambda (λ).

The **pterion** overlies the middle meningeal artery or its anterior branch and is an important neurosurgical landmark. It is the point at which the greater wing of the sphenoid bone meets both the parietal bone and the squamous part of the temporal bone.

Clinical Correlations . . . .

At birth, the calvarial bones (i.e., skull cap) are separated by fibrous sutures that permit the skull to enlarge during infancy. Most of the separations or fontanels close within 2 to 3 months; however, the anterior fontanel, being the largest, does not become fully closed until 18 to 24 months of age. Severely increased intracranial pressure prior to "mature" suture closure at 12 years of age may expand the calvarial bones and result in an enlarged head (i.e., macrocephaly) (page 10, discussion of enlarged ventricles [hydrocephalus]).

Bregma is used as a neuroradiologic point of reference to determine the location of certain intracranial structures such as the venous angle (page 13). **Lambda** also can be used as a neuroradiologic point of reference.

An epidural hematoma is a collection of blood between the dura and the skull. The most common **epidural hematoma** occurs in the temporal fossa due to damage to the middle meningeal artery where it underlies the **pterion.** As the hematoma pushes the temporal lobe medially, it causes the **uncal herniation syndrome** (pages 16 and 17).

Color the frontal bones red, the parietal bones blue, the occipital bone yellow, the temporal bone brown, the sphenoid bone purple, the maxilla orange, and the mandible green.

Absence lessens half-hearted passions, and increases great ones,
as the wind puts out candles and yet stirs up the fire. – Duc De La Rochefoucauld

6

Sutures and Fontanels in the Skull of a Neonate

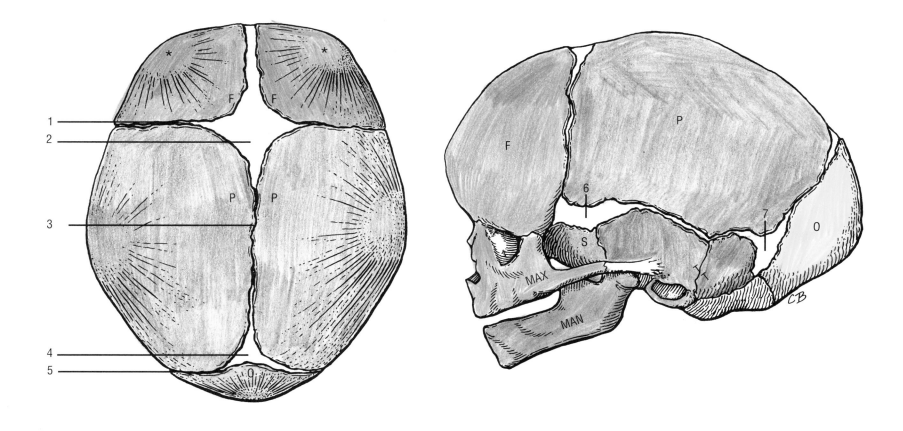

1. Coronal suture
2. Anterior fontanel (bregma)
3. Sagittal suture
4. Posterior fontanel (lambda)

5. Lambdoid suture
6. Left anterolateral fontanel (pterion)
7. Left posterolateral fontanel
   * Ossification centers

F.	Frontal bone
O.	Occipital bone
P.	Parietal bone
S.	Sphenoid bone
T.	Temporal bone
MAX	Maxilla
MAN	Mandible

Ventricles, Lateral View

Definition
Ventricles are irregularly shaped cavities within the brain that contain cerebrospinal fluid (CSF). An **aperture** is an opening such as a hole or gap.

Structural and Functional Features
CSF is continuously produced by the **choroid plexus** in the floor of the lateral ventricles and in the roof of the third and fourth ventricles. CSF circulates through the ventricles, exits the ventricular system through the apertures of the fourth ventricle, and fills the subarachnoid space. It is absorbed into the venous circulation via active and passive transport through the arachnoid villi, which project into the dural venous sinuses. The main site of the absorption is through the superior sagittal sinus and adjacent lacunae (lateral dilatations).

Clinical Correlations . . . .

A **cistern** (reservoir) is a widened part of the subarachnoid space where the arachnoid spans irregularities on the surface of the brain and in the vertebral canal caudal to the spinal cord. The volume of CSF ranges from **80 to 150 mL,** approximately **40 mL** of which is contained within the ventricles. Total replacement of CSF occurs several times daily. Normal pressure in the lumbar cistern (measured in the recumbent position) is **80 to 180 cm H₂O**. CSF is clear and colorless and contains very few cells, mainly lymphocytes. More than 10 cells per mL is usually indicative of disease.

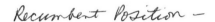

Recumbent Position —

Concentrate visually on the shape of the ventricles. Peruse the Imaging section in Chapter 7, directing your attention solely to the shape of the ventricles. Color the ventricles light blue in the direction of flow of the CSF, i.e., from lateral ventricles to the third ventricle and via the cerebral aqueduct to the fourth ventricle, and out through the exit apertures into the subarachnoid space. Only a ghost of the right lateral ventricle is apparent.

Ventricles, Lateral View

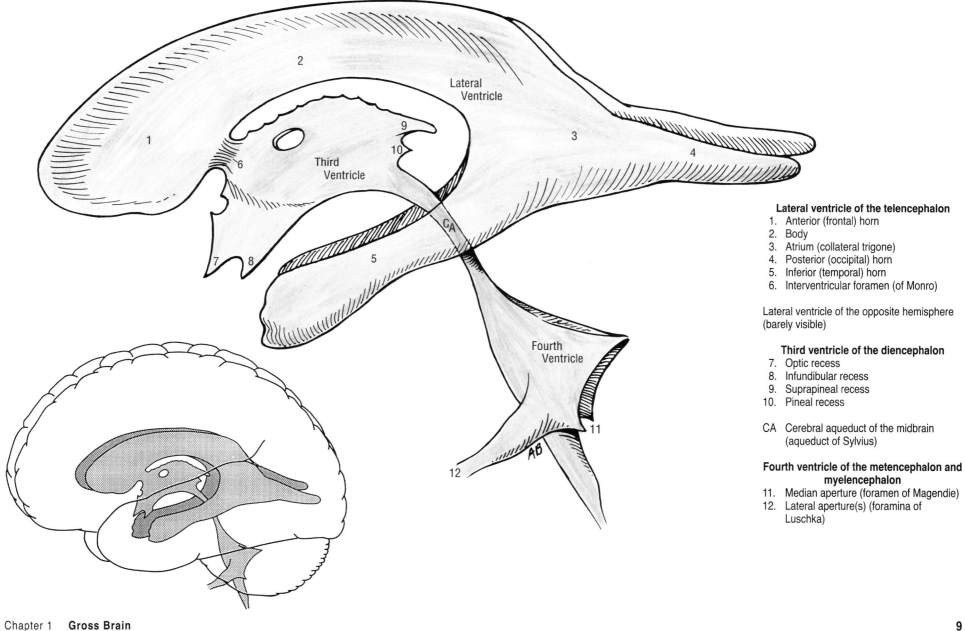

Lateral Ventricle

Third
Ventricle

CA

Fourth
Ventricle

Lateral ventricle of the telencephalon
1. Anterior (frontal) horn
2. Body
3. Atrium (collateral trigone)
4. Posterior (occipital) horn
5. Inferior (temporal) horn
6. Interventricular foramen (of Monro)

Lateral ventricle of the opposite hemisphere
(barely visible)

Third ventricle of the diencephalon
7. Optic recess
8. Infundibular recess
9. Suprapineal recess
10. Pineal recess

CA Cerebral aqueduct of the midbrain
(aqueduct of Sylvius)

Fourth ventricle of the metencephalon and
myelencephalon
11. Median aperture (foramen of Magendie)
12. Lateral aperture(s) (foramina of
Luschka)

Ventricles, Superior View

Definition
The lateral ventricles are located in the telencephalon, the third ventricle is in the diencephalon, and the fourth ventricle is dorsal to the pons and the rostral part of the medulla, and ventral to the cerebellum.

Structural and Functional Features
The lateral ventricles are essentially **symmetrical** except for the **posterior horns.** The reason for their asymmetry is unknown. Observe how much closer to the midline the anterior horns are than are the posterior horns.

Clinical Correlations . . . .

If the flow of CSF within the ventricles is obstructed, the fluid accumulates proximal to the blockage and causes a condition known as **internal (obstructive) hydrocephalus.** After complete ossification of the skull bones (20 years) and the fibrous sutures between the skull bones (12 years), the increased pressure may cause destruction of nervous tissue. In infants, the head may become greatly enlarged (**macrocephaly**). **External hydrocephalus** is seen in patients with senile atrophy of the brain, in which excess CSF is mainly in the subarachnoid space. There is, however, some dilation of the ventricles. All the ventricles are enlarged if the foramina (apertures) of the fourth ventricle (Magendie and Luschka) are occluded. If the cerebral aqueduct is obstructed, both of the lateral ventricles and the third ventricle are enlarged. Blockage of one interventricular foramen (a rare occurrence) results in dilation of only one lateral ventricle. Blood from subarachnoid hemorrhage may obstruct the absorption of CSF by the arachnoid villi. This results in a combination of **internal** and **external hydrocephalus (communicating hydrocephalus)**.

Causes of hydrocephalus include **stenosis of the cerebral aqueduct** (most common) and the **Arnold-Chiari malformation**. Most cases of stenosis seem to relate to a fetal viral infection or prematurity associated with interventricular hemorrhage. The cause of the Arnold-Chiari malformation is uncertain, although it is associated with spina bifida. In this condition, the medulla and part of the cerebellum are displaced downward into the upper cervical spinal canal.

Color CSF light blue, again giving attention to the direction of flow. Correlate the configuration of the ventricles in coronal sections through the anterior, inferior, and posterior horns as you color. Again, perusing the magnetic resonance imaging (MRI) in Chapter 7 is helpful in this regard.

True eloquence consists in saying all that is necessary,
and nothing but what is necessary. – Duc De La Rochefoucauld

10

Ventricles, Superior View

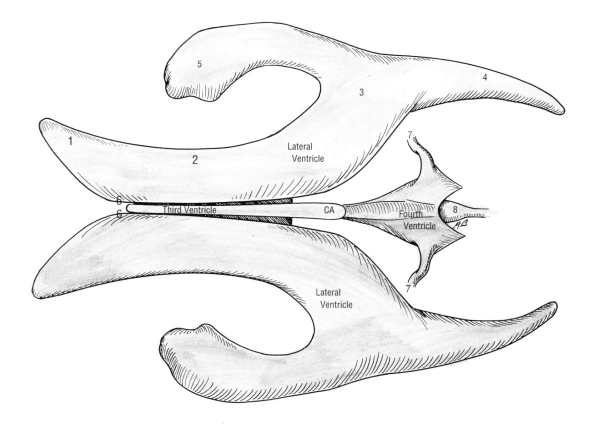

Lateral ventricles of the telencephalon
1. Anterior (frontal) horn
2. Body
3. Atrium (collateral trigone)
4. Posterior (occipital) horn
5. Inferior (temporal) horn
6. Interventricular foramina (of Monro)

Third ventricle of the diencephalon

CA Cerebral aqueduct of the midbrain
(aqueduct of Sylvius)

Fourth ventricle of the metencephalon and myelencephalon
7. Lateral apertures of Luschka
8. Median aperture of Magendie

Venous Sinuses of Dura Mater

Definitions

The **dura mater** (tough mother) is the outermost layer of the meninges (membranes) covering the brain and spinal cord. **Venous sinuses** are the valveless, endothelium-lined channels between the inner and outer layers of the dura mater. Within the cranium, venous blood ultimately drains to paired internal jugular veins via these channels. **Clivus** means slope or hill. It is the sloping bony anterior wall of the posterior cranial fossa from the dorsum sellae to the foramen magnum formed by parts of the sphenoid and occipital bones. The basilar venous plexus lies on the clivus.

Structural and Functional Features

The dorsolateral veins of the cerebral hemispheres drain to the **superior sagittal sinus**; those on the medial surface also drain to the **superior sagittal sinus.** The inferior sagittal sinus drians the falx cerebri, a sickle-shaped partition of the dura mater separating the right and left hemispheres. There are no large arteries in the depth or core of the brain, but there are large veins of clinical significance. The **thalamostriate vein** is continuous with the **internal cerebral vein** at the **venous angle.** The two internal cerebral veins are joined by the **basal veins (of Rosenthal)** to form the single **great cerebral vein (of Galen)** which drains into the **straight sinus**, as does the **inferior sagittal sinus.** The **confluence of sinuses** (torcular) is at the junction of the **straight sinus**, the **superior sagittal sinus** and the **left** and **right transverse sinuses.** Each **transverse sinus** makes an S-shaped turn as the **sigmoid sinuses**, which are continuous with the **internal jugular veins** at the jugular foramina. The **superior ophthalmic vein** and the **sphenoparietal sinus** drain to the **cavernous sinus**, which drains to the **basilar plexus, inferior petrosal sinus**, and **internal jugular vein.** The **superior petrosal sinus** drains to the upper end of the **sigmoid sinus.** The **inferior petrosal sinus** drains to the beginning of the **internal jugular vein.**

Clinical Correlations ·

Because there are no large arteries in the depth of the brain, the neuroradiologist uses the venous system to evaluate the deep structures of the hemispheres. The junction of the **thalamostriate vein** with the **internal cerebral vein,** at the level of the **interventricular foramen (of Monro**), forms the **venous angle.** On a frontal projection, the two angles can be used to fix the midline of the brain.

Blood in the veins and in the sinuses can be colored dark blue. Consider lumen size and direction of flow as you work.

When a man's hand touches the hand of a woman,
they both touch the heart of eternity. – Kahlil Gibran

Venous Sinuses of Dura Mater

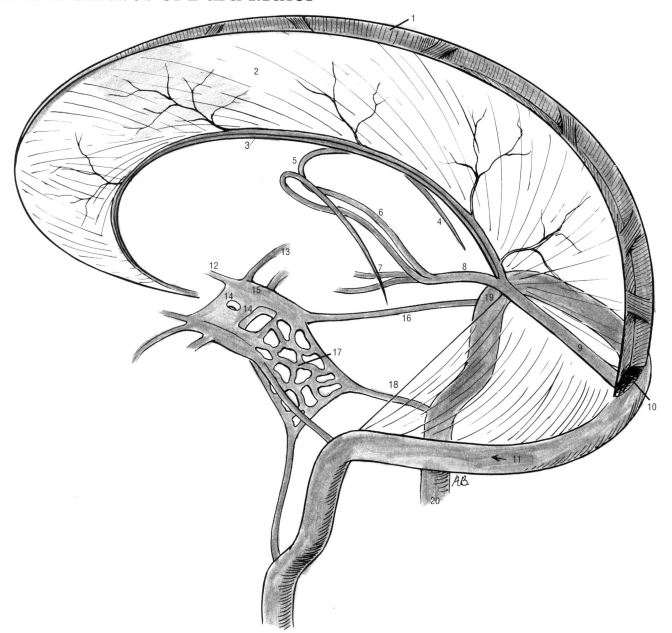

1. Superior sagittal sinus
2. Falx cerebri
3. Inferior sagittal sinus
4. Thalamostriate vein
5. Venous angle (at foramen of Monro)
6. Internal cerebral vein
7. Basal vein (of Rosenthal)
8. Great cerebral vein (of Galen) receives deep veins of the brain
9. Straight sinus
10. Confluence of sinuses (torcular)
11. Transverse sinus
12. Superior ophthalmic vein
13. Sphenoparietal sinus
14. Intercavernous sinuses
15. Right cavernous sinus (connects to left cavernous sinus by the intercavernous sinus)
16. Superior petrosal sinus
17. Basilar plexus on clivus
18. Inferior petrosal sinus
19. Sigmoid sinus
20. Internal jugular vein

Cranial Fossae, Dural Venous Sinuses, Tentorium Cerebelli

Definitions

The **planum sphenoidale** (jugum) is a flattened area of the sphenoid bone in the anterior cranial fossa. The **crista galli** is a bony ridge from the ethmoid bone that lies between the two olfactory bulbs. The **diaphragma sellae** is a dural partition through which the stalk of the pituitary gland in the **sella turcica** is connected to the brain, specifically to the hypothalamus of the diencephalon.

Structural and Functional Features

The **falx cerebri** attaches to the **crista galli** of the ethmoid bone; the axons of the **olfactory nerve** pass through its **cribriform** (sieve-like) **plate.** The **orbital plate** of the **frontal bone** is often very thin and therefore vulnerable to fracture. Both the **optic nerve** and the **ophthalmic artery** (not shown) traverse the **optic canal** whereas the **superior ophthalmic vein** passes through the superior orbital fissure. The drainage pattern and direction of flow of venous blood in the sinuses is detailed on page 12. The **oculomotor** and **trochlear nerves** and the **ophthalmic** and **maxillary divisions** of the **trigeminal nerve** are in the **lateral wall** of the cavernous sinus. The **internal carotid artery** and **plexus** and the **abducens nerve** run through the **cavernous sinus,** and the **superior ophthalmic vein** and **sphenoparietal sinus** drain into it. Details regarding the cranial fossae—two anterior, two middle, and one posterior—are presented in Chapter 3. The significant point to appreciate in this view is the "tent" or roof function of the tentorium cerebelli. It covers the brain stem and cerebellum in the posterior fossa and supports the occipital and posterior temporal lobes; the rostral brain stem and posterior cerebral artery traverse the tentorial notch (incisure; pages 16 and 17). The **medulla oblongata, meninges, vertebral arteries,** and **accessory nerves** pass through the **foramen magnum** at the base of the skull.

Clinical Correlations . . . .

Fractures of the thin orbital plate of the frontal bone in the anterior cranial fossa disrupt the meninges and subarachnoid space. **Leakage** of CSF through the nose and cribriform plate decreases CSF pressure. Disruption of the membranes indicates that the meninges may possibly become infected. The flat surface of the sphenoid bone, the **planum sphenoidale** (jugum), is important radiologically. **Meningiomas** sometimes occur in this region. Fractures of the **clivus** may disrupt the pituitary gland and damage the brain stem as well. Structures that run through the cavernous sinus, in contrast to those in the lateral wall, are most vulnerable in **thrombosis** of the sinus.

Color the ophthalmic vein dark blue. Color the sinuses dark blue in the direction of the venous blood flow. Color the optic nerve yellow. Indicate on the diagram the structures in the lateral wall of the cavernous sinus and the structures that run through it.

Cranial Fossae, Dural Venous Sinuses, Tentorium Cerebelli

Structures in lateral wall of the cavernous sinus:

- oculomotor & trochlear nerves
- opthalmic & maxillary divisions of the trigeminal nerve

Structures that run through the cavernous sinus:

- internal carotid artery & plexus
- abducens nerve

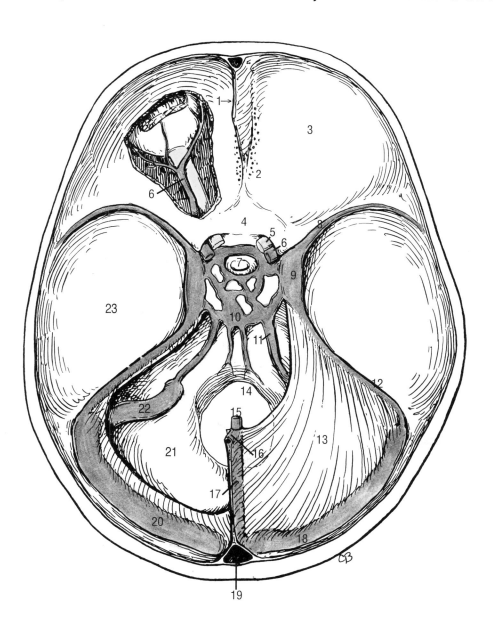

1. Falx cerebri attached to crista galli
2. Cribriform plate of ethmoid bone
3. Orbital plate of frontal bone and anterior cranial fossa (contains frontal lobe)
4. Planum sphenoidale (jugum)
5. Optic nerve in optic canal
6. Superior ophthalmic vein draining to cavernous sinus
7. Pituitary gland in sella turcica
8. Sphenoparietal sinus draining to cavernous sinus
9. Cavernous sinus
10. Basilar plexus on the clivus
11. Inferior petrosal sinus draining to the internal jugular vein
12. Superior petrosal sinus draining to the sigmoid sinus
13. Tentorium cerebelli (depicted only on the right)
14. Foramen magnum
15. Great cerebral vein (of Galen, cut)
16. Straight sinus
17. Cut edge of falx cerebri
18. Right transverse sinus; usually a continuation of superior sagittal sinus
19. Confluence of sinuses (torcular)
20. Left transverse sinus; usually a continuation of the straight sinus
21. Posterior cranial fossa (contains brain stem and cerebellum)
22. Sigmoid sinus (only left one is visible)
23. Middle cranial fossa (contains temporal lobe)

Tentorium Cerebelli, Descending Herniations

Definitions
The **tentorium cerebelli** is a dural partition under the occipital and posterior temporal lobes that confines the cerebellum and brain stem to the posterior cranial fossa. It lies within the **transverse fissure.**

Structural and Functional Features
The attachment of the **falx cerebri** elevates the tentorium cerebelli in the midline forming a tent-like configuration. The tentorium's peripheral attachments are along the petrous parts of the temporal bones and to the occipital bones along the sulci for the **transverse sinuses.** Anteriorly, it is anchored to the **anterior** and **posterior clinoid processes** of the sphenoid bones. The free border creates the **tentorial incisure** (**notch**), which accommodates both the midbrain and the posterior cerebral artery (PCA). The midbrain and the PCA begin in the posterior cranial fossa in an infratentorial position but continue in a position rostral to the tentorium, i.e., supratentorially.

Clinical Correlations . . . .

The basilar artery in the posterior cranial fossa bifurcates into the **posterior cerebral arteries,** which gain a **supratentorial position** by ascending over the unyielding free edge of the tentorium cerebelli. **Mass-occupying lesions** (e.g., **hemorrhage** or **tumor**) may cause a midline shift of the cranial contents and result in **herniation** of the uncus downward through the **tentorial notch.** The mass may be related to the **brain tissue** per se, to the **meninges** (meningioma) or to the **epidural space** (epidural hematoma). **Compression** of the posterior cerebral artery and of the third cranial nerve may be sequelae to **uncal herniation.** The medulla is compressed as a sequelae to cerebellar tonsilar herniation through the foramen magnum, which is seen after increased pressure in the posterior fossa. This causes disruption of respiratory and cardiac function. A third type of descending herniation is that of the cingulate gyrus under the falx cerebri (subfalcal).

Rapid action with a red pencil will simulate the speed with which an arterial hemorrhage creates a troublesome mass above the dura, i.e., an epidural hematoma. Use dark blue for venous blood in the sinuses.

Tentorium Cerebelli

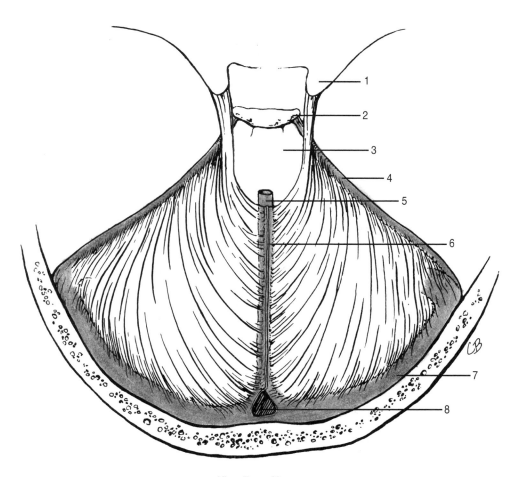

View From Above

1. Anterior clinoid process
2. Posterior clinoid process
3. Tentorial incisure or notch
4. Superior petrosal sinus
5. Great cerebral vein (of Galen) draining into straight sinus
6. Straight sinus and cut edge of falx cerebri
7. Transverse sinus
8. Confluence of sinuses (torcular)

Descending Herniations

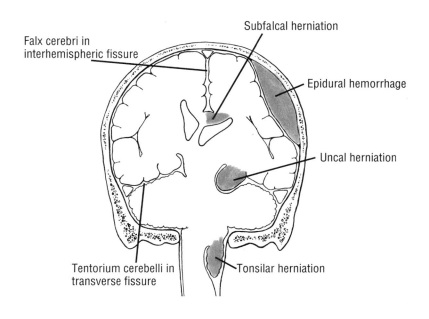

Coronal Section

Lobes of the Cerebral Hemisphere

Definitions

The left cerebral hemisphere is shown from the lateral surface and from the medial surface with the brain stem and cerebellum removed. Folding increases the surface area of the cerebral hemispheres. The elevations are **gyri**. The grooves between the gyri are **sulci**. There is considerable variation of surface markings from one brain to another and between the two hemispheres of the same brain. Nevertheless, sulci and gyri serve as a frame of reference for cortical functions.

Structural and Functional Features, Lateral Surface

The **lateral sulcus** (of Sylvius) and the **parieto-occipital sulcus** appear early in fetal development. These and the **central sulcus** (of Rolando) are the boundaries dividing the cerebral hemispheres into **frontal, parietal, temporal,** and **occipital lobes.** The central sulcus separates the frontal and parietal lobes. The lateral sulcus separates the frontal and parietal above from the temporal lobe below. A line drawn from the parieto-occipital sulcus to the **preoccipital notch** defines the occipital lobe on the lateral surface. Another line slanting posteriorly and somewhat downward from the posterior ramus of the lateral sulcus delineates the boundary between the posterior parts of the temporal and parietal lobes.

The **insula** (island of Reil) is a **central** lobe of the cerebrum not visible on the surface. It is composed of convolutions in the depth of the lateral sulcus.

Medial Surface

The **central sulcus**, although not very distinct, continues on the medial surface of the hemisphere and demarcates **frontal** and **parietal lobes.** The **parieto-occipital sulcus** separates the parietal and occipital lobes. An arbitrary line slanted upward and medially from the **preoccipital notch** to the parieto-occipital sulcus separates the occipital and **temporal lobes.**

Functional Correlations . . . .

Serial processing of unimodal (one stimulus or modality) and multimodal (polysensory) information proceeds from the parietal, temporal, and occipital lobes to the frontal lobe. The parietal lobe deals with external, soft tissue and joint stimuli as well as visceral sensations and spatial orientation. The temporal lobe processes olfactory and auditory stimuli, and the occipital lobe receives and integrates visual input. On receiving input from these sources within the same hemisphere and from the contralateral hemisphere, the frontal lobe further integrates and compares the present stimuli with past experience. If a motor response is warranted, executive command of motor function is largely the role of the frontal lobe. The anterior region of the frontal lobe (prefrontal cortex) makes decisions regarding motor activity that emanates from the posterior area of the frontal lobe (Brodmann's areas 4, 6, 8, 44, 45; page 29). These cortical areas that direct voluntary movement receive input via the ventral anterior and ventral lateral nuclei of the thalamus, and from subcortical motor areas, i.e., the basal ganglia and cerebellum.

Color the lobes as follows: frontal red, parietal blue, occipital yellow, and temporal green. Think about the boundaries as you work. Observe that both illustrations are of the **left** hemisphere and that the insula is not visible from the surface.

Everything should be made as simple as possible, but not simpler. – Albert Einstein

Lobes of the Cerebral Hemisphere

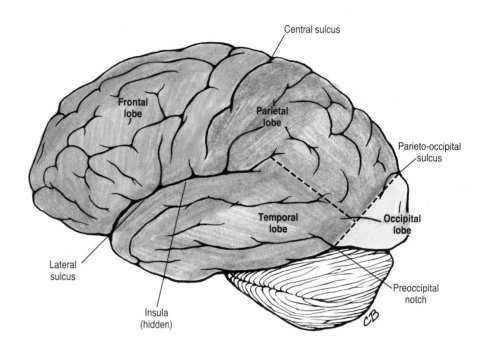

Central sulcus

Frontal lobe

Parietal lobe

Parieto-occipital sulcus

Temporal lobe

Occipital lobe

Lateral sulcus

Insula (hidden)

Preoccipital notch

CB

Lateral View, Left Hemisphere

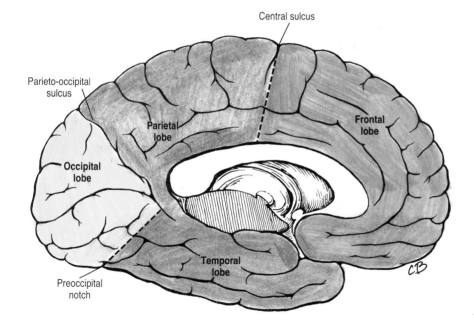

Central sulcus

Parieto-occipital sulcus

Parietal lobe

Frontal lobe

Occipital lobe

Temporal lobe

Preoccipital notch

CB

Medial View, Left Hemisphere

Sulci of the Cerebral Hemisphere

Structural and Functional Features, Lateral Surface

The deep stem of the **lateral sulcus** continues anteriorly as three shallow rami. The **posterior ramus** ascends in the parietal lobe whereas the **anterior horizontal** and **anterior ascending rami** (of the lateral sulcus) ascend a short distance into the frontal lobe. At the bottom of the lateral sulcus lies an area of cortex hidden from surface view, i.e., the insula (island of Reil).

Indenting the hemisphere between frontal and occipital poles is the **central sulcus.** It slopes downward and forward. The **precentral sulcus** runs anterior and parallel to the central sulcus and marks the anterior boundary of the precentral gyrus. Rostral (anterior) to the precentral sulcus, the **superior frontal** and **inferior frontal sulci** divide the remainder of the frontal lobe into superior, middle, and inferior gyri.

In the parietal lobe, the **postcentral sulcus** runs parallel to the center sulcus and bounds the postcentral gyrus posteriorly. An **intraparietal sulcus** extends posteriorly from the postcentral sulcus and separates superior and inferior parietal lobules.

Superior and **inferior temporal sulci** divide the temporal lobe into superior, middle, and inferior temporal gyri.

A short **lateral occipital sulcus** is sometimes apparent near the occipital pole.

Sulci of the Medial Surface

The **central sulcus** continues a short distance onto the medial surface of the cerebral hemisphere and projects into the paracentral lobule. Superior to the corpus callosum is the **callosal sulcus,** which delineates this mass of fibers connecting left and right hemispheres from the gyrus above. The cingulate gyrus, above the callosal sulcus, is bounded superiorly by the **cingulate sulcus.**

Posteriorly the **parieto-occipital sulcus** delineates the parietal and occipital lobes. In the occipital lobe, the **calcarine sulcus** runs anteriorly from the occipital pole to the parieto-occipital sulcus.

Inferior to the calcarine sulcus is the **collateral sulcus,** which is sometimes continuous anteriorly with the **rhinal sulcus.** These sulci define the lateral boundary of the parahippocampal gyrus. The **occipitotemporal sulcus** lies between the medial and lateral occipitotemporal gyri.

Clinical Correlations . . . .

The sulci become wider and more prominent with increasing age due to attrition of neurons that are not replaced. This feature is markedly apparent in certain CNS diseases characterized by atrophy that may be focal or somewhat generalized.

Color the sulci within each lobe as follows: frontal red, parietal blue, occipital yellow, and temporal green. The central, lateral, and parieto-occipital sulci are essential for delineating the lobes. You may choose to emphasize those boundaries by using the colors of each adjacent lobe on either side of those sulci.

Sulci of the Cerebral Hemisphere

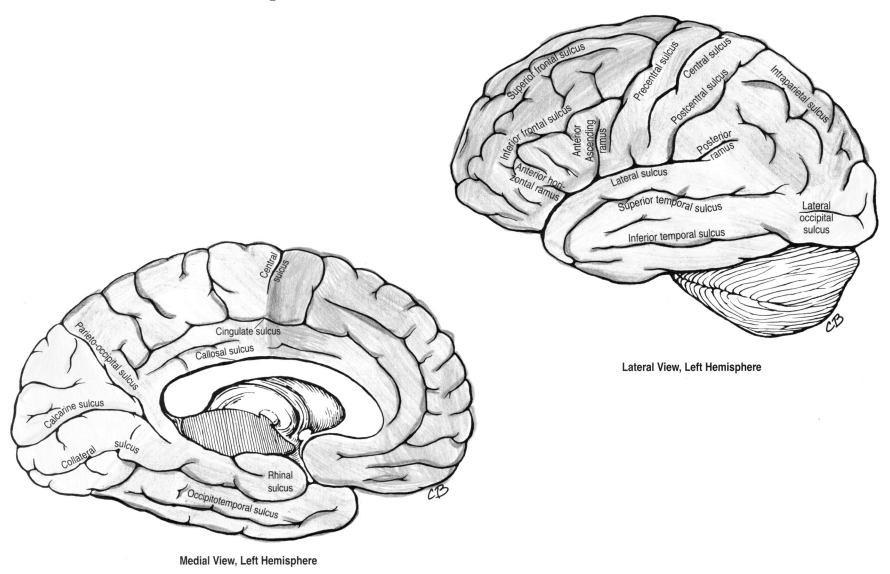

Lateral View, Left Hemisphere

Medial View, Left Hemisphere

Gyri of the Lateral Surface

Structural and Functional Features

On the lateral surface, the **frontal lobe** lies anterior to the central sulcus and above the lateral sulcus. It contains the following gyri:

Precentral gyrus, the primary motor area of the cerebral cortex;
Superior frontal and **middle frontal gyri,** which contain the premotor area and the frontal eye field;
Inferior frontal gyrus, that is divided into **opercular, triangular,** and **orbital** parts. The opercular and triangular areas in the left hemisphere make up the motor speech area.

The central and lateral sulci and two imaginary lines bound the **parietal lobe,** which contains the following gyri:

Postcentral gyrus is the primary general sensory (somatosensory) area of the cerebral cortex.
Superior and **inferior parietal lobules** are posterior to the postcentral gyrus. The **inferior lobule** consists of the gyri defined below.
Supramarginal and **angular gyri** surround the upturned ends of the lateral sulcus and superior temporal sulcus, respectively. In the left hemisphere, these gyri participate in the perception and the interpretation of the semantics of language. Their function in the right hemisphere is to interpret prosody and the intonation of speech.

The lateral sulcus and an arbitrary line drawn posteriorly and downward from the posterior ramus define the **temporal lobe.**

Superior temporal gyrus forms the floor of the lateral sulcus where the **transverse temporal gyri** are located. These gyri, also called **Heschl's convolutions,** mark the location of the primary auditory cortex.
Middle and inferior temporal gyri form areas of association cortex, especially auditory.

Note the inset, which shows the cortex of the **insula** in the depth of the lateral sulcus and the location of the transverse temporal gyri.

On the lateral surface of the hemisphere there are **lateral occipital gyri** in the **occipital lobe.**

Functional Correlations . . . .

(See page 28.)

In the frontal lobe, color the precentral, superior, and inferior frontal gyri red. Use vertical red lines to accentuate the location of the middle frontal gyrus. Color the postcentral gyrus and the superior parietal lobule blue. Use vertical blue lines for the inferior parietal lobule, which includes the angular and supramarginal gyri. Color the occipital gyri yellow. Color the superior and inferior temporal gyri green. Use vertical green lines to color the middle temporal gyrus.

Rule Number 1 is, don't sweat the small stuff. Rule Number 2 is, it's all small stuff.
And if you can't fight and you can't flee, flow. – Dr. Robert S. Eliot

22

Gyri of the Lateral Surface

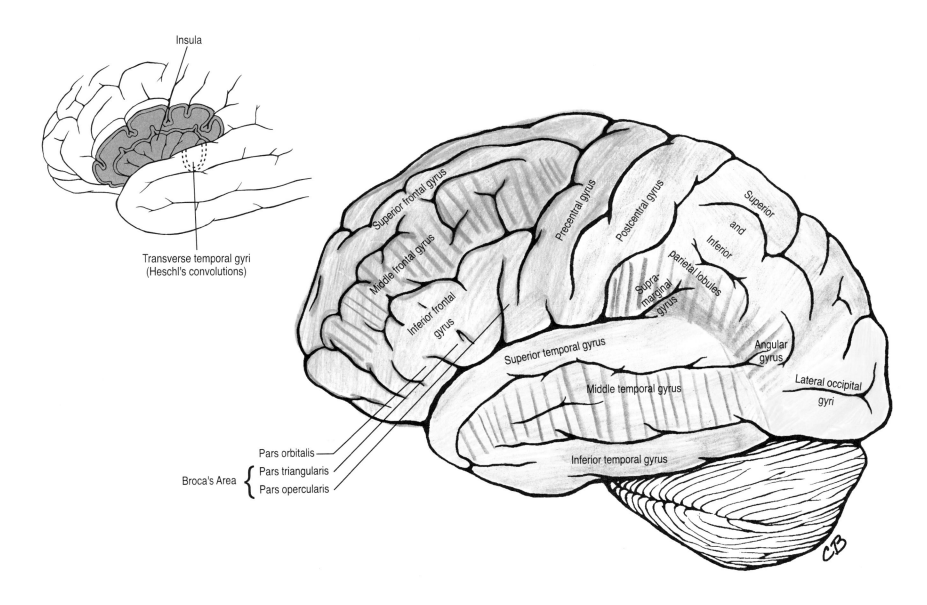

Insula

Transverse temporal gyri
(Heschl's convolutions)

Superior frontal gyrus

Middle frontal gyrus

Inferior frontal gyrus

Precentral gyrus

Postcentral gyrus

Superior and Inferior parietal lobules

Supra-marginal gyrus

Angular gyrus

Lateral occipital gyri

Superior temporal gyrus

Middle temporal gyrus

Inferior temporal gyrus

Pars orbitalis

Broca's Area { Pars triangularis

Pars opercularis

Gyri of the Medial Surface

Structural and Functional Features

Surface markings of the cerebral hemisphere into lobes are less apparent on the medial surface. The indentation made by the **central sulcus** on the medial surface is surrounded by extensions of the **precentral** and **postcentral** gyri from the lateral surface. These are motor and sensory areas, respectively. Their continuation on the medial surface creates the **paracentral lobule.** Posteriorly, and continuous with the superior parietal lobule of the lateral surface, is the **precuneus** of the parietal lobe.

The wedge-shaped gyrus bounded by the parieto-occipital and calcarine sulci is the **cuneus** of the occipital lobe. The **lingual gyrus** of the occipital lobe is inferior to the calcarine sulcus and continuous anteriorly with the **parahippocampal gyrus** of the temporal lobe. The latter hooks sharply backward as the **uncus.** An occipitotemporal sulcus delineates the **medial occipitotemporal gyrus** from the **lateral occipitotemporal gyrus,** which is continuous with the inferior temporal gyrus on the lateral surface of the hemisphere.

The **subcallosal area** is underneath the rostrum of the corpus callosum; the rostrum is that part between the genu and the lamina terminalis. The subcallosal area is a component of the limbic system. The **cingulate gyrus,** which lies above the corpus callosum, is also a part of the limbic system. The septal area is located anterior to the anterior commissure, between the medial surface of the frontal lobe and the anterior horn of the lateral ventricle, and consists of a number of nuclei. The **isthmus** of the cingulate gyrus is that part of the cerebral cortex posterior to the splenium of the corpus callosum, which connects the cingulate gyrus of the parietal lobe and the parahippocampal gyrus of the temporal lobe.

The **medial frontal gyrus** is continuous with the superior frontal gyrus of the lateral surface.

Functional Correlations . . . .

(See page 30.)

Color the anterior part of the paracentral lobule and the medial frontal gyrus red. Use red vertical lines to indicate the region of the cingulate gyrus that is in the frontal lobe. Color the posterior part of the paracentral lobule and the precuneus blue, and use vertical blue marks for the part of the cingulate gyrus in the parietal lobe. Note that the parietal is continuous with the temporal lobe via the isthmus. Color both gyri of the occipital lobe yellow. Color the parahippocampal and lateral occipitotemporal gyri green. Use green vertical lines to accentuate the medial occipitotemporal gyrus.

Build a better mousetrap and the world will beat a path to your door.
Build a better door and the mice can't get in anyhow. – Cal Tinney

24

Gyri of the Medial Surface

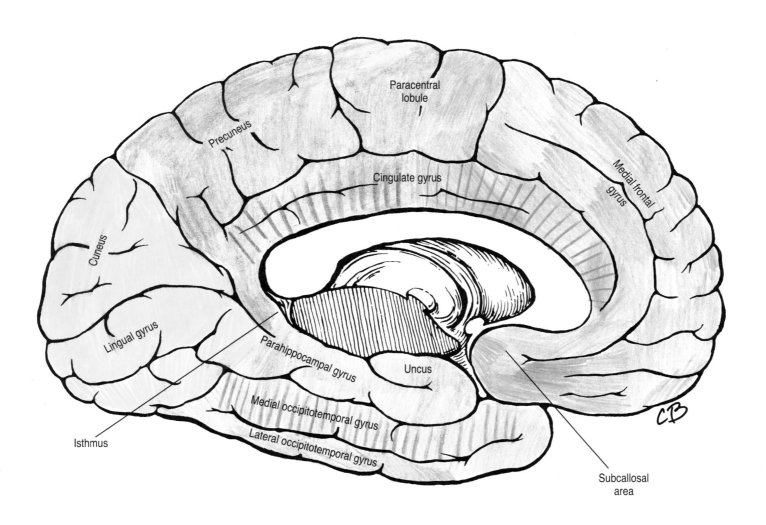

Paracentral lobule

Precuneus

Cingulate gyrus

Medial frontal gyrus

Cuneus

Lingual gyrus

Parahippocampal gyrus

Uncus

Medial occipitotemporal gyrus

Lateral occipitotemporal gyrus

Isthmus

Subcallosal area

Gyri and Other Structures of the Inferior Surface: Cerebellum and Brain Stem Removed

Definitions

The **interhemispheric (longitudinal) fissure** is a deep vertical fissure between the two cerebral hemispheres. The **anterior perforated substance** (space), perforated by many small blood vessels, is located posterior to the attachment of the olfactory tract and is bounded by the lateral olfactory stria dorsolaterally and the diagonal band of Broca and optic tract ventromedially. The diagonal band of Broca is a band of fibers that extends from the paraolfactory area on the medial surface of the frontal lobe ventrally to the lateral margin of the optic tract. The **posterior perforated substance** (space) is an area in the fossa between the bases of the two cerebral peduncles (interpeduncular fossa). **Tectum** means "roof." Collectively, the bilateral superior and inferior colliculi make up the tectum of the midbrain. The **gyrus rectus** (straight) lies on the ventral surface of the frontal lobe, medial to the olfactory sulcus.

Structural and Functional Features

The penetration of numerous central arteries from the circle of Willis (page 181) creates the perforations in the anterior and posterior perforated substances. These nonbranching "end" arteries are a crucial source of supply to the diencephalon, basal ganglia, and internal capsule.

This cross section through the midbrain at the level of the superior colliculus can be viewed to appreciate its division into the **tectum,** posterior to the aqueduct, and the cerebral peduncle. The latter contains the **tegmentum,** an area anterior to the aqueduct, and the basis pedunculi composed of the substantia nigra and pes pedunculi. The proximity of the **uncus** to the midbrain is apparent here.

Clinical Correlations . . . .

An **epidural hematoma** in the temporal fossa pushes the temporal lobe medially, causing herniation downward of the uncus and parahippocampal gyrus (uncal herniation). This syndrome is addressed on page 16. Bilateral **orbital lesions** of the orbital surfaces of the frontal lobes may result in **emotional indifference** (apathy). The parahippocampal and medial occipitotemporal gyri are involved in the recognition of familiar faces. Bilateral lesions of these gyri result in a rare disorder called prosopagnosia, i.e., face agnosia.

Color the orbital gyri of the frontal lobe red and use red horizontal lines to color the gyrus rectus. Color the parahippocampal and occipitotemporal gyri green. Use green horizontal lines to indicate the medial occipitotemporal gyrus. Color yellow the olfactory bulb and tract; the optic nerve, chiasm, and tract as well as the superior colliculus. Color the tuber cinereum, infundibulum, and mamillary body of the hypothalamus purple. Color the anterior and posterior perforated substances blue. Color the red nuclei and the basal region of the cerebral peduncles red. Observe that this orientation of the midbrain is opposite that in which it is usually presented; however, this orientation is as it appears in MRIs.

If it were not for our conception of weights and measures,
we would stand in awe of the firefly as we do before the sun. – Kahlil Gibran

26

Gyri and Other Structures of the Inferior Surface: Cerebellum and Brain Stem Removed

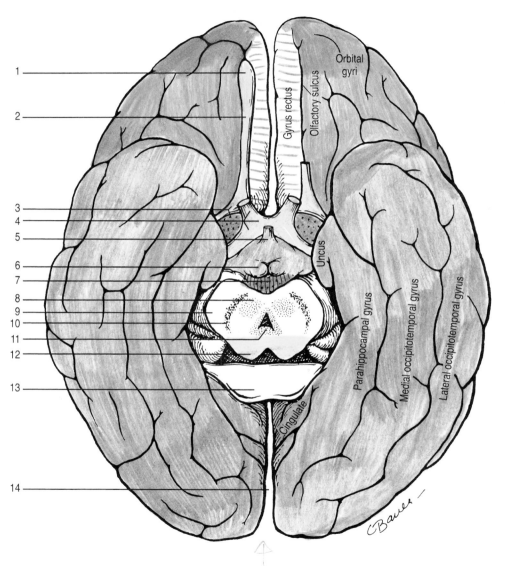

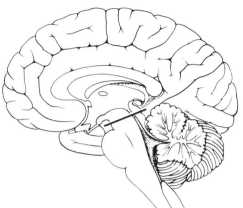

anterior

Orbital gyri

Gyrus rectus

Olfactory sulcus

Uncus

Parahippocampal gyrus

Medial occipitotemporal gyrus

Lateral occipitotemporal gyrus

Cingulate

CBauer

posterior

1. Olfactory bulb
2. Olfactory tract
3. Lateral stria of olfactory tract
    Olfactory tubercle
    Anterior perforated substance (space; area)
    (Medial stria of olfactory tract obscured by optic nerve)
4. Optic nerve
    Optic chiasma
    Optic tract
5. Tuber cinereum and infundibulum
6. Mamillary body of hypothalamus
7. Interpeduncular fossa and cistern
    Posterior perforated substance (space; area)
8. Red nucleus
9. Cerebral peduncles of midbrain
10. Substantia nigra
11. Cerebral aqueduct and periaqueductal gray
12. Superior colliculus of midbrain
13. Splenium of corpus callosum
14. Interhemispheric (longitudinal) fissure

Selected Brodmann's Areas, Lateral Surface

Definitions

Cortical areas vary in overall thickness, in thickness of different laminae (layers), in neuronal morphology, and in fiber lamination. On the basis of these criteria, investigators have parceled the cortex into from 20 to 200 cytoarchitectonic areas. The most widely used classification is that of **Brodmann**, which contains 52 numbered areas. A few of the areas of known functional significance are of interest to the beginning student.

Structural and Functional Features

Somesthetic, visual, and auditory areas are three of the five primary sensory areas. (The remaining areas, taste and olfaction, are discussed with the cranial nerves). Each area is surrounded by a larger zone of association cortex. Motor and associational areas are dependent on sensory input; therefore, the functional **classification** of cortical areas as **motor, sensory,** or **associational** is somewhat arbitrary. The left hemisphere is concerned with the right sides of the lower face, body, and visual field, whereas the right hemisphere controls the left sides of the lower face, body, and visual field.

Color 4 dark red, and 6 and 8 light red. Designate 44 and 45 with horizontal red lines. Color 3, 1, 2 dark blue. Color 5 and 7 light blue. Designate 43 with vertical yellow lines. Color 41 and 42 dark green. Color 22 light green. Designate the posterior area of 22 with green vertical lines and areas 39 and 40 with horizontal blue lines. Color 17, 18, and 19 yellow. Color the insula orange.

Table 1–1. Selected Brodmann's Areas, Lateral Surface

Brodmann's Areas	Location	Synonyms	Function
Frontal Lobe			
4	Precentral gyrus	Primary motor area	Motor control of face, upper limb, trunk and thigh
6	Premotor area	Premotor cortex	Motor control of proximal joints
8	Frontal lobe	Frontal eye field	Conjugate eye movements
44,45	Inferior frontal gyrus	Anterior language area[a,b]	Left hemisphere; motor speech control. Right hemisphere; imparting prosody and emotional intonation of speech
Parietal Lobe			
3,1,2	Postcentral gyrus	Primary somesthetic area	Recognition of somesthetic stimuli
5,7	Superior parietal lobe	Somesthetic association cortex	Understanding somesthetic input
39	Angular gyrus (plus posterior part 22)	Posterior language area	Left hemisphere; understanding semantics
40	Supramarginal gyrus		Right hemisphere; understanding prosody and emotional intonation of speech
43	Postcentral gyrus and parainsular cortex	Taste (gustatory) area	Recognition of taste
Temporal lobe			
41,42	Transverse temporal gyri	Primary auditory cortex[a,c]	Recognition of auditory stimuli
22	Superior temporal gyrus	Auditory association cortex[a,d]	Understanding auditory input
Occipital lobe			
17	Calcarine area	Primary visual cortex	Recognition of visual stimuli
18,19	Occipital cortex	Visual association cortex	Understanding visual input

[a]Eponyms.
[b]Broca's area.
[c]Heschl's convolutions.
[d]Wernicke's area (posterior 22, 39, 40).

To act is easy: to think is hard. – Goethe

Selected Brodmann's Areas, Lateral Surface

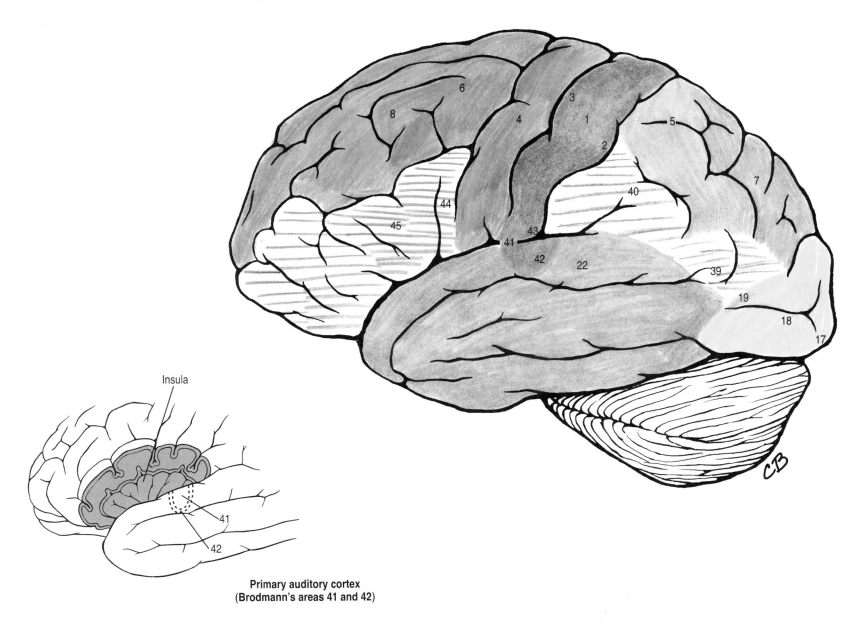

Insula

41
42

Primary auditory cortex
(Brodmann's areas 41 and 42)

Selected Brodmann's Areas, Medial Surface

Definitions

The **paracentral lobule** is the area surrounding the continuation of the central sulcus on the medial surface. The area anterior to the sulcus is a continuation of the **motor gyrus,** whereas the posterior area is the continuation of the **primary somesthetic gyrus.**

 Color 4 dark red and 6 and 8 light red. Color 3, 1, 2 dark blue, and 5 and 7 light blue. Color 17, 18, 19, and 34 yellow.

Table 1–2. Selected Brodmann's Areas, Medial Surface

Brodmann's Areas	Location	Synonyms	Function
Frontal Lobe			
4	Anterior paracentral lobule	Primary motor area	Motor control of lower limb
6	Medial frontal gyrus	Supplementary motor area	Planning and control of movement
Parietal Lobe			
3,1,2	Posterior paracentral lobule	Primary somesthetic cortex	Recognition of somesthetic stimuli, lower limb, and genitals
5,7	Precuneus	Somesthetic association cortex	Understanding somesthetic stimuli, lower limb
Temporal Lobe			
34	Medial temporal area	Uncus	Recognition of olfactory stimuli
Occipital Lobe			
17	Calcarine area	Primary visual cortex (striate)	Recognition of visual stimuli
18	Surrounds calcarine area	Visual association cortex	Understanding visual input
19	Surrounds area 18	Visual association cortex	Understanding visual input

Our life is frittered away by detail . . . simplify, simplify, symplify. – Henry David Thoreau

Selected Brodmann's Areas, Medial Surface

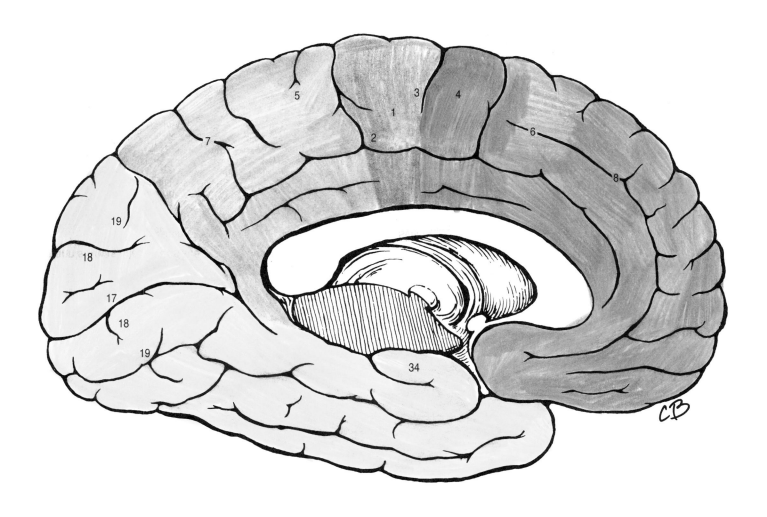

Fibers of the Cerebral Hemispheres

Definitions and Structural and Functional Features

Associational fibers connect cortical areas within the same hemisphere. Examples are:

Cingulum, which connects frontal, parietal, and temporal areas medially;

Arcuate fibers, which interconnect neighboring gyri;

Inferior occipitofrontal fasciculus, which interconnects temporal, occipital, and frontal lobes;

Superior longitudinal fasciculus (arcuate fasciculus), which interconnects frontal, parietal, occipital, and temporal lobes laterally;

Uncinate fasciculus, which interconnects the rostral temporal lobe with the orbital area and part of the lateral surface of the frontal lobe.

Commissural fibers cross the midline and sometimes, but not always, interconnect corresponding cortical areas of the two hemispheres. These include:

Corpus callosum, which interconnects neocortical areas in all lobes;

Anterior commissure, which crosses the midline anterior to the fornix columns and interconnects the temporal lobes;

Hippocampal commissure (not shown), which interconnects the two hippocampal formations. (It lies beneath the splenium of the corpus callosum.)

Projectional fibers pass in both directions between cortex and subcortical centers. Examples are:

Lateral corticospinal fibers, which originate in one hemisphere, descend, decussate, and terminate on contralateral motor neurons of the spinal cord. A **decussation** is a place where nerve fibers cross the median plane.

Thalamocortical fibers, which originate in the thalamus and ascend to the cortex.

Clinical Correlations . . . .

Interruption of the **superior longitudinal fasciculus** disconnects the **posterior sensory language area (Wernicke's area)** from the **anterior motor language area (Broca's area).** This results in **conduction aphasia** in which there is relatively good comprehension and spontaneous speech but poor repetition of a sentence spoken by the examiner.

General Classification of Fibers

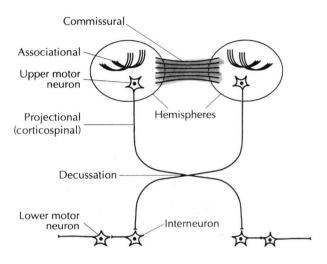

Color the superior longitudinal fasciculus blue. Color the inferior occipitofrontal fasciculus purple. Color the uncinate fasciculus orange. Color the arcuate fibers green. Color the cingulum yellow. Color the corpus callosum brown and the anterior commissure red.

Fibers of the Cerebral Hemispheres

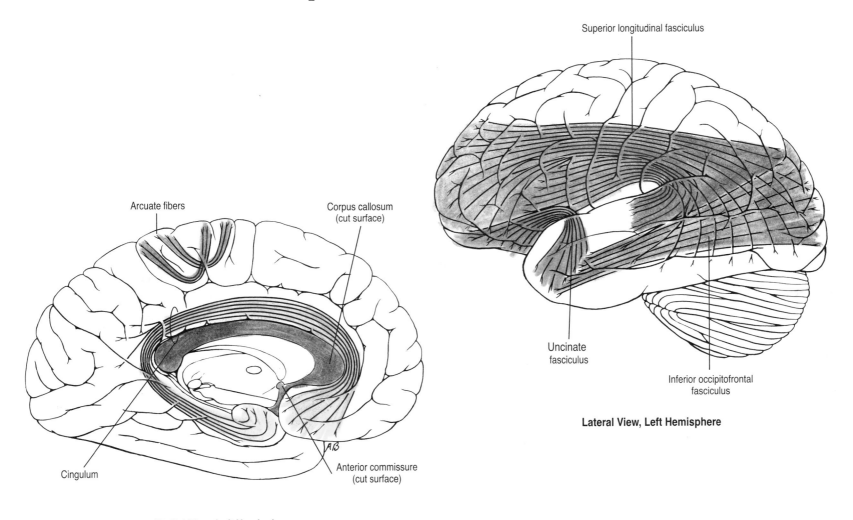

Superior longitudinal fasciculus

Arcuate fibers

Corpus callosum
(cut surface)

Cingulum

Anterior commissure
(cut surface)

Medial View, Left Hemisphere

Uncinate
fasciculus

Inferior occipitofrontal
fasciculus

Lateral View, Left Hemisphere

Superior View of the Cerebrum

Definitions

In an unstained brain, **neuronal elements,** whether in layers or clusters, appear **gray** in contrast to the **white** matter comprising myelinated and unmyelinated **fibers.** The **myelin** covering of the axons is responsible for the **white** appearance of **fibers** in the fresh specimen. In the intact hemisphere, a bark-like covering of gray is distinguished from the sponge-like appearance of the core of white matter in the dissected hemisphere.

Structural and Functional Features

The **cerebral cortex** is intact in the left hemisphere. It is a convoluted sheath of gray substance that varies regionally in thickness from 2 to 4 mm and consists of **horizontally layered** cells ranging from three to five layers in a few areas and six layers in 90% of the human cortex.

The cortex has been dissected away in the right hemisphere to expose the underlying core of **white matter.** The cortical cells are intricately connected to subcortical centers and to areas within the same hemisphere as well as across the midline to corresponding areas in the opposite hemisphere. The white matter exposed on the right is an intricate mixture of **connecting** fibers classified as **associational** (within the same hemisphere), **commissural** (to and from the opposite hemisphere), and **projectional** (to and from subcortical centers). Diagrams of these fibers are on pages 32 and 33.

This view reveals the convolutions (gyri) whose configuration is determined by growth spurts during development. The various gyri are subdivisions within a lobe demarcated by depressions (sulci). Studying every brain in such detail so as to define every crook and turn is a futile exercise. It is useful, however, to learn the general pattern in a typical brain in order to discuss function relative to a particular gyrus.

The configuration in this brain is typical and one can see that the **central sulcus** (5) and the **precentral** (6) and **postcentral** (4) **gyri** are distinguished by coursing in a plane that is more **vertical** than horizontal. This is likewise true of the **precentral** (7) and the **postcentral** (3) **sulci.** Note that the "central" sulcus is posterior to the center. Recall that the central sulcus is the boundary between the **frontal lobe** anteriorly and the **parietal lobe** posteriorly. The region anterior to the central sulcus contains the **precentral gyrus** and the **superior** (10), **middle** (9), and **inferior** (8) **frontal gyri.**

In the parietal lobe, posterior to the **postcentral gyrus** and **sulcus,** the **intraparietal sulcus** (2) demarcates a boundary between the **superior parietal lobule** (1) and the inferior parietal lobule.

The falx cerebri, contained within the **interhemispheric fissure** (11), abuts the corpus callosum.

Clinical Correlations . . . .

The gyri are thinner and the sulci wider in an aging brain. This reflects a **generalized attrition** of neurons over time, which is accompanied by some enlargement of the ventricles. The **overall atrophy** of a **senile brain,** i.e., global atrophy, is in contrast to similar but grossly accentuated **focal changes** limited, for example, to the frontal and temporal lobes as in Pick's disease. Atrophy of the brain of a patient with Alzheimer's disease is usually generalized on gross inspection; however, there are specific cholinergic pathways that seem to be affected (and possibly other transmitters as well).

Superior View of the Cerebrum

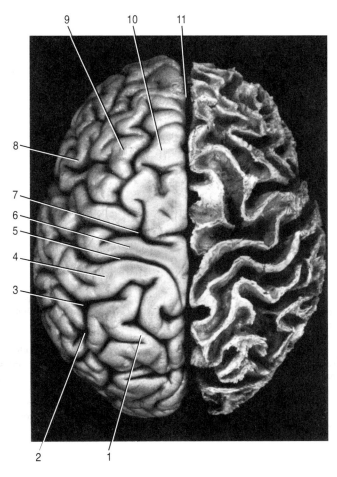

1. Superior parietal lobule
2. Intraparietal sulcus
3. Postcentral sulcus
4. Postcentral gyrus
5. Central sulcus
6. Precentral gyrus
7. Precentral sulcus
8. Inferior frontal gyrus
9. Middle frontal gyrus
10. Superior frontal gyrus
11. Interhemispheric fissure

(Reprinted with permission from Ludwig E, Klingler J. Atlas Cerebri Humani. Basel, Switzerland: S. Karger, 1956, Table 1.)

Medial Surface of the Brain With Blood Vessels Removed Showing Sulci, Gyri, and Median Features

Definitions

The **inferomedial subdivision** of the forebrain, i.e., diencephalon, is shown in this median or mid-sagittal plane as the **thalamus** (29) and **hypothalamus** (30). Understanding the three-dimensionality of this region and its relationship to the basal ganglia of the telencephalon is important. Coronal sections through the anterior telencephalon and transverse sections through the mesencephalon, metencephalon, and myelencephalon are more easily understood in contrast.

Structural and Functional Features

Features of the medial aspect of the cortex are rather straightforward. The medial frontal **gyrus** (7) is anterior to the paracentral lobule and superior to the **cingulate gyrus** (9). The paracentral lobule is located by finding the central sulcus on the dorsolateral surface and following it over the convexity of the hemisphere. It is a continuation on the medial surface of the precentral and postcentral gyri. This important cortical area is unlabeled because one identifies it by following the central sulcus over the convexity onto the medial surface.

Between the **callosal** (10) and **cingulate** (8) sulci lies the cingulate gyrus. The continuation of the cingulate gyrus posterior and inferior to the **splenium** (13) provides continuity among frontal and parietal cortices and the parahippocampal gyrus of the temporal lobe. This posterior region is the **isthmus** (14). The **parieto-occipital sulcus** (16) marks the boundary between the parietal and occipital lobes, and the **calcarine sulcus** (18) divides the occipital lobe into the **cuneus** (17) and the **lingual gyri** (19). The **precuneus** (15) is in the parietal lobe. Cortical visual pathways are discussed and shown in Chapter 3 (pages 90, 91).

Prominent here is the sectioned **corpus callosum** (11). Its parts include the **rostrum** (5), **genu** (6), **trunk** (11) (body), and **splenium** (13). Together with the underlying fornices, the corpus callosum forms the roof over the body of the lateral ventricles. Stretching sagittally between the corpus callosum and the fornices is a thin sheet of tissue, the **septum pellucidum** (3), which forms the medial wall of the anterior horns of the lateral ventricles. The interventricular foramina lead from the lateral ventricles of the two cerebral hemispheres into the single third ventricle, which is in the midline and is bordered laterally by the thalamus and hypothalamus, ventrally by the hypothalamus and optic chiasm, anteriorly by the lamina terminalis, and posteriorly by the pineal gland. In this view, the interventricular foramen is unlabeled; however, it is immediately posterior to the column of the **fornix** (1). The **anterior commissure** (2) is anterior to the interventricular foramen. It consists of nerve fibers interconnecting the temporal lobes.

Connecting the third ventricle to the **fourth ventricle** (25) is the cerebral aqueduct, which is covered by the tectum (roof) of the midbrain composed of the bilateral **superior** (21) and **inferior** (22) **colliculi**. The **pulvinar** (12) of the thalamus is superior to the colliculi. The bulbous portion of the brain stem is the pons, with the **medulla oblongata** (26) lying more caudally, continuous with the spinal cord at the foramen magnum. **Corticospinal fibers** (27) descend in the base of the pons. In the median plane of the cerebellum is the **vermis** (23), which, with the **superior medullary velum** (24) and the inferior medullary velum, forms the roof of the fourth ventricle. The inferior medullary velum is not apparent in this section.

Diencephalic structures include the **habenulae**, rostral to the **pineal gland** (20), and the **stria medullaris thalami** (28) as a narrow ridge on each side. The latter extends from the interventricular foramen to the habenula and arches along the dorsal extent of the thalamus. The **interthalamic adhesion** (29) (massa intermedia, anterior leader) spans the third ventricle, whereas the **thalamus** (29) (posterior leader) and **hypothalamus** (30) form the wall of the third ventricle. The optic "nerve" is a tract of the brain, specifically an outgrowth of the diencephalon. Ventral and anterior to the hypothalamus lies the optic chiasm. This view clearly shows the **septal area** (4).

Connecting the habenulae across the midline is the habenular commissure (rostral to the pineal gland). The posterior commissure interconnects the pretectal and other nuclei caudal to the pineal at the junction of the diencephalon and the midbrain.

Clinical Correlations . . . .

The anterior portion of the paracentral lobule (frontal lobe) is the site of **motor control** of the **contralateral leg**, whereas the strip posterior to the central sulcus (parietal lobe) is the **primary somesthetic cortex** of the **contralateral leg**.

Pineal tumors may press against the superior colliculi and result in **paralysis** of **upward gaze**, "sunset eyes." Midline **meningiomas** of the falx cerebri may affect functional areas in one or both hemispheres. For example, symptoms of a tumor of the falx in the region of the paracentral lobule could include motor or sensory deficits or both, in one or both legs, depending on the size and symmetry of the tumor.

Medial Surface of the Brain With Blood Vessels Removed Showing Sulci, Gyri, and Median Features

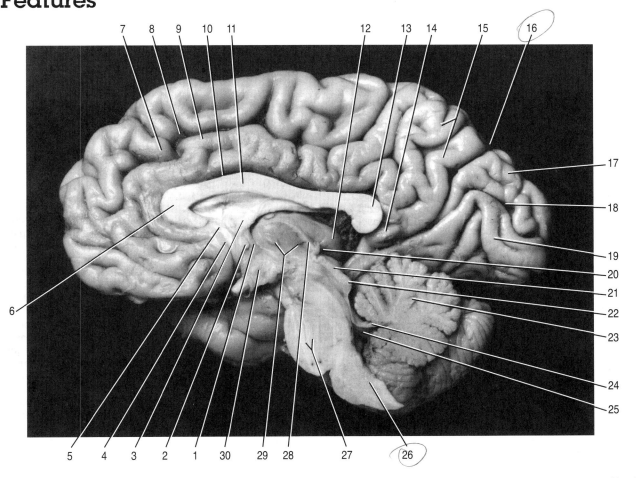

1. Fornix, column
2. Anterior commissure
3. Septum pellucidum
4. Septal area
5. Rostrum of corpus callosum
6. Genu of corpus callosum
7. Medial frontal gyrus
8. Cingulate sulcus
9. Cingulate gyrus
10. Callosal sulcus
11. Trunk (body) of corpus callosum
12. Pulvinar of thalamus
13. Splenium of corpus callosum
14. Isthmus of cingulate gyrus
15. Precuneus
16. Parieto-occipital sulcus
17. Cuneus
18. Calcarine sulcus
19. Lingual gyrus
20. Position of pineal gland
21. Superior colliculus
22. Inferior colliculus
23. Vermis of cerebellum
24. Superior medullary velum
25. Fourth ventricle
26. Medulla oblongata
27. Corticospinal fibers in base of pons
28. Stria medullaris thalami
29. Interthalamic adhesion (anterior leader) and thalamus (lateral to third ventricle)
30. Hypothalamus

Lateral Surface of the Left Cerebral Hemisphere Showing Sulci and Gyri

Definitions
Compare the **precentral** (7) and **postcentral gyri** (13) in this brain with those shown on page 23. The **transverse fissure** (20) contains the tentorium cerebelli.

Structural and Functional Features
The **inferior** (1) and **superior** (2) **temporal sulci** demarcate the **inferior** (3), **middle** (4), and **superior** (5) **temporal gyri.** Two small gyri on the superior surface of the temporal lobe within the lateral sulcus make up the transverse temporal gyri, where auditory radiations from the medial geniculate nucleus of the thalamus terminate in the primary auditory cortex (Heschl's convolutions; areas 41, 42). These two gyri are functionally important but are not labeled here because they are hidden within the **lateral sulcus** (18).

In this particular specimen, the supramarginal and angular gyri of the **inferior parietal lobule** (16) are difficult to discern in relation to the lateral sulcus and superior temporal sulcus, respectively; therefore they are not labeled. The left angular and supramarginal gyri plus the posterior part of area 22 in the left superior temporal gyrus make up the sensory or receptive speech area (Wernicke's area). Lobes, gyri, and sulci were first presented in line drawings showing typical topography, because they are landmarks difficult to discern. Just as surface anatomy of the body shows variations, so do internal structures, including the brain.

Broca's area includes the **pars opercularis** (8) (area 44) and **pars triangularis** (9) (area 45). These areas are immediately anterior to the precentral sulcus and gyrus. The pars opercularis, pars triangularis, and **pars orbitalis** (6) are all parts of the inferior frontal gyrus. The **inferior frontal sulcus** (10) borders the **middle frontal gyrus** (11).

Thalamocortical radiations relaying information from sensory pathways of the contralateral side of the face and body terminate somatotopically on neurons in the postcentral gyrus. The **postcentral sulcus** (14) separates the postcentral gyrus anteriorly from the **superior** (15) and **inferior parietal lobules** posteriorly. The postcentral sulcus borders the superior parietal lobule anteriorly.

The **precentral gyrus** (7) lies between the **central** (12) and **precentral sulci** (7) and contains the motor cortex (area 4). Large neurons here (predominantly) give rise to axons that descend ipsilaterally through the internal capsule and brain stem. Most of these axons cross the midline in the pyramidal decussation in the medulla.

Lateral occipital gyri (17) are seen posterior to the **preoccipital notch** (19).

Clinical Correlations . . . .

Corticospinal fibers terminate on interneurons or anterior motor horn cells in the spinal cord and exert voluntary control of limb muscles contralateral to their hemispheric site of origin. Some fibers (corticobulbar fibers) end in relation to motor nuclei in the brain stem for voluntary control of muscles supplied by cranial nerves. Lesions of the descending motor fibers between the cortex and the medulla result in motor deficits that are most pronounced in the limbs contralateral to the lesion; following lesions below the crossover in the medulla, the motor deficits are ipsilateral to the lesion. Vascular insults, traumatic injuries, and disease processes usually occur in predictable sites, based on anatomical, topographical, and physiologic parameters.

The postcentral gyrus is referred to as somesthetic (sensory) cortex or areas 3,1,2. Beginning at the lateral sulcus, somatic localization is mouth, tongue, face, hand, arm, trunk, and hip on the convexity of the hemisphere. The leg area continues over the medial surface in the paracentral lobe. In summary, **the perception of sensory stimuli and the control of voluntary motor function of one side of the face and body are largely controlled by the contralateral hemisphere.**

In the left hemisphere, **Broca's area** is synonymous with the **motor** or **expressive speech area**. **Wernicke's area** is synonymous with the **sensory** or **receptive speech area**. Language disorders are discussed on pages 32 and 40.

He who is firm in will, moulds the world to himself. – Goethe

Lateral Surface of the Left Cerebral Hemisphere Showing Sulci and Gyri

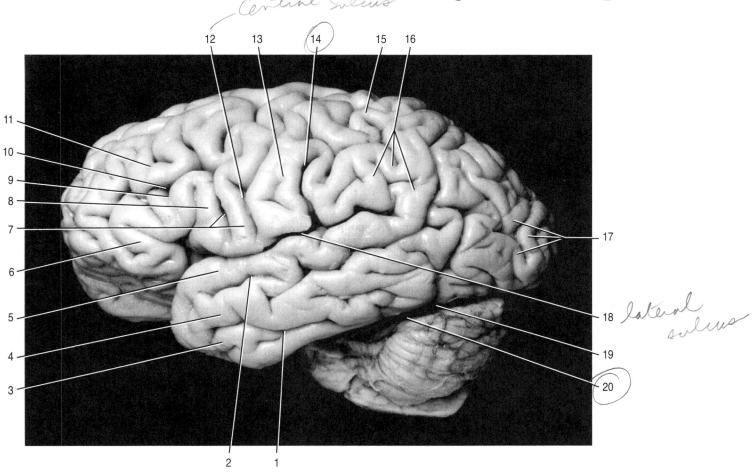

1. Inferior temporal sulcus
2. Superior temporal sulcus
3. Inferior temporal gyrus
4. Middle temporal gyrus
5. Superior temporal gyrus
6. Pars orbitalis
7. Precentral sulcus and gyrus
8. Pars opercularis
9. Pars triangularis
10. Inferior frontal sulcus
11. Middle frontal gyrus
12. Central sulcus
13. Postcentral gyrus
14. Postcentral sulcus
15. Superior parietal lobule
16. Inferior parietal lobule
17. Lateral occipital gyri
18. Lateral sulcus
19. Preoccipital notch
20. Transverse fissure

Dissection of the Left Hemisphere from the Lateral Surface

Definitions

The **insula** (1) is a lobe of the cerebral cortex that forms the floor of the lateral sulcus. It is covered by the opercula (lid), parts of the cerebrum that overlie the insula and form the lips of the lateral sulcus. When the cortex of the frontal, parietal, and temporal lobes is dissected as shown, associational fiber bundles are exposed.

Structural and Functional Features

The most superficial feature of cerebral white matter is the **superior longitudinal fasciculus** (2) (**arcuate fasciculus**) located lateral to the insula. It interconnects the cortices of the frontal, parietal, occipital, and temporal lobes.

The **inferior occipitofrontal fasciculus** (3) interconnects the inferolateral cortex of the frontal lobe to the cortex of the occipital lobe and also to the inferior temporal and medial occipitotemporal gyri of the temporal lobe. The hook-shaped association bundle, the **uncinate fasciculus** (4), is an anterior subdivision of the inferior occipitofrontal fasciculus. The cortices of the temporal pole and middle frontal gyrus are joined by the dorsal division of the uncinate fasciculus, and the ventral division joins the cortex of the parahippocampal gyrus with the orbital surface of the frontal lobe.

The **optic chiasm** (5) of the diencephalon and the **olfactory tract** (6) of the telencephalon are both located on the ventral surface.

Clinical Correlations . . . .

Aphasia is defined as a language disorder: loss of the ability to comprehend or express the signs and symbols of communication. **Lesions** of the **superior longitudinal fasciculus** in the left hemisphere **disconnect** the **receptive (sensory) posterior language area** from the **expressive (motor) anterior area.** Stated another way, the area for language comprehension becomes disconnected from the area for language expression (page 32). The following description is an oversimplification of the components of language, presented in this manner merely to emphasize the importance of anatomy in contributing to language complexity.

Global aphasia results from lesions of both the anterior and posterior language areas in which all aspects of speech and language are severely disturbed. **Motor (Broca's) aphasia** (areas 44, 45) is the loss of ability to express ideas by speech or writing and is associated with a lesion, often vascular, of the inferior frontal gyrus of the dominant hemisphere. Due to the proximity of Broca's area to the precentral gyrus, motor or nonfluent aphasia is usually accompanied by right-sided hemiparesis. **Sensory (Wernicke's) aphasia** (posterior portion of area 22 and areas 39, 40) is associated with a lesion in the temporal lobe of the dominant hemisphere in the region near the primary auditory area, or in the inferior parietal lobule (angular and supramarginal gyri), or both. Sensory aphasia or difficulty in comprehending spoken language is also associated with disturbances in reading (alexia, dyslexia) and writing (agraphia, dysgraphia).

Dissection of the Left Hemisphere from the Lateral Surface

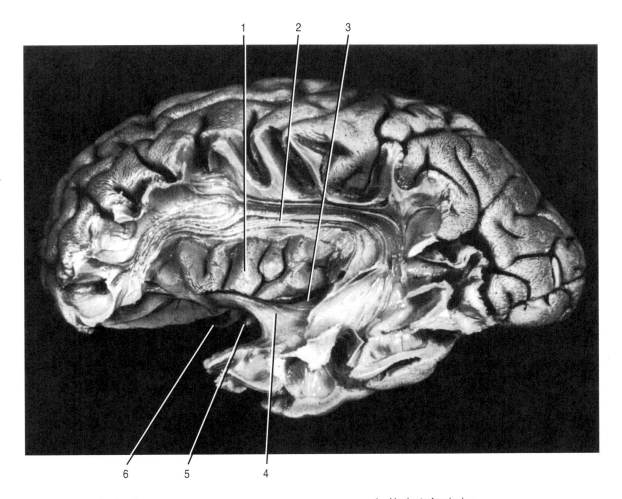

1. Insula
2. Superior longitudinal fasciculus
3. Inferior occipitofrontal fasciculus
4. Uncinate fasciculus
5. Optic chiasm
6. Olfactory tract

(Reprinted with permission from Ludwig E, Klingler J. Atlas Cerebri Humani. Basel, Switzerland: S. Karger, 1956, Table 5.)

Chapter One Study Questions

Questions 1–11
Directions: Each question below contains four or five suggested answers. Choose the one best response to each question.

1. **All of the following are located in the diencephalon except the**
   (a) Epithalamus
   (b) Putamen
   (c) Hypothalamus
   (d) Subthalamus
   (e) Thalamus

2. **Incomplete fusion at the rostral neuropore results in**
   (a) Spina bifida cystica
   (b) Meningomyelocele
   (c) Myelocele
   (d) Meningocele
   (e) None of the above

3. **The following statements regarding CSF are correct except**
   (a) The ventricles contain about 40 mL of CSF.
   (b) Together the ventricles and the subarachnoid space contain about 150 mL of CSF.
   (c) A count of 30 cells in each milliliter of CSF is normal.
   (d) Production and absorption results in replacement of CSF several times daily.
   (e) In the recumbent posture, normal CSF pressure in the lumbar cistern is 80–180 cm H_2O.

4. **CSF enters the venous circulation via**
   (a) Active transport through the arachnoid villi
   (b) Passive transport through the arachnoid villi
   (c) The superior sagittal sinus
   (d) All of the above

5. **Through which of the following foramina does CSF flow from the lateral ventricle into the third ventricle?**
   (a) Hypoglossal foramen
   (b) Interventricular foramen
   (c) Foramen of Magendie
   (d) Foramen of Luschka
   (e) Cerebral aqueduct

6. **In an adult, blockage of the foramina leading from the fourth ventricle results in**
   (a) Dilation of only the lateral ventricles
   (b) Internal hydrocephalus of the ventricular system
   (c) External hydrocephalus
   (d) Macrocephaly
   (e) Internal hydrocephalus involving only the third and fourth ventricles

7. **The most frequent site of blockage of CSF circulation is the**
   (a) Cerebral aqueduct
   (b) Left interventricular foramen
   (c) Right interventricular foramen
   (d) Foramen of Magendie
   (e) Right foramen of Luschka

8. **The inferior sagittal sinus lies in the free margin of the**
   (a) Diaphragma sellae
   (b) Tentorium cerebelli
   (c) Falx cerebri
   (d) Falx cerebelli
   (e) None of the above

9. **Which of the following patterns describes the typical continuous, sequential direction of flow of venous blood?**
   (a) Superior sagittal sinus, straight sinus, left transverse sinus, left sigmoid sinus
   (b) Internal cerebral vein, straight sinus, right transverse sinus, sigmoid sinus
   (c) Thalamostriate vein, internal cerebral vein, great cerebral vein, left sigmoid sinus
   (d) Internal cerebral vein, great cerebral vein, straight sinus, left transverse sinus
   (e) Superior sagittal sinus, straight sinus, right transverse sinus, right sigmoid sinus

10. **Which of the following are either in the cavernous sinus per se or in the wall of the cavernous sinus?**
    (a) Abducens, oculomotor and trochlear nerves
    (b) Internal carotid artery and plexus
    (c) Ophthalmic division of the trigeminal nerve
    (d) Maxillary division of the trigeminal nerve
    (e) All of the above

11. **In mass-occupying lesions, the structure most likely to herniate through the tentorial incisure (notch) is the**
    (a) Cingulate gyrus
    (b) Uncus
    (c) Tonsils of the cerebellum
    (d) Hypothalamus
    (e) Occipital lobe

Answers and Explanations for Chapter One Study Questions

1. **b** [page 2] The putamen, one of the basal ganglia, is a telencephalic structure. One can easily identify the thalamus and hypothalamus in the median plane. The epithalamus is the posterior part of the diencephalon and comprises the habenula and its fiber bundles, the pineal gland, part of the posterior commissure, and the tela choroidea of the third ventricle. The subthalamus (ventral thalamus) contains the subthalamic nucleus, which is involved in motor circuits.

2. **e** [page 4] Failure of the cerebral hemispheres to develop is termed anencephaly. Anencephaly occurs due to a lack of fusion of the rostral neuropore. Spina bifida cystica, meningomyelocele, myelocele, and meningocele are abnormalities associated with incomplete fusion at the caudal neuropore.

3. **c** [page 8] Normal CSF is clear and colorless and contains very few cells. More than 10 cells per milliliter is usually indicative of disease.

4. **d** [page 8] CSF exits the brain via the apertures of the fourth ventricle into the subarachnoid space, which encloses the CNS. Through arachnoid villi, which project into the superior sagittal sinus, CSF moves via passive and active transport into the venous circulation.

5. **b** [page 8] The interventricular foramen allows the CSF to flow from the lateral ventricle into the third ventricle. The hypoglossal foramen (of the skull) transmits the hypoglossal nerve, the foramina of Magendie and Luschka are apertures related to the fourth ventricle, and the cerebral aqueduct connects the third and fourth ventricles.

6. **b** [page 10] Internal hydrocephalus refers to enlargement of either one or all of the four ventricles as well as the cerebral aqueduct. External hydrocephalus refers to excess CSF in the subarachnoid space. When elements of both phenomena occur, the condition is called communicating hydrocephalus.

7. **a** [page 10] Stenosis of the narrow cerebral aqueduct is the most common cause of blockage of CSF circulation and, therefore, of internal hydrocephalus. Occlusion of either the left or right interventricular foramina is a rare occurrence. If the foramen of Magendie (midline) and the foramina of Luschka (lateral), which are apertures of the fourth ventricle, are blocked, there is dilatation of the ventricles upstream (i.e., the entire ventricular system becomes enlarged).

8. **c** [page 12] The falx cerebri abuts the corpus callosum in the interhemispheric fissure, which separates the cerebral hemispheres. The inferior sagittal sinus lies in its free border and receives venous blood from the falx cerebri. The diaphragma sellae covers the sella turcica. The falx cerebelli is midline within the posterior cranial fossa, whereas the tentorium cerebelli forms the roof of the posterior fossa.

9. **d** [page 12] The usual pattern of venous blood flow is from the superior sagittal sinus to right transverse sinus and from the inferior sagittal sinus straight to left transverse sinus.

10. **e** [page 14] The oculomotor and trochlear nerves and the ophthalmic and maxillary divisions of the trigeminal nerve are in the lateral wall. The internal carotid artery and plexus and the abducens nerve run through the cavernous sinus and are most vulnerable to thrombosis of the sinus.

11. **b** [page 16] The uncus is the anteriomedial part of the parahippocampal gyrus of the temporal lobe, which lies in a medial position, superior to the tentorial incisure. Mass-occupying lesions in the middle cranial fossa push the uncus downward through the incisure into the posterior fossa.

Chapter One Study Questions (*continued*)

Directions: Matching Exercises. For each numbered item, select the **one** lettered choice with which it is the **most** closely associated. Each lettered choice may be used once, more than once, or not at all.

12–18: Match each mature brain structure with the correct subdivision of the brain.

12. **Tectum**

13. **Pons**

14. **Cerebral peduncles**

15. **Medulla oblongata**

16. **Lateral ventricles**

17. **Cerebellum**

18. **Third ventricle**
    (a) Metencephalon
    (b) Telencephalon
    (c) Myelencephalon
    (d) Diencephalon
    (e) Mesencephalon

19–21: Match each description with the correct topographical site.

19. **Closes between 18 and 24 months of age**

20. **Overlies the middle meningeal artery**

21. **Site of the posterior fontanel**
    (a) Bregma
    (b) Lambda
    (c) Pterion

22–24: Match each boundary between lobes with the correct sulcus.

22. **Boundary between the parietal and occipital lobes**

23. **Separates frontal from temporal lobe**

24. **Boundary between frontal and parietal lobes**
    (a) Calcarine
    (b) Postcentral
    (c) Central
    (d) Lateral
    (e) None of the above

25–30: Match each gyrus or area with the correct function or corresponding Brodmann's area.

25. **Precentral gyrus**

26. **Recognition of auditory stimuli**

27. **Broca's area**

28. **Paracentral lobule**

29. **Recognition of taste**

30. **Heschl's convolutions**
    (a) Brodmann's areas 41, 42
    (b) Surrounds the central sulcus above the cingulate gyrus
    (c) Brodmann's area 43
    (d) Anterior (motor) speech area
    (e) Primary motor cortex

12. **e** [pages 4 and 5] The tectum is that part of the mesencephalon dorsal to the cerebral aqueduct and comprising the superior and inferior colliculi. (syn: quadrigeminal plate; corpora quadrigemina)

13. **a** [pages 4 and 5] The word "pons" means bridge. A part of the metencephalon, it is that part of the brain stem **between** the mesencephalon and the open medulla.

14. **e** [pages 4 and 5] The cerebral peduncles are the ventral part of each half of the mesencephalon, exclusive of the tectum. It consists of a dorsal part, the tegmentum, and a ventral part, the basis pedunculi or crus cerebri.

15. **c** [pages 4 and 5] The medulla oblongata is the caudal division of the brain stem interposed between the spinal cord and the pons. Its two subdivisions are the open medulla bordering on the fourth ventricle and the closed medulla, which surrounds the rostral part of the central canal.

16. **b** [pages 4 and 5] The lateral ventricles are irregularly shaped cavities in each cerebral hemisphere of the telencephalon. Each lateral ventricle communicates with the third ventricle through its own interventricular foramen.

17. **a** [pages 4 and 5] The cerebellum (little brain) is derived from the alar plates of the metencephalon. It consists of a median part, the vermis, and two laterally placed cerebellar hemispheres. It is located in the posterior cranial fossa and is concerned with equilibrium, coordination, and the regulation of muscle tone.

18. **d** [pages 4 and 5] The third ventricle is a midline cavity between the two halves of the diencephalon that extends rostrally to the lamina terminalis. Caudally it is continuous with the cerebral aqueduct.

19. **a** [pages 6 and 7] Bregma is the largest of the fontanels in the skull and is the point where the coronal and sagittal sutures meet: the juncture of the frontal bone with the two parietal bones.

20. **c** [pages 6 and 7] The pterion is the point at which the greater wing of the sphenoid bone meets the parietal bone and the squamous part of the temporal bone. Fractures in this area often damage the underlying artery and result in an epidural hematoma.

21. **b** [pages 6 and 7] Lambda is the point of juncture of the occipital bone and the two parietal bones of the skull; here the lambdoid and sagittal sutures meet in the form of the Greek letter lambda.

22. **e** [pages 18 and 19] The parieto-occipital sulcus is the boundary between the parietal and occipital lobes on the medial surface of the cerebral hemisphere. On the lateral surface, a line from the parieto-occipital sulcus to the preoccipital notch defines the anterior limits of the occipital lobe.

23. **d** [pages 18 and 19] The lateral sulcus lies below the frontal and parietal lobes and above the temporal lobe.

24. **c** [pages 18 and 19] The central sulcus is about midway between the frontal and occipital poles mostly on the lateral surface of the cerebral hemisphere, and it separates the frontal and parietal lobes. Its upper end extends a short distance into the paracentral lobule on the medial surface of the hemisphere.

25. **e** [pages 22 and 23] The precentral gyrus (area 4) on the lateral surface of the frontal lobe extends from the lateral sulcus to the superior border of the hemisphere. It is the primary motor cortex.

26. **a** [pages 28 and 29] Transverse gyri in the floor of the lateral sulcus (located posteriorly and superiorly in the superior temporal gyrus) function as primary auditory cortex for recognition of auditory stimuli.

27. **d** [pages 28 and 29] Broca's area (44, 45) in the inferior frontal gyrus is the anterior speech area. Lesions of this area interfere with language expression, therefore, the deficit is termed "expressive aphasia."

28. **b** [pages 24 and 25] The central sulcus on the dorsolateral surface of the hemisphere continues a short distance into the paracentral lobule on the medial surface. Areas 3,1,2 continue posterior to the sulcus and area 4 continues anterior to the sulcus in the paracentral lobule on the medial surface of the hemisphere. These are cortical areas of lower limb sensation and motor control, respectively.

29. **c** [pages 28 and 29] The cortical area for taste is area 43, located just above the lateral sulcus.

30. **a** [pages 28 and 29] Heschl's convolutions are synonymous with the transverse temporal gyri, the primary auditory cortex (areas 41,42).

CHAPTER 2 The Relation of the Spinal Cord and Spinal Nerves to the Meninges and Vertebral Column

Definitions

Neurons in the spinal cord make up the **central gray matter,** which is surrounded by ascending and descending fibers in the **dorsal, lateral, and ventral funiculi** of **white matter. Dorsal** and **ventral horns** of gray matter indicate the presence of continuous columns of sensory and motor neurons, respectively. The **lateral horn** of gray matter indicates the presence of preganglionic autonomic neurons.

Dorsal roots transmit sensory information from dorsal root ganglia (collections of sensory neurons within the intervertebral foramina) to neurons in the dorsal horn. **Ventral roots** transmit motor information from neurons in the ventral horn to striated muscle. Dorsal and ventral roots join at the intervertebral foramen to form a mixed **spinal nerve.** A **nerve** is defined as a bundle of fibers connecting the brain or spinal cord with the eyes, ears, muscles, glands, and other parts of the body. Nerves are elements of the peripheral nervous system (PNS); 31 pairs of spinal nerves supply all parts of the body. Cranial nerves similarly innervate the face and head and additionally mediate the special senses. The spinal cord is not segmented; rather, the distribution of the spinal nerves gives it a **functional segmentation.** The spinal cord, roots, and meningeal coverings lie within the **vertebral canal** collectively formed by the vertebral foramina of all the vertebrae.

Structural and Functional Features

There are seven cervical vertebrae and eight cervical nerves; nerves C1–C7 leave the vertebral canal above the vertebrae with the corresponding number and C8 passes through the foramen between the seventh cervical and the first thoracic vertebrae. From that point caudally, each spinal nerve exits the vertebral canal below the corresponding vertebrae.

The tapered end of the spinal cord (**conus medullaris**) lies at L3 at birth; however, it ends at L2 in the adult. The diameter and shape of the nearly cylindrical spinal cord is dependent on the tissue mass of the area innervated by the spinal nerves of the region. For example, there are cervical (C3–T1) and lumbosacral (L1–S2) enlargements due to the innervation of the upper and lower limbs. However, the thoracic central gray matter is thin because thoracic segments (except T1) do not contribute to the innervation of the limbs. Conversely, the thoracic lateral horn is prominent at T1–L2 because those levels provide preganglionic sympathetic (thoracolumbar) innervation. Preganglionic parasympathetic neurons are located in a similar position at S2–S4 (sacral component of craniosacral system).

The cross-sectional area of the white matter is greatest at rostral cervical levels because ascending and descending fibers from, and to, more caudal levels pass through cervical funiculi. It follows that the smallest cross-sectional area of fibers are present in the caudal sacral regions.

Surface indentations visible in cross sections and subtle intrinsic differences characterize spinal cord levels as cervical, thoracic, lumbar, or sacral. The deep **ventral median fissure,** bounded ventrally by the single **anterior spinal artery** (ASA), and a less distinct **dorsal medium septum** are present at all levels. The **dorsal intermediate septum** is present only at and above T6. Its presence distinguishes ascending fibers subserving the upper limb from those of the lower limb, which are located medial to the dorsal intermediate septum. The bilateral **posterior spinal arteries** descend along the entry zone of the dorsal root fibers.

Within the vertebral canal, the spinal cord is also protected by ligaments, cerebrospinal fluid (CSF), and meninges. The microscopic innermost meningeal layer, the **pia mater,** adheres to the surface of the cord. The **arachnoid** layer bridges over the surface irregularities to form the outer boundary of the subarachnoid space. Below the conus medullaris, the spinal nerves descend in the **subarachnoid space,** which makes up the **lumbar cistern.** The outermost meningeal covering, the **dura mater,** extends from the base of the skull to the level of the second sacral vertebra. It is continuous with the **epineurium** of spinal nerves at the intervertebral foramen. The spinal meninges are continuous with those of the brain through the foramen magnum at the base of the skull.

Clinical Correlations . . . .

Spinal taps (lumbar puncture) into the lumbar cistern are made to withdraw CSF for analysis and to inject anesthetic agents. Safe needle entry into the cistern is indicated at L3–L4 below the conus medullaris.

Meningiomas, tumors of the meninges, are more common than tumors within the spinal cord. Compression of the spinal cord within the vertebral canal affects ascending and descending tracts as well as segmental nerve roots. A skilled clinician often ascertains the level of a suspected mass by the dermatomes and movements affected and relies on technical procedures to confirm the level. Early surgical intervention is desirable to prevent irreversible damage.

In the figure on the left, color the cervical spinal cord yellow, the thoracic segments green, the lumbar region blue, and the sacral area red. Note the termination of the spinal cord at L2. In the figure on the right, color the pia mater blue, the arachnoid green, and the dura mater red.

The Relation of the Spinal Cord and Spinal Nerves to the Meninges and Vertebral Column

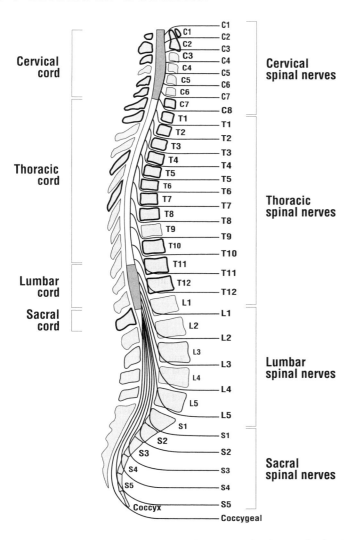

Cervical cord

Thoracic cord

Lumbar cord

Sacral cord

| C1 | C2 | C3 | C4 | C5 | C6 | C7 |

Cervical spinal nerves

C1 · C2 · C3 · C4 · C5 · C6 · C7 · C8

T1 · T2 · T3 · T4 · T5 · T6 · T7 · T8 · T9 · T10 · T11 · T12

Thoracic spinal nerves

L1 · L2 · L3 · L4 · L5

Lumbar spinal nerves

S1 · S2 · S3 · S4 · S5 · Coccygeal

Sacral spinal nerves

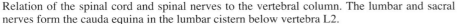

Relation of the spinal cord and spinal nerves to the vertebral column. The lumbar and sacral nerves form the cauda equina in the lumbar cistern below vertebra L2.

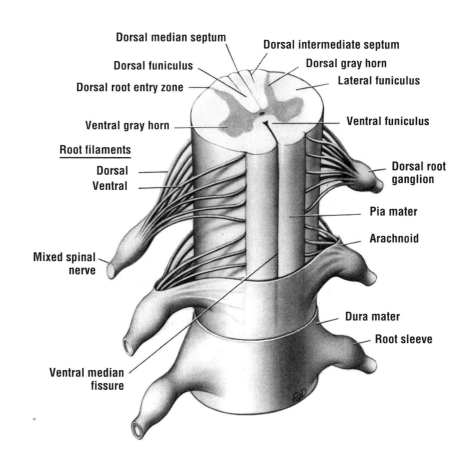

Dorsal median septum

Dorsal funiculus

Dorsal root entry zone

Ventral gray horn

Root filaments
Dorsal
Ventral

Mixed spinal nerve

Ventral median fissure

Dorsal intermediate septum

Dorsal gray horn

Lateral funiculus

Ventral funiculus

Dorsal root ganglion

Pia mater

Arachnoid

Dura mater

Root sleeve

Relation of the meninges to the spinal cord and nerve roots. (Reprinted with permission from Carpenter MB. Core Text of Neuroanatomy. 4th ed. Baltimore: Williams and Wilkins, 1991.)

Transverse Section of the Spinal Cord Showing a Somatic Reflex Arc

Sensory   The dorsal portion of the neural tube and, later, the **alar** plate derivatives transmit sensory information. Cells that bring information from the periphery to the central nervous system (CNS) are **afferent** or **sensory** neurons. A **dermatome** is the cutaneous area innervated by the afferent fibers of a particular spinal nerve. The first order neuron is located within the dorsal root ganglia (DRG) of spinal nerves or within ganglia of cranial nerve (CN) **V, VII, VIII, IX**, and **X** (Details of **CN I, II**, and **VIII** are below). The peripheral process extends to somatic or visceral sensory receptors; the central process enters the CNS and terminates on association neurons or directly on second order neurons in sensory pathways. First order sensory neurons in DRG of spinal nerves are derivatives of neural crest. First order sensory neurons of CN V, VII, IX, and X are derived from neural crest. Sensory neurons in CN I are derived from the olfactory placode, in CN II from the optic cup, and in CN VIII from the otic placode. Bipolar neurons of CN I, located in the olfactory epithelium in each nasal cavity, serve as receptors for the sense of smell. Receptor cells for CN II are located in the retina. Auditory receptors for CN VIII are hair cells located in the organ of Corti in the inner ear, and the vestibular receptors are hair cells in the semicircular ducts and in the vestibular portion of the labyrinth, also located in the inner ear.

Motor   The ventral portion of the neural tube and, later, the **basal** plate derivatives give rise to neurons whose axons leave the CNS to innervate the appropriate target organ. Nerve impulses traveling from the cell body along the axon elicit a response in the target organ, therefore, these are **efferent** or **motor** neurons. A **motor unit** is an alpha motor neuron (anterior motor horn cell) and the muscle fibers it innervates. The number varies from as few as 10 to as many as several hundred, depending on the precision required.

Association   These neurons (interneurons) serve a "connector" function in the spinal cord, brain stem, and diencephalon. Those of the cerebral hemisphere establish connections with other cortical nerve cells in the same hemisphere.

Modality   Sensations consciously perceived from the skin are known as modalities. In medical practice, the five somatic modalities easily tested by clinical examination include fine (discriminative) touch, vibration, light touch, temperature (warmth or cold), and pain. The pathways that process these are well defined. Transmission of other modalities—itch, tickle, firm pressure, and rubbing—are less well understood.

Somatotopic   Representation of parts of the body in corresponding parts of the brain. Fibers in a tract are orderly layered (laminated) to faithfully relay messages relative to their site of origin. **Retinotopic** and **tonotopic** connote a similar meaning regarding information from the eyes and ears, respectively.

General Organization   It is an understatement to say that the nervous system is, including spinal mechanisms, immensely complex. The spinal cord is probably the least complex, mainly because the 8 cervical, 12 thoracic, 5 lumbar, 5 sacral, and 1 coccygeal spinal nerves are all similarly organized. Modalities and functional components categorize the ways in which the spinal and cranial nerves transmit sensory information to various levels of the neuraxis. The result is either an immediate reflex response or a conscious experience that may lead to an immediate or delayed behavioral response. Nerves contain fibers designated as **general** if they are distributed throughout the head and body. **Somatic** refers to the body wall and limbs; **visceral** describes innervation of the viscera. Each spinal nerve contains four functional components: **general somatic afferent** (GSA), **general somatic efferent** (GSE), **general visceral afferent** (GVA), and **general visceral efferent** (GVE). (Exceptions are the first cervical nerve, which lacks a dorsal root and the coccygeal nerve, which may be absent.) Cranial nerves may contain only one afferent component, only one efferent component, or as many as five components. In addition to the four functional components contained in spinal nerves, cranial nerves may have special components: these are designated as **special somatic afferent** (SSA), **special visceral afferent** (SVA), and **special visceral efferent** (SVE). "Special" refers to the senses of olfaction, gustation (taste), vision, audition, and equilibrium and to the muscles of branchiomeric origin.

The somatic motor system innervates voluntary skeletal (striated) muscle, whereas the **autonomic nervous system** (ANS) influences involuntary smooth muscle, cardiac muscle, and glands. Somatic motor axons from ventral horn cells go directly through the ventral root and spinal nerve to striated muscle. Visceral innervation involves two neurons. The preganglionic neuron in the lateral horn gives rise to a myelinated axon that goes through the ventral root and white ramus communicans to terminate on a postganglionic neuron in a sympathetic ganglion, which gives rise to an unmyelinated axon that joins the spinal nerve through the gray ramus communicans to reach visceral target organs in the body wall. The autonomic nervous system is described and illustrated in Chapter 4 (pages 144–147)

Clinical Correlations . . . .

Herpes zoster (shingles), a viral infection of the DRG, is characterized by pain and an eruption of groups of vesicles on one side of the body following the course of a nerve. It commonly occurs in the thoracic region and is usually limited to one or two dermatomes. The segmental skin lesions confined to one half of the body are a hallmark of this condition.

Color the dorsal horns blue and the ventral horns red. Color the sensory fiber blue from the receptor to its synapse in the dorsal horn. Color the axon of the motor neuron red. Distal to the DRG, observe that the spinal nerve contains GSA and GSE components. (GVA and GVE components are not pictured.)

Transverse Section of the Spinal Cord Showing a Somatic Reflex Arc

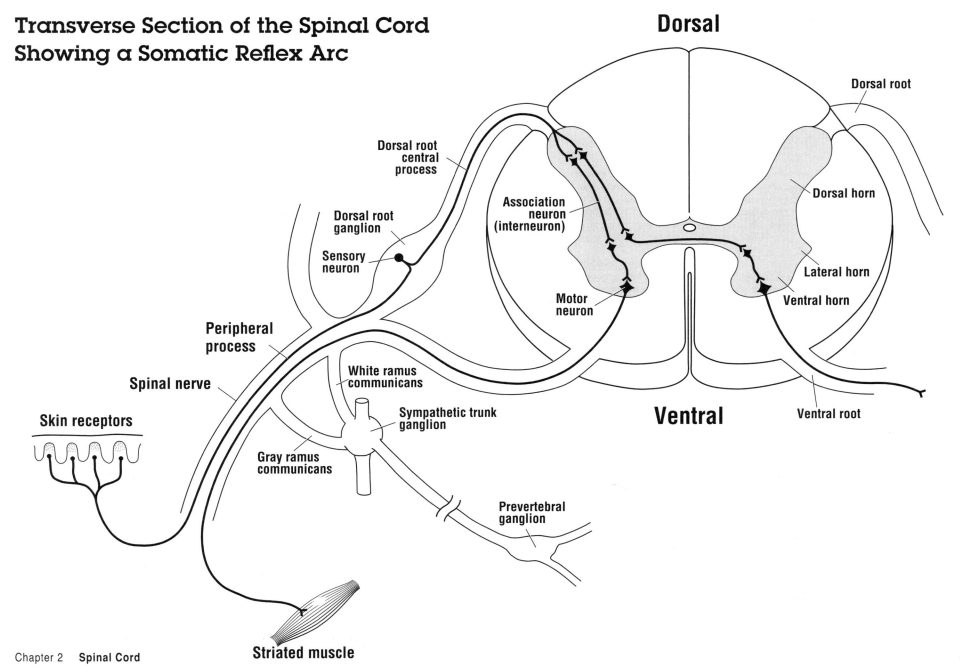

Dorsal

Dorsal root

Dorsal root central process

Dorsal horn

Dorsal root ganglion

Association neuron (interneuron)

Sensory neuron

Lateral horn

Motor neuron

Ventral horn

Peripheral process

Spinal nerve

White ramus communicans

Skin receptors

Sympathetic trunk ganglion

Gray ramus communicans

Ventral

Ventral root

Prevertebral ganglion

Striated muscle

Spinal Cord at Lumbosacral Enlargement (S1)

Definitions

Terms used for a bundle of fibers in the CNS include **tract, fasciculus, brachium, peduncle, lemniscus, ansa,** and **capsule. Decussation** and **commissure** connote fibers that cross the midline. A **funiculus** is one of the large masses of white matter of the spinal cord, set off by the dorsal and ventral horns of the gray matter, the dorsal median septum, and the ventral median fissure. The dorsal funiculus varies in size and shape at lower and upper spinal cord levels. (Note that **fasciculus** is a tract in a funiculus.) The **gracile** (slender) **fasciculus** occupies the dorsal funiculus of the cord below T6. The **cuneate** (wedge-shaped) **fasciculus** lies lateral to the gracile fasciculus at, and above T6 and is visually definable due to the presence of the dorsal intermediate septum.

Propriospinal fibers (fasciculus proprius; spinospinal) surround the gray matter and arise and terminate within the spinal cord. Fibers in the **ventral white commissure** cross ventral to the **central canal,** an ependyma-lined cavity that extends throughout the spinal cord and to the obex of the medulla, where it opens into the fourth ventricle.

Structural and Functional Features

Relative amounts of gray and white matter, the presence or absence of particular nuclei, and the overall shape of this cross section characterizes this level as sacral.

Characteristics of the S1 level are as follows:

- A circular form in cross section
- Massive dorsal and ventral horns
- An extensive substantia gelatinosa
- Less white matter than at higher spinal cord levels
- A gracile fasciculus
- The absence of a dorsal intermediate septum
- The absence of a cuneate fasciculus
- The absence of the dorsal nucleus of Clarke

At all levels, the butterfly-shaped gray matter of the dorsal horn contains the posteromarginal nucleus, the substantia gelatinosa, and the nucleus proprius. Dorsally a thin layer of large cells in the **posteromarginal nucleus** gives rise to intrinsic (propriospinal) fibers and to some axons that join the spinothalamic pathway. The **substantia gelatinosa** is composed of small cells in the outer part of the dorsal horn and is largely a synaptic zone of interneurons that receive incoming and descending messages. The densely packed cells with finely branched dendrites make up a prominent unstained area in myelin-stained sections. The **nucleus proprius,** an area ventral to the substantia gelatinosa, contains both large and small cells including the cells of origin of numerous ascending fibers, many of which are spinothalamic. The long dendrites of tract cells ramify into laminae II and III. In contrast to the substantia gelatinosa, which is unstained, the nucleus proprius is conspicuous in myelin-stained sections. There are no GVE–ANS neurons present at this level. The **dorsal nucleus of Clarke** (nucleus dorsalis) is prominent more rostrally; however, it does not extend below midlumbar level.

The **lumbosacral enlargement** (L1–S2) has extensive gray matter and a well-developed substantia gelatinosa due to the innervation of the lower limb. Medial and lateral cell columns in the ventral horn innervate trunk and limb muscles, respectively. The dorsal funiculus contains only the gracile fasciculus, an uncrossed tract that transmits proprioception, vibration, pressure, and discriminative touch from the leg (at this level). The S1 level does not contain parasympathetic neurons, which are located laterally at S2–S4 levels in the intermediate zone between the dorsal and ventral horns.

Clinical Correlations . . . .

Flexion injuries of the spine, coupled with existing degenerative changes in the intervertebral disc, result in **posterolateral herniation** of the disc into the vertebral canal, which, in turn, results in **root** or **spinal nerve compression.** If **dorsal** or **ventral roots** are independently involved, **sensory** or **motor symptoms** occur, respectively. **Spinal nerve** disorders involve both **sensory** and **motor** disturbances, either of which affects the stretch reflex. Disc prolapse tends to occur in the freely mobile lumbar and cervical regions of the vertebral column. Herniation is most prevalent at lumbar levels L4–L5 and L5–S1 and cervical levels C5–C6 and C6–C7.

The dotted line surrounding the gray matter demarcates the position of the propriospinal fibers. They interconnect spinal cord segments. Use alternating blue (sensory) and red (motor) slash marks to fill the PS region in **all** funiculi, indicating ascending and descending fibers interconnecting various levels of the spinal cord.

Spinal Cord at Lumbosacral Enlargement (S1)

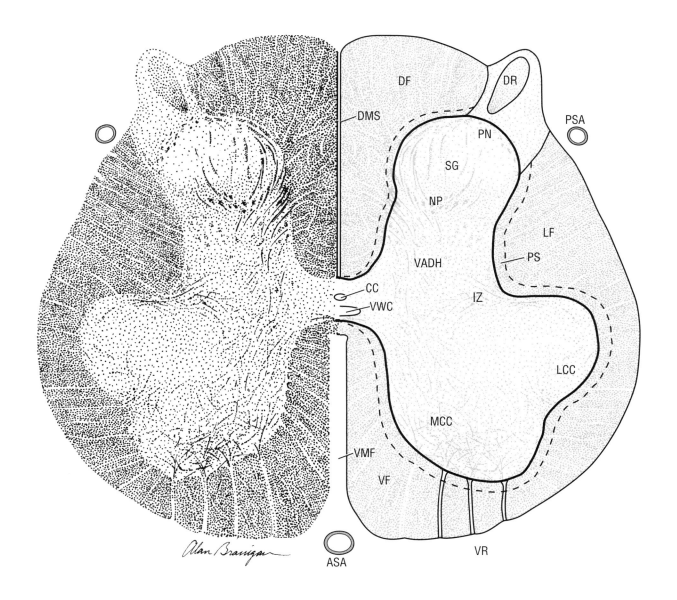

White Matter (fiber pathways)
DF Dorsal funiculus containing gracile fasciculus
LF Lateral funiculus
VF Ventral funiculus
PS Propriospinal fibers
DR Dorsal root entry zone has medial and lateral (Lissauer's zone) divisions
VR Ventral root exit
VWC Ventral white commissure

Gray Matter
PN Posteromarginal nucleus
SG Substantia gelatinosa
NP Nucleus proprius
VADH Ventral area of dorsal horn
IZ Intermediate zone
MCC Medial cell column
LCC Lateral cell column

Other
DMS Dorsal median septum
CC Central canal
VMF Ventral median fissure
PSA Posterior spinal arteries
ASA Anterior spinal artery

Spinal Cord at High Lumbar Level (L2)

Definitions

In the intermediate zone or **ventral area of the dorsal horn** (VADH), the **intermediomedial** and **intermediolateral cell columns** receive and give rise to GVA and GVE messages, respectively. The presence of sympathetic (thoracolumbar) preganglionic motor neurons creates the prominent **lateral horn** at T1–L2 levels.

Pathways are often named relative to their origin and termination. Thus, **spinothalamic** describes an ascending tract that is sensory, whereas **corticospinal** refers to a descending pathway that originates in the cortex and terminates at spinal levels.

Structural and Functional Features

Characteristics of the L2 level are as follows:

- The transverse diameter is greater than the sagittal diameter.
- The ventral horns contain robust medial and lateral motor nuclei (lumbosacral enlargement; L1–S2).
- The dorsal nucleus of Clarke (nucleus dorsalis) is prominent.
- A lateral horn containing GVE neurons is present.
- A dorsal intermediate septum is absent.
- A cuneate fasciculus is absent.

The white matter is more extensive in the lumbar region than in the sacral region; however, lumbar and sacral segments contribute innervation to the lower limb, therefore, the gray matter at the lumbar level is similar to that of the sacral level. A major difference is the presence of the **dorsal nucleus of Clarke** (nucleus dorsalis) in the dorsal horn at segments C8–L3. This nucleus contains large neurons with eccentric nuclei, which give rise to myelineated axons that ascend in the same side of the cord in the **dorsal spinocerebellar tract** (DSCT) and enter the **inferior cerebellar peduncle** (ICP) to terminate in the ipsilateral cerebellar cortex. There are three conduit peduncles to the cerebellum: The inferior one links the spinal cord and medulla to the cerebellum. The dorsal nucleus of Clarke receives incoming fibers from DRG at C8–L3 levels as well as from DRG below L3. Above C8, fibers from the DRG ascend ipsilaterally to terminate in the **accessory** (lateral) **cuneate nucleus** in the medulla, which functions homologous to the dorsal nucleus of Clarke. Like the DSCT from Clarke's nucleus, the accessory cuneate nucleus projects through the ICP (cuneocerebellar fibers) to transmit proprioceptive messages to the cerebellum.

Cells in laminae V, VI, and VII as well as spinal border cells on the edge of the ventral gray matter in the lumbar segments give rise to fibers that cross and ascend in the ventral funiculus as the **ventral spinocerebellar tract** (VSCT). This tract takes an aberrant route to the cerebellum through the **superior cerebellar peduncle** (SCP), a conduit that generally relates the cerebellum to more rostral structures in the diencephalon and telencephalon. (Page 59 shows the position of the DSCT and VSCT in the periphery of the lateral funiculus.)

Clinical Correlations . . . .

A traumatic, complete **transverse lesion** of the spinal cord results in the sudden loss of all sensations and all **voluntary** movement caudal to the level of injury. Demyelinating and degenerative **diseases** cause variable symptoms over time and may selectively involve ascending pathways (tabes dorsalis), descending pathways (vascular lesions of corticospinal fibers in the internal capsule), DRG and **dorsal roots** (DR) (herpes zoster), or motorneurons (poliomyelitis) or combinations of these involvements. For example, in **subacute combined degeneration**, demyelination of nerve fibers in the dorsal and dorsolateral funiculi results in the loss of position and vibration senses and discriminative touch as well as ataxia and spastic paresis. The patient's gait is ataxic (incoordinated) but is improved when the patient looks at the position of the feet (sensory ataxia). This phenomenon is due to lack of dorsal column and spinocerebellar input. The spastic paresis is due to demyelination of the corticospinal tracts. It is important to diagnose subacute combined degeneration because the causative factor, a **vitamin B$_{12}$ deficiency**, is remediable.

Diagonal lines can indicate lesions. On the labeled half of the cord, draw blue diagonal lines through the dorsal funiculus and along the peripheral edge of the dorsal region of the lateral funiculus (position of ascending fibers, page 59). Draw red diagonal lines in the dorsal region of the lateral funiculus to represent a lesion of the lateral corticospinal tract (page 59). You have created a visual representation of the loss of sensory input and voluntary motor control involved in pernicious anemia (B$_{12}$ deficiency). Be aware that systemic demyelinating diseases cause **bilateral** damage, whereas trauma and vascular insults can result in **unilateral** demyelination.

Spinal Cord at High Lumbar Level (L2)

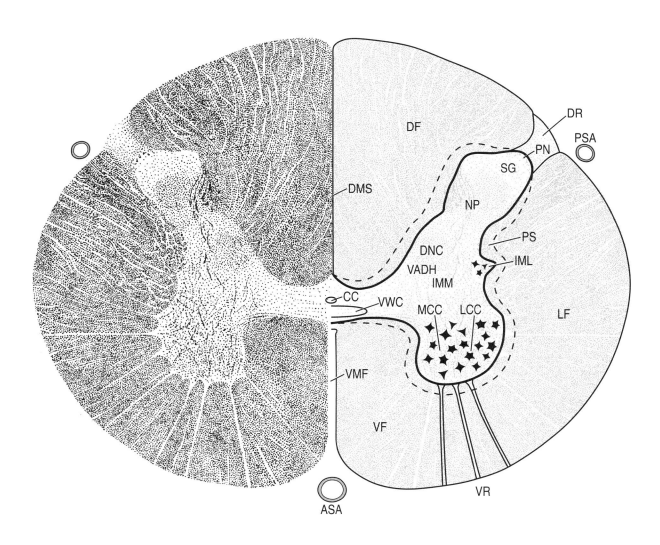

White Matter (fiber pathways)

DF	Dorsal funiculus containing gracile fasciculus
LF	Lateral funiculus
VF	Ventral funiculus
PS	Propriospinal fibers
DR	Dorsal root entry zone has medial and lateral (Lissauer's zone) divisions
VR	Ventral root exit
VWC	Ventral white commissure

Gray Matter

PN	Posteromarginal nucleus
SG	Substantia gelantinosa
NP	Nucleus proprius
VADH	Ventral area of dorsal horn
DNC	Dorsal nucleus of Clarke
IMM	Intermediomedial cell column
IML	Intermediolateral cell column
MCC	Medial cell column
LCC	Lateral cell column

Other

DMS	Dorsal median septum
CC	Central canal
VMF	Ventral median fissure
PSA	Posterior spinal arteries
ASA	Anterior spinal artery

Spinal Cord at High Thoracic Level (T2)

Definitions

Primary or first order (1°) sensory fibers arise from cells in the DRG. The dorsal root entry zone has a **lateral** division containing small fibers and a **medial** division composed of myelinated fibers, many of which are of large caliber. Fibers in the lateral division transmit sensations of pain and temperature, whereas those in the medial division transmit vibration, touch, pressure, and proprioceptive modalities. Lemniscus refers to a fiber bundle composed of **secondary** or second order (2°) sensory fibers that terminate in the thalamus.

Dorsal column refers to the dorsal funiculus (DF) of the spinal cord because it contains two "columns" of fibers (gracile and cuneate). Neurons in the gray matter also form columns. Therefore, this terminology can be confusing. Nonetheless, it is an entrenched, useful clinical term, especially in describing the **dorsal column–medial lemniscal** system (below).

Structural and Functional Features

Characteristics of the T2 level are as follows:

- The transverse diameter is greater than the sagittal diameter.
- The amount of white matter is greater than the gray matter.
- The thin dorsal and ventral horns are H-shaped.
- The dorsal nucleus of Clarke is prominent.
- A prominent intermediolateral cell column (lateral horn) is present, which contains sympathetic GVE neurons.
- All levels at and above T6 show a dorsal intermediate septum defining the gracile fasciculus medially and the cuneate fasciculus laterally.
- A lateral cell column (lamina IX) is absent in the ventral horn because only trunk muscles are supplied at this level.

Group C (unmyelinated) fibers and group A (thinly myelinated) fibers in the lateral division of the dorsal root divide into ascending and descending branches that course in the dorsolateral fasciculus (of Lissauer). Many fibers terminate within the segment of entry; others extend as far as four segments rostral or caudal. Their collateral branches terminate on cells in the substantia gelatinosa and on interneurons or tract cells in the nucleus proprius, whose axons mediate sensations of pain, temperature, and touch. The fibers cross and ascend in the spinothalamic tract together with spinoreticular and spinotectal fibers making up the **ventrolateral system** (spinal lemniscus). The crossing and contralateral ascent of the spinothalamic fibers have significant clinical relevance. Pain transmission is altered by both incoming and descending fibers; the modulation or "editing" of pain sensation occurs largely through excitatory and inhibitory interneurons in the substantia gelatinosa.

The large, rapidly conducting dorsal root fibers in the medial division also divide into ascending and descending branches. The descending branches form fasciculi adjacent to the dorsal median septum (**fasciculus septomarginalis**) and between the gracile and cuneate fasciculi (**fasciculus interfascicularis**). Descending branches enter the dorsal horn at various levels. Ascending branches below T6 make up the gracile fasciculus (lower trunk and limb); those branches at and above T6 form the cuneate fasciculus (upper trunk and limb). Many fibers enter the dorsal horn as they ascend. About one fourth of the fibers reach the medulla and terminate ipsilaterally in the gracile and cuneate nuclei in the medulla. These nuclei give rise to fibers that cross and ascend in the brainstem as the **medial lemniscus.** These fibers convey vibration, discriminative touch and pressure and position sense (proprioception) to the contralateral thalamus. This clinically important **dorsal column–medial lemniscal** pathway is ipsilateral in the spinal cord and contralateral in the brain stem.

Clinical Correlations . . . .

Interruption of the **gracile** and **cuneate fasciculi** in the dorsal column of the spinal cord interrupts the transmission of vibration, pressure, position sense, and discriminative touch ipsilateral to the lesion. For example, a traumatic hemisection of the **spinal cord** above the lumbar enlargement impairs the above sensations and causes incoordination of the leg on the **side of the lesion** (ataxic gait). However, in the **brain stem**, a total lesion of the **medial lemniscus** interrupts the same modalities on the side of the body **contralateral to the lesion**. Furthermore, sensory ataxia is apparent in the arm as well. When executing the command to touch the finger to the nose, the patient's hand makes jerky movements that miss the mark.

The **pathway** involvement of fibers in the dorsal funiculus should be appreciated in contrast to the **segmental pathology** exemplified by herpes zoster (discussed on page 48).

Color to Learn

Encircle and color the PN, SG, NP, and DNC with blue to indicate GSA function. Encircle and color the IMM cell column with purple to indicate GVA function. Encircle and color IML cell column with orange for GVE function. Finally, encircle and color MCC with red to connote its GSE function.

Spinal Cord at High Thoracic Level (T2)

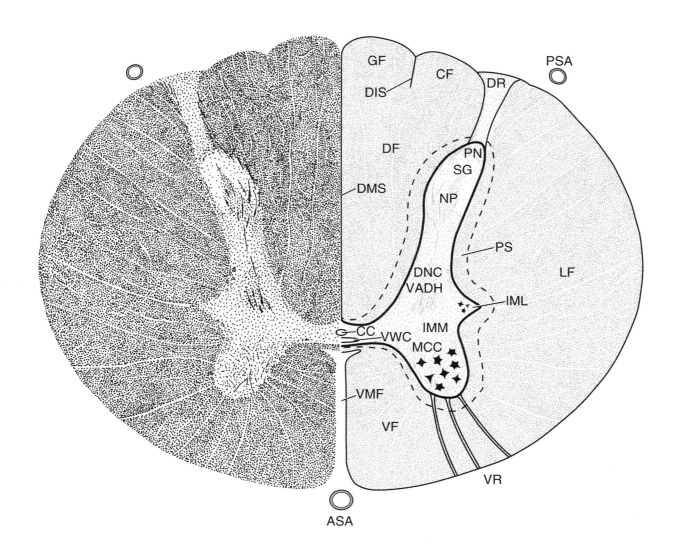

White Matter (fiber pathways)

DF   Dorsal funiculus containing gracile fasciculus (GF) and cuneate fasciculus (CF) demarcated by dorsal intermediate septum
LF   Lateral funiculus
VF   Ventral funiculus
PS   Propriospinal fibers
DR   Dorsal root entry zone has medial and lateral (Lissauer's zone) divisions
VR   Ventral root exit
VWC   Ventral white commissure

Gray Matter

PN   Posteromarginal nucleus
SG   Substantia gelantinosa
NP   Nucleus proprius
VADH   Ventral area of dorsal horn
DNC   Dorsal nucleus of Clarke
IMM   Intermediomedial cell column
IML   Intermediolateral cell column
MCC   Medial cell column

Other

DMS   Dorsal median septum
DIS   Dorsal intermediate septum
CC   Central canal
VMF   Ventral median fissure
PSA   Posterior spinal arteries
ASA   Anterior spinal artery

Spinal Cord at Cervical Enlargement (C7)

Definitions

The **laminae** of **Rexed** is a numerical designation of continuous columns of cells in the spinal cord gray matter. These columns are identified consecutively from dorsal to ventral by **Roman numerals I–X**. This numerical method reflects recently acquired data and is rather precise relative to the segmental variations. Some cell columns are continuous, i.e., present at all levels, whereas other columns are present at very specific levels.

Structural and Functional Features

Characteristics of the C7 level are as follows:
- The transverse diameter greatly exceeds the sagittal diameter.
- The dorsal horns are not as extensive as the ventral horns, which contain robust medial and lateral motor nuclei. This level is part of the cervical enlargement (C3–T1) for innervation of the upper limb.
- The dorsal intermediate septum is well defined as are the gracile and cuneate fasciculi.
- The amount of white matter is greatest at this level.
- Sympathetic GVE neurons are absent.
- The dorsal nucleus of Clarke is absent.

Rexed's laminae are shown at the C7 level only. Although these subdivisions of the gray matter are based on the **Nissl** (cell soma) staining method, they reflect functional properties that vary considerably even within the cervical segments. Details are given below for only laminae that have not been discussed in connection with the verbal nomenclature because there is considerable overlap. (Compare page 57.)

Lamina I and **Lamina II** are the posteromarginal nucleus and the substantia gelatinosa, respectively.

Lamina III functions similar to Lamina II but contains fewer neurons (interneurons). It receives many dorsal root fibers. **Lamina IV** contains a nucleus proprius that is distinct because of neurons whose myelinated axons course transversely to reach the white matter, i.e., tract cells of the spinoreticular, spinotectal, and spinothalamic pathways (below). **Laminae V** and **VI** contain medium-sized cells in the base of the dorsal horn. These cells receive some primary afferent fibers and many descending fibers including most of the corticospinal fibers. This area is also the source of many propriospinal fibers interconnecting other segmental levels.

Lamina VII, the VADH and largest of the laminae, lies in the **intermediate zone** between the dorsal and ventral horns. Many propriospinal fibers arise from cells in lamina VII. It also contains the following well-known cell columns: the intermediomedial, which receives primary afferents from visceral structures; the intermediolateral sympathetic neurons, which form the lateral horn at T1–L2; the parasympathetic neurons at S2–S4; and the dorsal nucleus of Clarke at segments C8–L3.

Lamina VIII contains a variety of cells. Many of the fibers descending in the ventral funiculus, e.g., vestibulospinal and reticulospinal, terminate on cells in this lamina whose axons project to laminae VII and IX of both sides.

Lamina IX contains motor neurons of varying sizes including gamma neurons whose fibers are efferent to muscle spindles (intrafusal). Lamina IX also contains small neurons whose axons extend up and down in the adjacent propriospinal fasciculus. Ventromedial motor neurons innervate trunk and neck muscles, and dorsolateral neurons supply limb musculature. The **phrenic nucleus** (C3–C5) is ventromedially located in the cervical cord and innervates the diaphragm. The **(spinal) accessory nucleus** is located laterally in segments C1–C5. The nerve rootlets emerge from the cord between the dorsal and ventral roots and form the (spinal) accessory nerve, which ascends into the cranium through the foramen magnum and exits through the jugular foramen to supply the sternocleidomastoid and trapezius muscles.

Lamina X contains small cells surrounding the central canal.

The spinothalamic pathway is clinically important. Its primary afferents enter the lateral division of the dorsal root and terminate on interneurons or tract cells in lamina IV, whose axons cross in the ventral white commissure. These fibers form the spinothalamic tract, which ascends in the ventrolateral white matter en route to the contralateral thalamus and parietal lobe. It transmits sensations of pain, temperature, and touch.

Clinical Correlations . . . .

Syringomyelia is a cavitation around the central canal, usually in the low cervical cord, which initially interrupts the crossing spinothalamic fibers in the ventral white commissure. A segmental or **yoke-like** (bilateral) loss of **pain** and **temperature** sensations in the hands is the hallmark of this rare but instructive condition. Touch is preserved in alternate pathways. As the cavitation (syrinx) enlarges, it encroaches on the neurons that supply motor innervation to the upper limb and, additionally, causes **paresis** (weakness).

Like herpes zoster, **syringomyelia** emphasizes the **segmental nature** of the **spinal nerves.** Interruption of the crossing fibers involves segmental levels bilaterally in contrast to a lesion of the tract in the ventrolateral region of the cord. The latter results in loss of pain and temperature caudal and contralateral to the lesion.

A **complete transection** of the high cervical cord abolishes sensations caudal to the lesion, paralyzes upper and lower limbs (**quadriplegia**), and inactivates the diaphragm if the lesion is above the phrenic nucleus (C3–C5). **Paraplegia**, paralysis of the lower limbs, results from lesions below the cervical limb enlargement and above the lumbosacral enlargement (L1–S2). **Hemiplegia**, paralysis of one side of the body, is one component of the **Brown-Séquard syndrome**, which is caused by a hemisection of the spinal cord. A hemisection above the upper limb innervation causes ipsilateral hemiplegia (descending motor fibers), ipsilateral loss of dorsal column input, and contralateral loss of pain and temperature.

Use blue to color laminae I–VI, all of which receive or send sensory input. Use red to color the clusters of neurons in lamina IX. Be aware that medial and lateral cell clusters of lamina IX supply motor innervation to trunk and limb muscles, respectively. Note that, at this level, lamina VII does not contain ANS neurons.

Spinal Cord at Cervical Enlargement (C7)

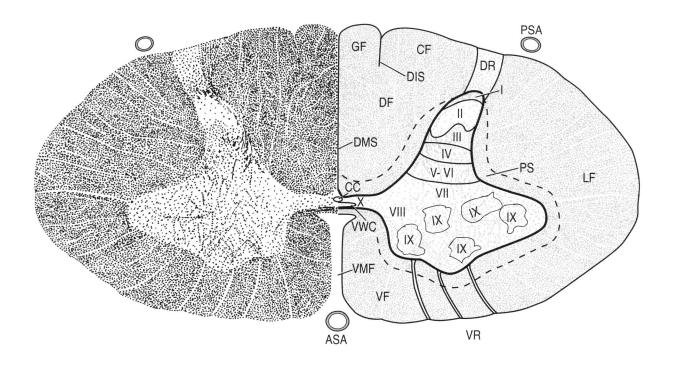

White Matter (fiber pathways)

DF Dorsal funiculus containing gracile fasciculus (GF) and cuneate fasciculus (CF) demarcarted by dorsal intermediate septum

LF Lateral funiculus

VF Ventral funiculus

PS Propriospinal fibers

DR Dorsal root entry zone has medial and lateral (Lissauer's zone) divisions

VR Ventral root exit

VWC Ventral white commissure

Rexed's Laminae of Gray Matter

I Posteromarginal nucleus

II Substantia gelatinosa

III Contains interneurons

IV Nucleus proprius

V, VI Ventral area of dorsal horn

VII Intermediate zone

VIII Integrative cell column

IX Motor cell columns, medial and lateral

X Surrounds central canal

Other

DMS Dorsal median septum

DIS Dorsal intermediate septum

CC Central canal

VMF Ventral median fissure

PSA Posterior spinal arteries

ASA Anterior spinal artery

Spinal Cord Summary Including Blood Supply

Observe the overall shape of the spinal cord; the amount and shape of the gray matter; and the relative amounts of gray and white matter at sacral, lumbar, thoracic, and cervical levels.

Regions, S1
The sacral (S1) cross section shows the topographic **regions** of white matter surrounding the central gray matter. The entry of the dorsal root fibers and the exit of the ventral roots demarcate a hemisection of the cord into **dorsal, lateral,** and **ventral funiculi.** The dorsal funiculi contain only sensory fibers, whereas both sensory and motor tracts ascend and descend in the lateral and ventral funiculi.

Color the dorsal funiculi blue to represent the ipsilateral ascent of these fibers. Consult the tract diagram below and add and color the lateral corticospinal red bilaterally (and label LCST) and add and color the ventrolateral system (VLS) blue bilaterally. You have created a visual representation of the three most clinically relevant pathways in the spinal cord.

Tracts, T2
Motor tracts are depicted on one half of the spinal cord and sensory tracts on the other half at a thoracic (T2) level. The **lateral corticospinal tract** (LCST), the **rubrospinal tract** (RST), and the **medullary (lateral) reticulospinal tract** (RTST) descend in the lateral funiculus. The ventral funiculus contains the **vestibulospinal tract** (VST), the **pontine (medial) reticulospinal tract** (RTST), the **ventral corticospinal tract** (VCST), and the **tectospinal tract** (TST). **Gracile fasciculus** (GF) and **cuneate fasciculus** (CF) ascend in the dorsal funiculus, whereas the **ventrolateral system's fibers** (VLS) ascend in the ventrolateral region of the cord. Both the **dorsal spinocerebellar tract** (DSCT) and the **ventral spinocerebellar tract** (VSCT) ascend in the periphery of the lateral funiculus.

Color the ascending tracts on the right side of the diagram blue and the descending tracts on the left side red. These are all bilateral, of course, but are depicted unilaterally as sensory and motor for visual simplicity.

Blood Supply, L2
A cross section of the lumbar cord (L2) depicts the **blood supply. Bilateral posterior spinal arteries** arise from either the vertebral or posterior inferior cerebellar artery, exit through the foramen magnum, and descend along the entry of the dorsal root fibers. They anastomose with the posterior radicular artery, a branch of the segmental spinal artery, and supply the posterior one third of the spinal cord. A branch from each vertebral artery joins to form a **single anterior spinal artery** that descends along the ventral median fissure. It anastomoses with the anterior radicular branch of the segmental artery and supplies the anterior two thirds of the cord. Contributions from certain segmental arteries are of special significance; e.g., the **artery of Adamkiewicz** is the **main** arterial source from T8 to the conus medullaris.

Consider the direction of flow, the size of the blood vessel, and the effect of lumen size on rate of flow as you color the arteries red.

Fiber Arrangement, C7
Somatotopic fiber layering facilitates the efficient organization of neuronal connections. Note that the layering of cervical (C), thoracic (T), lumbar (L), and sacral (S) fibers is such that cervical fibers tend to surround the central gray matter and sacral fibers are toward the periphery. Thus, pathology involving the central gray matter initially encroaches on cervical levels, whereas extrinsic tumors initially create pressure at sacral levels (Lateral corticospinal tract [LCST] and ventrolateral system [VLS]).

Color the LCST red. Color the VLS and dorsal column fibers blue. Observe the proximity of the cervical fibers to the gray matter.

Spinal Cord Summary Including Blood Supply

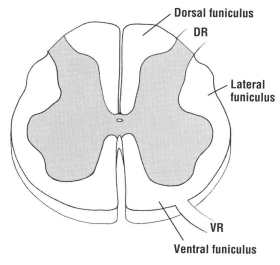

Dorsal funiculus
DR
Lateral funiculus
VR
Ventral funiculus

Regions, S1

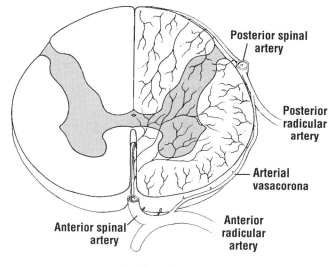

Posterior spinal artery
Posterior radicular artery
Arterial vasacorona
Anterior spinal artery
Anterior radicular artery

Blood Supply, L2

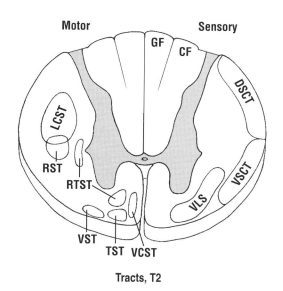

Motor Sensory
GF CF
DSCT
LCST
RST
RTST
VSCT
VLS
VST
TST VCST

Tracts, T2

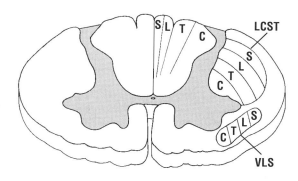

S L T C
LCST
S
L
T
C
C T L S
VLS

Fiber Arrangement, C7

Chapter Two Study Questions

Directions: Following each question below are four or five suggested answers. Choose the **one best** response to each question.

1. Which of the following spinal cord levels contains both gracile and cuneate fasciculi?
   - (a) S2
   - (b) T2
   - (c) T10
   - (d) L1
   - (e) L5

2. Which of these fibers ascend and descend adjacent to the gray matter in all funiculi and are intrinsic to the spinal cord?
   - (a) Ventral spinocerebellar
   - (b) Spinothalamic
   - (c) Corticospinal
   - (d) Propriospinal
   - (e) Dorsal spinocerebellar

3. The prominent nucleus of the dorsal horn that is unstained in myelin sections and is largely a synaptic zone for incoming and descending fibers is the
   - (a) Substantia gelatinosa
   - (b) Dorsal nucleus of Clarke
   - (c) Nucleus proprius
   - (d) Posteromarginal nucleus
   - (e) Laminae V and VI of Rexed

4. Neurons of the sympathetic and parasympathetic components of the autonomic system lie at these spinal cord levels, respectively.
   - (a) T1–L2, L3–S2
   - (b) T6–T10, S2–S4
   - (c) C1–T2, S2–S4
   - (d) T1–L5, S1–S2
   - (e) T1–L2, S2–S4

5. Which spinal levels contain the least amount of white matter?
   - (a) Sacral
   - (b) Cervical
   - (c) Lumbar
   - (d) T1–T5
   - (e) T6–T12

6. The safest vertebral level from which CSF can be withdrawn from the lumbar cistern in an adult is
   - (a) L1–L2
   - (b) T10–T11
   - (c) L3–L4
   - (d) L2–L3
   - (e) S1–S2

7. The cross-sectional area of the central gray matter is largest in the segments
   - (a) Containing preganglionic sympathetic neurons
   - (b) Innervating the limbs
   - (c) Containing preganglionic parasympathetic neurons
   - (d) Containing the phrenic nucleus
   - (e) Containing the dorsal nucleus of Clarke

8. The pathway that transmits pain, temperature, and touch from the nucleus proprius to the thalamus is the
   - (a) Propriospinal
   - (b) Dorsal spinocerebellar tract
   - (c) Spinothalamic
   - (d) Gracile fasciculus
   - (e) Dorsal column

9. Which spinal cord region has more spinal nerves than vertebrae?
   - (a) Sacral
   - (b) Lumbar
   - (c) Thoracic
   - (d) Cervical

10. Neurons in the DRG are embryologically derived from the
    - (a) Alar plate
    - (b) Basal plate
    - (c) Otic placode
    - (d) Neural crest

11. Which of the following is not a functional component of spinal nerves?
    - (a) GSA
    - (b) GSE
    - (c) SVE
    - (d) GVA
    - (e) GVE

Case History

A forty-year-old right-handed housewife burned her right hand by grasping the handle of a frying pan. She did not recall pain with the incident. Two months later, she experienced weakness in her hands and noticed wasting (atrophy) of the muscles of both hands. At that point she was aware of a lack of pain and temperature sensation in her hands.

Explain whether these symptoms suggest segmental or long tract deficits and describe the anatomy involved.

Answers and Explanations for Chapter Two Study Questions

1. **b** [pages 46, 50, and 54] At and above T6, the dorsal intermediate septum lies between the gracile fasciculus located medially and the cuneate fasciculus located laterally. They contain ascending fibers from the lower trunk and limb and upper trunk and limb, respectively. These uncrossed fibers transmit sensations of discriminative touch, pressure, vibration, and proprioception. The other levels listed lie below T6.

2. **d** [page 50] Spinospinal is a synonym for propriospinal. Tracts are often named relative to their origin and termination. Two of the incorrect answers terminate in the cerebellum, one terminates in the thalamus and one originates in the cortex.

3. **a** [pages 50 and 54] Incoming and descending fibers modulate the activity of excitatory and inhibitory interneurons in the substantia gelatinosa, especially in regard to pain. The dorsal nucleus of Clarke contains the neurons whose axons form the dorsospinocerebellar tract. The nucleus proprius contains tract cells including those giving rise to the spinothalamic tract. The posteromarginal nucleus is a thin layer that caps the dorsal horn. Rexed laminae V and VI receive some primary afferent and many descending fibers but are not distinguished by being unstained in myelin preparations.

4. **e** [page 46] A synonym for the sympathetic nervous system is thoracolumbar because its preganglionic neurons lie at those levels. Craniosacral describes the location of parasympathetic neurons, which are at S2–S4 levels and in the brain stem within the cranium.

5. **a** [page 46] The cross-sectional area of white matter is minimal in the most caudal spinal cord level, i.e., the sacral, where there are fewer ascending and descending fibers.

6. **c** [page 46] Although the spinal cord ends at vertebral level L2 in most adults, there is some variability. It is therefore safer to do a spinal tap at L3–L4 than at L2–L3. The lumbar cistern is not present at T10–T11 (the spinal cord is). The fusion of the sacral vertebrae precludes that route of entry at sacral levels.

7. **b** [pages 46 and 47] ANS motor neurons are smaller than alpha motor neurons in the lateral cell column of lamina IX of the ventral horn. Generally, the cell size correlates with the length of the axon, and motor cells innervating the limbs are larger than those to trunk muscles.

Neither the phrenic nucleus (motor) nor the dorsal nucleus of Clarke (sensory) cause any appreciable gross differences in the size of the spinal cord.

8. **c** [page 56] The propriospinal fibers are intrinsic to the spinal cord; the dorsal spinocerebellar tract transmits proprioceptive sensations to the cerebellum, not the thalamus. The gracile fasciculus is in the dorsal column and is not involved in pain transmission.

9. **d** [page 46] There are seven cervical vertebrae and eight cervical nerves. The significance of this is that each of the spinal nerves 1–7 exits through intervertebral foramina above the corresponding vertebra; however, caudal to the C8 nerve, each nerve exits in the foramen below the vertebra with the same number. There are 12 thoracic, 5 lumbar; 5 sacral (fused) vertebrae, and 1 coccyx; and 12 thoracic, 5 lumbar, 5 sacral and 1 coccygeal nerves, though the coccygeal is sometimes absent.

10. **d** [page 48] Additionally, sensory neurons of CN V, VII, IX, and X are also derived from neural crest. The alar plate, basal plate, and otic placode give rise to neurons in the dorsal horn, ventral horn, and CN VIII, respectively.

11. **c** [page 48] Three functional components are unique to cranial nerves, each of which begins with the word "special." Cranial nerves may have general functional components but spinal nerves do not have special components.

Case History
This history is typical in women with syringomyelia [page 56]. The cause is a syrinx around the central canal, usually in the low cervical cord. Interruption of the pain and temperature fibers in the ventral white commissure caused **bilateral segmental** loss of these modalities. (Injury of only the right hand reflects right-handedness.) As the syrinx enlarges, it destroys ventral horn cells, which innervate the muscles of the hand, causing **bilateral** weakness and wasting in this patient. Sometimes the enlargement of the syrinx is asymmetrical and results in unilateral motor symptoms. The cause is unknown and there is no cure; it occurs in women more often than in men.

CHAPTER 3 Medial View of Brain Stem Nuclei Excluding Cranial Nerve Nuclei

Definitions

The superior (1) and inferior (2) colliculi are prominent nuclei dorsal to the cerebral aqueduct of the midbrain. (They are discussed on pages 84 and 82.) Other midbrain nuclei are located in the tegmentum or in the **periaqueductal gray** (PAG) (15). The tegmentum is the part of the cerebral peduncle between the cerebral aqueduct and the basis pedunculi, and between the fourth ventricle and the basal region of the pons. The PAG surrounds the cerebral aqueduct and extends less conspicuously into the pons and rostral medulla, and can be recognized as a clear area in the left half of the myelin-stained sections (pages 83–85).

The **nucleus of Darkschewitsch** (3), which is also called the ventral nucleus of the posterior commissure, is a small nucleus in the PAG. The **interstitial nucleus of Cajal** (3) is a subdivision of the nucleus of Darkschewitsch and consists of cells intermingled with the fibers of the posterior commissure. The **dorsal tegmental nucleus** (4) is in the PAG of the caudal midbrain and pontine isthmus.

The **red nucleus** (5) is in the rostral midbrain tegmentum. The **substantia nigra** (6) is a nucleus of pigmented cells in the ventral midbrain. The **interpeduncular nucleus** (7) is a median nucleus in the caudal midbrain tegmentum between the bases of the two cerebral peduncles.

Pontine nuclei (8), intermingled with bundles of nerve fibers in the base of the pons, receive corticopontine fibers. The **superior olivary nucleus** (9) is an auditory nucleus in the caudal and ventral part of the **pontine tegmentum.**

The **inferior olivary nucleus** (10) in the ventrolateral medulla is shaped like a crumpled bag. The **arcuate nucleus** (11) on the surface of the pyramid is similar to pontine nuclei. The **accessory** (lateral, external) **cuneate nucleus** (12) is lateral to the **cuneate nucleus** (13). The **gracile nucleus** (14) and cuneate nucleus project to the thalamus and are distinctive features of the caudal medulla. The **reticular formation** (16) is an intricate network of neurons and fibers that makes up the central core of the brain stem.

Structural and Functional Features

Some authors consider the propriospinal tract between the gray and white matter in the spinal cord to be a caudal component of the reticular formation. The projection neurons in the brain stem reticular formation have extensively branched dendritic trees oriented in a transverse plane; their axons branch and then ascend and descend for considerable distances. The reticular formation consists of **three zones: lateral, medial,** and **midline (raphe)**. The lateral "sensory" zone has small cells with short axons that terminate in the medial "motor" zone. The lateral zone receives input from the spinal cord, cranial nerves, cerebellum, and cerebrum. The medial motor zone is composed of large projection neurons whose numerous axons ascend and descend to make connections caudally to the spinal cord, posteriorly to the cerebellum, laterally to the cranial nerve nuclei, and rostrally to the hypothalamus and thalamus. The spatial arrangement of the network provides an ideal anatomic substrate for receiving converging multimodality input and providing widespread diverging output.

Reticular pathways ascend and descend in the **central tegmental tract** of this intricate and highly organized neural network. Fibers of the ascending reticular activating system (ARAS) relay mainly in the intralaminar nuclei of the thalamus en route to widespread regions of the cerebral cortex. The function of the ARAS is to create a state of arousal or general alertness.

Reticular mediated messages that reach the **hypothalamus** are integrated into the regulation of visceral activity via fibers in the **dorsal longitudinal fasciculus** that reach brain stem and spinal autonomic neurons. Regulation of the respiratory and circulatory systems is, in part, through "vital" reticular centers in the pons and medulla.

Reticular nuclei related to the cerebellum are chiefly concerned with somatomotor activity, as are the medial (pontine) and lateral (medullary) reticulospinal tracts. Several reticular nuclei involved in the control of eye movement interconnect through the medial longitudinal fasciculus.

Among the biochemically defined reticular nuclei are the **locus ceruleus (norepinephrine)**, the **raphe nuclei (serotonin)**, the **ventral tegmental area (dopamine)**, and the **pedunculopontine** and **laterodorsal tegmental nuclei (acetylcholine)**. Extensively dispersed terminals from the locus ceruleus reach the tectum, thalamus, hypothalamus, hippocampus, cerebral cortex, cerebellum, medulla, and spinal cord. These adrenergic projections act to modulate synaptic activity of other neurotransmitters by either suppressing or enhancing their effect.

Axons from serotonergic raphe neurons are likewise diffusely distributed throughout the brain and spinal cord. **Serotonin** has a widespread inhibitory action in the thalamus and cerebral cortex and plays a role in actively **inducing sleep. Serotonin** modulates the **transmission of pain.** Activation of raphe serotonergic neurons in the PAG or in the medulla (raphe spinal tract) inhibits the activity of neurons in the dorsal horn and spinal trigeminal nucleus that mediate the transmission of pain impulses.

Clinical Correlations

A possible explanation for the mechanism of pain relief afforded by **acupuncture** is that the needle-induced painful stimuli activate peripheral nerves. These signals in turn induce the release of endorphins (morphine-like peptides), which inhibit pain transmission. Serotonergic projections from midbrain raphe neurons to the dorsal horn are clinically important because this activity suppresses the conscious awareness of pain.

Color the superior (1) and inferior (2) colliculi and the superior olivary nuclei (9) yellow. Color the accessory cuneate (12), cuneate (13), and gracile (14) nuclei blue. Color the nucleus of Darkschewitsch (3), the dorsal tegmental (4), the interpeduncular (7), and the PAG (15) nuclei orange. Color the red (5), pontine (8), inferior olivary (10), and arcuate (11) nuclei red. Draw red and blue diagonal marks through the reticular formation (16). Color the substantia nigra (6) brown.

Medial View of Brain Stem Nuclei Excluding Cranial Nerve Nuclei

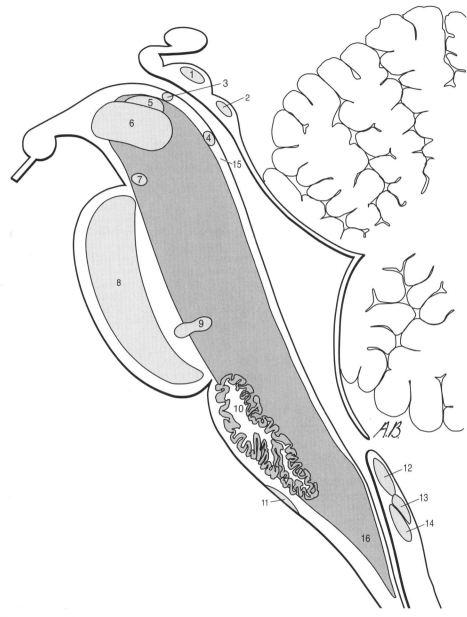

Mesencephalon
1. Nucleus of superior colliculus
2. Nucleus of inferior colliculus
3. Nucleus of Darkschewitsch and interstitial nucleus of Cajal
4. Dorsal tegmental nucleus
5. Red nucleus
6. Substantia nigra
7. Interpeduncular nucleus

Pons
8. Diffuse pontine nuclei in basal pons
9. Superior olivary nucleus

Medulla
10. Inferior olivary nucleus and accessory olivary nuclei
11. Arcuate nucleus of medulla oblongata
12. Accessory (lateral, external) cuneate nucleus
13. Cuneate nucleus
14. Gracile nucleus

Mesencephalon, Pons, Medulla
15. Periaqueductal gray
16. Reticular formation

(The locus ceruleus is shown on the cross-section of the pons, page 79.)

Cross-Sectional Levels

Definitions
The transition from the spinal cord to the medulla is defined by the decussation of the pyramids. The **tegmentum** is the portion of the brain stem composed of reticular formation, tracts, and nuclei. It lies in the dorsal part of the midbrain and pons but is ventral to the cerebral aqueduct and fourth ventricle. It is dorsal to the pyramids of the medulla. A **lemniscal** pathway is composed of 2° sensory axons.

Structural and Functional Features
There are basic similarities and basic differences between spinal cord and brain stem topography.

Basic Similarities
- The medial longitudinal fasciculus (MLF) is located ventral to the central canal in the spinal cord, and ventral to the fourth ventricle and cerebral aqueduct in the brain stem.
- The spinothalamic tract, dorsal and ventral spinocerebellar tracts, spinotectal tract, and spinal nucleus and tract of the trigeminal are located laterally in the spinal cord and laterally in the medulla.

Basic Differences
- Basal plate derivatives are located ventrally in the spinal cord but medially in the medulla due to the enlargement of the fourth ventricle.
- Alar plate derivatives are located dorsally in the spinal cord and laterally in the open medulla.
- The dorsal column–medial lemniscus pathway undergoes a major shift in the brain stem. First order fibers ascend in the dorsal funiculus (column) in the spinal cord; second order fiber bundles are medial and vertical in the medulla and become horizontal and ventrolateral in the midbrain.
- Corticospinal fibers are located laterally in the spinal cord but ventrally in the medulla.

General Organization of the Brain Stem Roof
- Tectum in midbrain
- Cerebellum in pons and medulla

Ventricular Cavity
- Caudal (closed) medulla—central canal
- Rostral (open) medulla—fourth ventricle
- Pons—fourth ventricle
- Midbrain—cerebral aqueduct

Tegmentum
- Motor nuclei of cranial nerves
- Sensory nuclei (2° neurons) of cranial nerves with sensory components
- Long ascending (specific) lemniscal pathways
- Motor pathways excluding those listed below under "Basal Region"; these include the MLF, tectospinal, rubrospinal, reticulospinal, and vestibulospinal tracts and others
- Reticular formation and its ascending (nonspecific) and descending pathways in the central tegmental tract (CTT)

Basal Region
- Cerebral peduncles of midbrain, ventral region of the pons, and ventral region of the medulla;
- Corticobulbar fibers to cranial nerve nuclei;
- Corticospinal fibers to anterior motor horn cells at spinal levels;
- Corticopontine fibers to pontine nuclei;
- Pontocerebellar fibers.

These particular drawings are representative of Weigert-stained tissue. The levels were selected to show cross-sections where there is a significant change in the topography of the brain stem. Observe that three levels are through the forebrain (depicted in Chapter 5, pages 154–159).

Clinical Correlations . . . .

Lesions of the brain stem that interrupt the descending corticospinal fibers in the **basal region** may disrupt volitional control of the contralateral limbs. Lesions in the **tegmentum** may disrupt ascending (sensory) pathways as well as descending pathways in the tegmentum and the cranial nerves.

Color the area ventral to the broken lines red to indicate the basal region. Draw red and blue longitudinal lines through the tegmentum—the region between the broken line and the ventricular cavities.

Cross-Sectional Levels

page 155

page 157

page 159

page 85

page 83

page 81

page 79

page 77

page 75

page 73

page 71

page 69

page 67

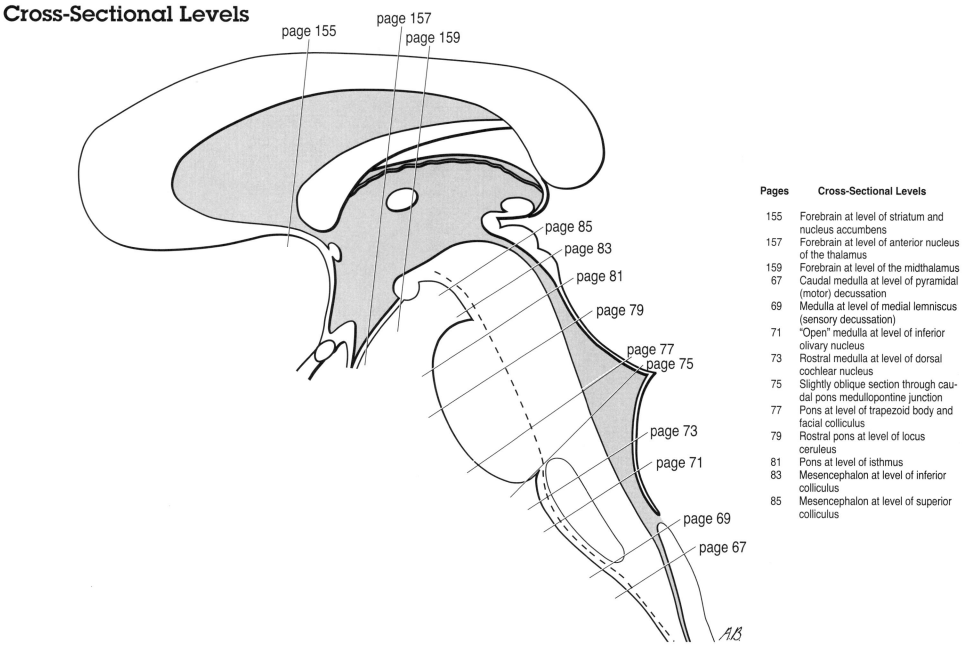

Pages	Cross-Sectional Levels
155	Forebrain at level of striatum and nucleus accumbens
157	Forebrain at level of anterior nucleus of the thalamus
159	Forebrain at level of the midthalamus
67	Caudal medulla at level of pyramidal (motor) decussation
69	Medulla at level of medial lemniscus (sensory decussation)
71	"Open" medulla at level of inferior olivary nucleus
73	Rostral medulla at level of dorsal cochlear nucleus
75	Slightly oblique section through caudal pons medullopontine junction
77	Pons at level of trapezoid body and facial colliculus
79	Rostral pons at level of locus ceruleus
81	Pons at level of isthmus
83	Mesencephalon at level of inferior colliculus
85	Mesencephalon at level of superior colliculus

Caudal Medulla at Level of Pyramidal (Motor) Decussation

Characteristics of the Level of the Motor Decussation

- Prominent gracile and cuneate nuclei "capped" dorsally by the gracile and cuneate fasciculi;
- Prominent spinal trigeminal nucleus and tract that lie lateral to the dorsal column nuclei and tracts;
- The absence of the pyramids due to the decussation of 85% of the corticospinal fibers from a ventral position in the brain stem to a dorsolateral position in the spinal cord (arrows indicate direction);
- The absence of the ventral median fissure due to pyramidal decussation (the most conspicuous feature of the spinomedullary transition area);
- The absence of the inferior olivary nuclei, which are prominent at more rostral levels of the medulla.

Clinical Correlations . . . .

A lesion of the upper spinal cord or of the caudal lateral medulla may interrupt first order (uncrossed) pain and temperature fibers in the spinal trigeminal tract and second order (crossed) pain and temperature fibers in the spinothalamic tract. Loss of these modalities on **one side of the face** and on the **opposite side of the body** is therefore indicative of a lesion at this level.

Color blue the afferent pathways (GF, CF, STT, DSCT, VSCT, STET, and STHT). Draw blue diamonds to represent neurons in the gracile, cuneate, and spinal trigeminal nuclei. Draw green diamonds to represent neurons in the accessory nucleus. Color red those pathways related to efferent outflow (VSCT, VST, TST, MLF, RST, LCST). Finally, beginning medially, color red the decussating pyramidal fibers. Observe that via the decussation these fibers become dorsolateral in the spinal cord.

Caudal Medulla at Level of Pyramidal (Motor) Decussation

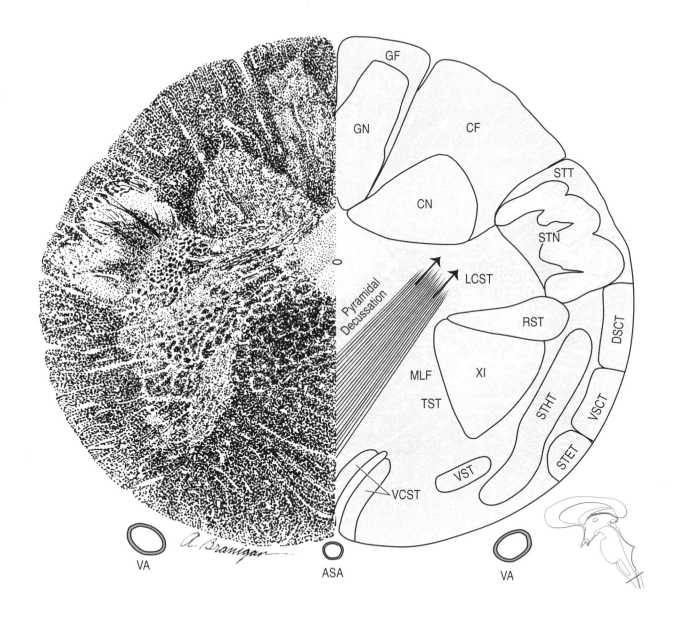

Structures Related to Afferent Input
- **GN, GF** Gracile nucleus and fasciculus
- **CN, CF** Cuneate nucleus and fasciculus
- **STN, STT** Spinal trigeminal nucleus and tract
- **DSCT** Dorsal spinocerebellar tract
- **VSCT** Ventral spinocerebellar tract
- **STHT** Spinothalamic tract
- **STET** Spinotectal tract

Structures Related to Efferent Outflow
- **RST** Rubrospinal tract
- **LCST** Lateral corticospinal tract
- **VCST** Ventral corticospinal tract
- **VST** (Lateral) vestibulospinal tract
- **MLF** Medial longitudinal fasciculus
- **TST** Tectospinal tract
- **XI** (Spinal) accessory nucleus

Arteries
- **ASA** Anterior spinal artery
- **VA** Vertebral artery

Medulla at Level of Decussation of Medial Lemniscus (Sensory Decussation)

Characteristics of the Level of the Sensory Decussation

- Internal arcuate fibers arise from gracile and cuneate nuclei and sweep across to the ventral raphe (sensory decussation) to form the medial lemniscus. The homunculus shows the body areas served by the gracile, cuneate, and spinal trigeminal nuclei. Fibers from gracile neurons relay general somatic afferent (GSA) information from the lower limb and trunk, whereas those fibers arising from cuneate neurons relay GSA input from the upper limb and neck. Note the somatotopic position of "leg ventral, arm dorsal" in the medial lemniscus. Through a relay in the ventral posterolateral (VPL) nucleus of the thalamus, the information reaches the parietal lobe. This system for touch, pressure, proprioception, and vibration is the most discriminative of the general sensory systems and serves as a prototype for conscious awareness of sensation.
- The pyramid contains mainly corticospinal fibers. Most of the corticobulbar fibers reach their destination rostral to this level.
- Dorsal and ventral spinocerebellar tracts mediate proprioceptive input to the cerebellum.
- The accessory cuneate nucleus projects proprioceptive input to the cerebellum via the cuneocerebellar tract (pages 120 and 121).
- The arcuate nucleus is homologous to pontine nuclei and projects to the cerebellum via the ventral external arcuate fibers and the striae medullares of the fourth ventricle.
- The solitary tract contains fibers from VII, IX, and X. These SVA fibers mediating taste terminate in the rostral part of the solitary nucleus. The cell bodies lie in the geniculate ganglion of VII and in inferior ganglia of IX or X. Other cells in the inferior ganglia of IX or X mediate GVA sensations from pharynx, larynx, trachea, esophagus, thoracic, and abdominal viscera. Cranial nerve VII also has a small GVA component. GVA fibers terminate in the caudal part of the solitary nucleus.
- The spinal trigeminal tract contains fibers from V (primarily), VII, IX, and X, which relay pain and temperature and nondiscriminative touch to 2° sensory neurons in the spinal trigeminal nucleus. The spinal trigeminal nucleus emits predominantly crossed fibers, which relay this GSA input from the face to the ventral posteromedial (VPM) nucleus of the thalamus. The VPM projects to the "face" area of the parietal lobe.

- The hypoglossal nucleus is a medial column of neurons. Its GSE axons course ventrally through the preolivary sulcus and exit the hypoglossal canal to innervate intrinsic and extrinsic tongue muscles.
- The dorsal motor nucleus of the vagus is the parasympathetic component of the vagus (DMX). These GVE fibers exit the postolivary sulcus; pass through the jugular foramen; and innervate cardiac muscle, smooth muscle, and glands of the viscera.
- The nucleus ambiguus (NA) furnishes the SVE component of IX and X. Fibers exit in the postolivary sulcus; pass through the jugular foramen; and innervate the larynx, pharynx, and palate. Axons from spinal neurons in the upper cervical levels that make up the (spinal) accessory nerve (XI) ascend through the foramen magnum, exit the jugular foramen, and supply SVE innervation to the sternocleidomastoid and trapezius muscles.
- All of the above nuclei extend from the "closed" medulla to near the rostral limit of the "open" medulla. Medial to lateral they are XII, DMX, and NA.

Clinical Correlations . . . .

The **nucleus ambiguus** innervates the efferent limb of the gag reflex as well as the laryngeal and pharyngeal muscles. A destructive lesion of the nucleus ambiguus (lateral medullary syndrome, page 122) results in **dysphagia**, **dysarthria**, and **dysphonia**.

Color the afferent related structures (per instructions on page 66), noting that the internal arcuate fibers form the medial lemniscus contralaterally. Color this caudal part of the solitary tract and nucleus purple, and the dorsal motor nucleus of X orange. Color red the hypoglossal nucleus, MLF, and TST, the medial lemniscus blue, and the pyramid and arcuate nucleus red. Color the nucleus ambiguus green.

Medulla at Level of Decussation of Medial Lemniscus (Sensory Decussation)

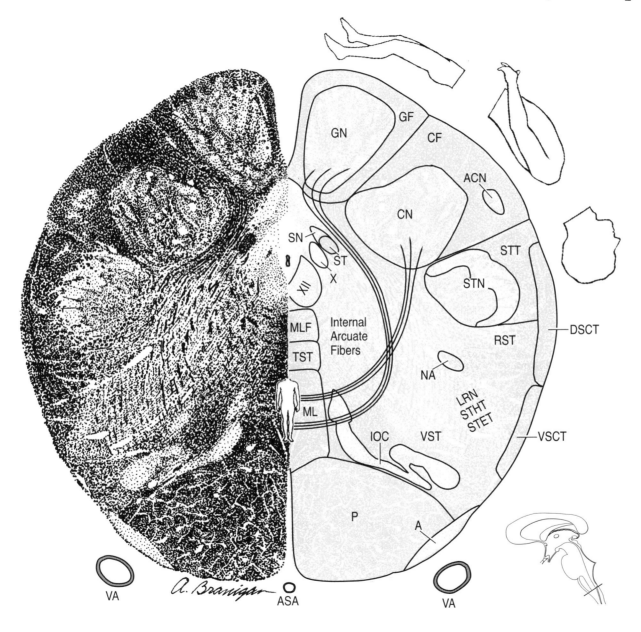

Structures Related to Afferent Input

GN, GF	Gracile nucleus and fasciculus
CN, CF	Cuneate nucleus and fasciculus
ACN	Accessory cuneate nucleus (similar to Clarke's nucleus)
STN, STT	Spinal trigeminal nucleus and tract
DSCT	Dorsal spinocerebellar tract
VSCT	Ventral spinocerebellar tract
STHT	Spinothalamic tract
STET	Spinotectal tract
SN, ST	Solitary nucleus and tract
ML	Medial lemniscus

Structures Related to Efferent Outflow

RST	Rubrospinal tract
P	Pyramid
VST	(Lateral) vestibulospinal tract
MLF	Medial longitudinal fasciculus
TST	Tectospinal tract
XII	Hypoglossal nucleus
X	Dorsal motor nucleus of vagus
NA	Nucleus ambiguus

Arteries and Integrative Structures

ASA	Anterior spinal artery
VA	Vertebral artery
A	Arcuate nucleus
IOC	Inferior olivary complex
LRN	Lateral reticular nucleus

"Open" Medulla at Level of Inferior Olivary Nucleus

Characteristics of the Medulla at the Level of the Inferior Olivary Nucleus

- The central canal "opens"into the fourth ventricle.
- A highly convoluted configuration in the ventral tegmentum, the inferior olivary nucleus (ION) receives input from the spinal cord and from the cerebral cortex via the corticobulbar tract; and from the basal ganglia, periaqueductal gray, and red nucleus via the central tegmental tract. Olivocerebellar fibers sweep from the hilus of the ION to enter the contralateral inferior cerebellar peduncle and terminate as "climbing" fibers on Purkinje cell dendrites.
- The pyramid contains corticospinal fibers and the corticobulbar fibers that terminate in the caudal (closed) medulla.
- A massive inferior cerebellar peduncle (ICP) contains numerous tracts into the cerebellum from the spinal cord, the medulla, and a medial component of cerebellovestibular fibers.
- Medial and inferior vestibular nuclei are lateral to the sulcus limitans (SL).
- The solitary nucleus and tract are ventral to the vestibular nuclei. The rostral part of the solitary nucleus receives first order SVA (taste) fibers from cranial nerves VII, IX, and X.
- Fibers of the hypoglossal nucleus emerge from the preolivary sulcus.
- The anatomically ill-defined nucleus ambiguus lies dorsolateral to the olivary complex. Special visceral efferent (SVE) fibers arise from the nucleus ambiguus and emerge with other vagal and glossopharyngeal fibers in the postolivary sulcus to innervate striated muscles of branchiomeric origin.
- The central tegmental tract (CTT) is more apparent at pontine and midbrain levels (and is defined on page 82). Many CTT fibers end in the inferior olivary nucleus.

Clinical Correlations . . . .

In animals, the corticospinal fibers can be experimentally severed in the pyramids. The result is **paralysis** of the **flaccid type** of the **contralateral limbs** (if the lesion is of **only one pyramid**), which indicates that **only excitatory fibers are located** in the **pyramids**. Therefore, inhibition of the lower motor neurons occurs via descending fibers other than the glutaminic excitatory fibers in the pyramids. Classically, in naturally occurring lesions in the human nervous system, inhibitory circuits are interrupted as well as excitatory corticospinal fibers. A decrease of inhibitory input onto lower motor neurons accounts for the excessive tone, hyperreflexia, and eventual spasticity characteristic of most "strokes" (upper motor neuron lesions) that cause spastic hemiparesis or hemiplegia. Clinically, the term hemiplegia is often used when hemiparesis would be a more accurate description inasmuch as proximal joint muscles usually remain functional.

Color the ML, ACN, STT, STN, ICP, VSCT, STHT, and STET blue. Color XII, MLF, TST, RST, and the pyramid red. Color the vestibular nuclei (MVN and IVN) yellow and the NA green. This **rostral** level of the solitary tract and nucleus (ST and SN) transmit taste sensations; color them brown.

"Open" Medulla at Level of Inferior Olivary Nucleus

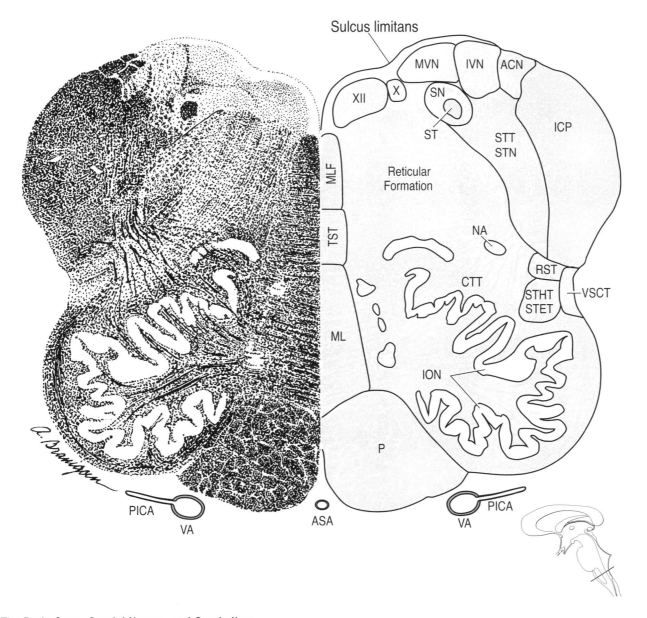

Sulcus limitans

MVN   IVN   ACN

XII   X   SN

ST   STT
STN

ICP

MLF

Reticular
Formation

TST

NA

RST

CTT

STHT
STET

VSCT

ML

ION

P

PICA

VA

ASA

PICA

VA

Structures Related to Afferent Input

STN, STT	Spinal trigeminal nucleus and tract
SN, ST	Solitary nucleus and tract
ML	Medial lemniscus
ACN	Accessory cuneate nucleus
VSCT	Ventral spinocerebellar tract
MVN	Medial vestibular nucleus
IVN	Inferior vestibular nucleus
ICP	Inferior cerebellar peduncle
STHT	Spinothalamic tract
STET	Spinotectal tract

Structures Related to Efferent Outflow

RS	Rubrospinal tract
P	Pyramid
MLF	Medial longitudinal fasciculus
TST	Tectospinal tract
XII	Hypoglossal nucleus
X	Dorsal motor nucleus of vagus
NA	Nucleus ambiguus
ICP	Inferior cerebellar peduncle

Arteries and Integrative Structures

ASA	Anterior spinal artery
VA	Vertebral artery
PICA	Posterior inferior cerebellar artery
IOC	Inferior olivary complex
CTT	Central tegmental tract

Rostral Medulla at Level of Dorsal Cochlear Nucleus

Characteristics of the Medulla at the Level of the Dorsal Cochlear Nucleus

- An extensive "open" rhomboid fossa of the fourth ventricle.
- The fibers of VIIIv (vestibular), IX, and X are all essentially in the same position relative to the ICP. VIIIv and IX are apparent in this section ventral to the ICP. Note that VIIIc (cochlear; auditory) fibers travel dorsal to the ICP to reach the dorsal cochlear nucleus. Vestibular and auditory components of CN VIII are classified as SSA.
- Dorsal and ventral cochlear nuclei are named with respect to their position to the ICP. Schematically both are shown at this level; however, in stained sections the ventral cochlear nucleus is distinct in a more rostral section. Cochlear nuclei receive central fibers from ganglion cells whose peripheral fibers terminate in the organ of Corti. Although projections from these nuclei are predominantly contralateral, the ipsilateral projection is remarkable in number and ensures bilateralism of auditory input from this point rostrally.
- The vestibular nuclei and the midline tegmental structures, pyramids, and inferior olivary nuclei are similar to a more caudal "open" medulla. In addition to the ventrally located pyramids, midline tracts include, dorsal to ventral, the medial longitudinal fasciculus, tectospinal tract, and medial lemniscus.
- The massive ICP is an afferent route to the cerebellum from the spinal cord and medulla. Moreover, the ICP provides efferent links with structures in the medulla, notably the vestibular nuclei and reticular formation.

- Parasympathetic fibers in the glossopharyngeal nerve arise from the inferior salivatory nucleus (GVE) and exit in the postolivary sulcus, with other components of IX, to supply the parotid and pharyngeal glands.

Clinical Correlations . . . .

The posterior inferior cerebellar artery usually supplies the lateral medulla. It has a long, tortuous course and is subject to occlusion by emboli or thrombi. The medial medulla is supplied either by the anterior spinal artery or medullary branches of the vertebral artery. (A complete description of these vascular syndromes is found on pages 122 and 123.)

 Color yellow the DCN, VCN, VIIIc, MVN, IVN, and VIIIv. Note the different routes of VIIIc and VIIIv to reach their respective nuclei. Color blue the ICP, STT, STN, VSCT, STHT, STET, and ML. Color red the PN, MLF, TST, RST, and the pyramid. Color ST and SN brown and NA green.

Rostral Medulla at Level of Dorsal Cochlear Nucleus

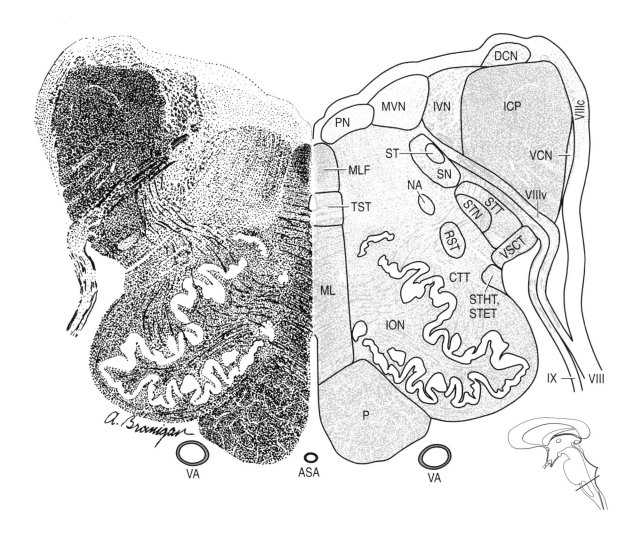

Structures Related to Afferent Input

STN, STT	Spinal trigeminal nucleus and tract
SN, ST	Solitary nucleus and tract
ML	Medial lemniscus
VSCT	Ventral spinocerebellar tract
MVN	Medial vestibular nucleus
IVN	Inferior vestibular nucleus
DCN	Dorsal cochlear nucleus
VCN	Ventral cochlear nucleus
VIII	Vestibulocochlear nerve
VIIIc	Central fibers of cochlear
VIIIv	Central fibers of vestibular
IX	Glossopharyngeal nerve
STHT	Spinothalamic tract
STET	Spinotectal tract

Structures Related to Efferent Outflow

RST	Rubrospinal tract
P	Pyramid
MLF	Medial longitudinal fasciculus
TST	Tectospinal tract
PN	Perihypoglossal nucleus
NA	Nucleus ambiguus
ICP	Inferior cerebellar peduncle

Arteries and Integrative Structures

ASA	Anterior spinal artery
VA	Vertebral artery
ION	Inferior olivary nucleus
CTT	Central tegmental tract

Oblique Section Through Caudal Pons Medullopontine Junction

Characteristics at the Level of the Medullopontine Junction

- The massive middle cerebellar peduncle (MCP) of transversely coursing pontocerebellar fibers connects the basal pons with the cerebellum.
- The ventrolateral intraaxial course of facial nerve fibers around the abducens nucleus creates the internal genu. These SVE fibers course posteriorly and medially to loop around the abducens nucleus and then descend to emerge in the cerebellopontine angle, enter the internal auditory meatus, and exit the skull through the stylomastoid foramen. The superior salivatory nucleus provides parasympathetic fibers in the nervus intermedius of VII to innervate lacrimal and nasopalatine glands as well as submaxillary and sublingual salivary glands. The facial colliculus is an elevation in the medial eminence on the floor of the fourth ventricle, medial to the sulcus limitans and overlying the abducens nucleus and the internal genu of the facial nerve.

- The central tegmental tract (CTT), positioned dorsal in the tegmentum, conveys fibers from the basal ganglia and midbrain to the inferior olivary nucleus. Fibers from reticular neurons also ascend and descend in the CTT (page 82).

Clinical Correlations . . . .

A tumor, e.g., an **ependymoma**, in the floor of the fourth ventricle may exert pressure on the facial colliculus and impair the function of both the abducens and the facial nerves. Also, **cerebellopontine angle tumors** sometimes involve the facial nerve.

Color red the MLF, TST, CN VI, RST, and the pyramid. Color blue the ML, STHT, STET, STT, STN, VSCT, and MCP. (The fibers in the MCP are afferent to the cerebellum.) Color the VN yellow and the CN VII nucleus and fibers green. Use both red and blue to color diagonal lines through CTT.

Oblique Section Through Caudal Pons Medullopontine Junction

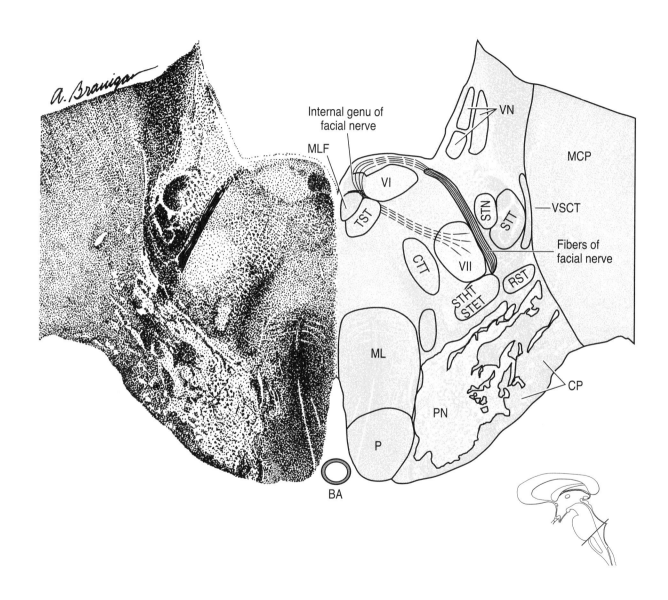

Internal genu of
facial nerve

MLF

VN

MCP

VI

TST

STN

STT

VSCT

CTT

VII

Fibers of
facial nerve

STHT
STET

RST

ML

CP

PN

P

BA

Structures Related to Afferent Input

STN, STT	Spinal trigeminal nucleus and tract
STHT	Spinothalamic tract
STET	Spinotectal tract
ML	Medial lemniscus
VSCT	Ventral spinocerebellar tract
VN	Vestibular nuclei (medial, superior, and lateral)

Structures Related to Efferent Outflow

RST	Rubrospinal tract
P	Pyramid
MLF	Medial longitudinal fasciculus
TST	Tectospinal tract
VI, VII	Abducens and facial nuclei
VN	Vestibular nuclei

Arteries and Integrative Structures

BA	Basilar artery
CTT	Central tegmental tract
CP	Corticopontine fibers
PN	Pontine nuclei
MCP	Middle cerebellar peduncle

Pons at Level of Trapezoid Body and Facial Colliculus

Characteristics of the Pons at the Level of the Trapezoid Body and Facial Colliculus

- The trapezoid body defines the ventral limit of the tegmentum and the dorsal limit of the basal region of the pons. It engulfs the medial lemniscus and contains decussating fibers coursing transversely from the cochlear nuclei.
- Auditory fibers aggregate in the ventrolateral tegmentum as the lateral lemniscus en route to the inferior colliculus and to the medial geniculate nucleus (MGN) of the thalamus.
- The intraaxial course of the abducens nerve is apparent. It emerges at the medullopontine junction and enters the superior orbital fissure to innervate the lateral rectus muscle of the eye.
- The internal genu of the facial nerve "loops" the abducens nucleus and creates an elevation in the floor of the rhomboid fossa (the facial colliculus). The external genu is in the facial canal (page 100).
- The basal pons contains perpendicularly coursing corticobulbar and corticospinal fibers as well as scattered pontine nuclei, which receive corticopontine fibers and emit transversely coursing pontocerebellar fibers. These fibers cross the midline and enter the cerebellum through the contralateral middle cerebellar peduncle (MCP).

- The superior olivary nucleus in the pontine tegmentum receives collaterals of fibers from the ventral cochlear nucleus and contributes fibers to the trapezoid body and the lateral lemniscus for conduction of auditory stimuli. It is involved in sound localization. The superior olivary nucleus projects to the organ of Corti via the olivocochlear bundle.

Clinical Correlations . . . .

A basal pontine lesion involves the abducens nerve (pages 122 and 123).

Color red the MLF, TST, VI (nucleus and fibers), RST, CBT, and CST. Color blue the ML, STHT, STET, STT, STN, VSCT, ICP, and MCP. Color the VN, TB, SON, and LL yellow. Color the nucleus and fibers of VII green. Also, color SCP red, indicating that it predominantly contains fibers that are efferent to the cerebellum.

Life is a festival only to the wise. Seen from the nooks and chimney-side of prudence,
it wears a ragged and dangerous front. – Ralph Waldo Emerson

76

Pons at Level of Trapezoid Body and Facial Colliculus

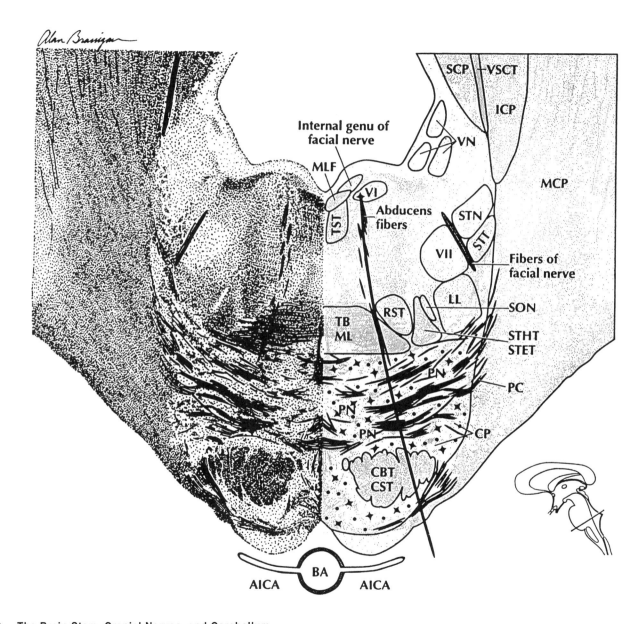

Internal genu of facial nerve

MLF

Abducens fibers

TST

VI

STN

VII

STT

Fibers of facial nerve

LL

RST

SON

TB
ML

STHT
STET

PN

PC

PN

PN

CP

CBT
CST

SCP — VSCT

ICP

VN

MCP

BA

AICA   AICA

Structures Related to Afferent Input

STN, STT	Spinal trigeminal nucleus and tract
STHT	Spinothalamic tract
STET	Spinotectal tract
VSCT	Ventral spinocerebellar tract
VN	Vestibular nuclei (medial, superior, and lateral)
LL	Lateral lemniscus
SON	Superior olivary nucleus
TB	Trapezoid body
ICP, SCP	Inferior and superior cerebellar peduncles
ML	Medial lemniscus

Structures Related to Efferent Outflow

RST	Rubrospinal tract
MLF	Medial longitudinal fasciculus
TST	Tectospinal tract
VI, VII	Abducens and facial nuclei
VN, ICP	See above
SCP	Superior cerebellar peduncle
CBT, CST	Corticobulbar and corticospinal tracts

Arteries and Integrative Structures

AICA	Anterior inferior cerebellar artery
BA	Basilar artery
CP	Corticopontine fibers
PN	Pontine nuclei
PC	Pontocerebellar fibers
MCP	Middle cerebellar peduncle

Rostral Pons at Level of Locus Ceruleus

Characteristics of the Rostral Pons at the Level of the Locus Ceruleus

- The superior cerebellar peduncle (SCP) borders the fourth ventricle laterally. It contains some cerebellar afferent fibers but mainly conveys efferent outflow from the intracerebellar nuclei to the red nucleus and thalamus.
- The mesencephalic nucleus and tract of the trigeminal nerve lie medial to the SCP.
- The pigmented locus ceruleus is visible on the floor of the fourth ventricle even in unstained sections due to its melanin-containing cells. These neurons, rich in norepinephrine, distribute fibers diffusely, extending from the cerebral cortex to the spinal cord. As a component of the extrathalamic corticopetal modulatory systems, they are said to influence blood vessels, respiration, micturition, paradoxical (rapid eye movement) sleep, arousal, and response to stress.
- The crossed ventral trigeminothalamic tract (VTT) is the principal pathway from the chief sensory and spinal trigeminal nuclei to the thalamus (VPM). Both crossed and uncrossed fibers ascend to the thalamus from the chief sensory nucleus. Uncrossed fibers ascend in the dorsal trigeminothalamic tract (DTT).
- The medial lemniscus, spinothalamic tract, and lateral lemniscus traverse the ventral and ventrolateral tegmentum.

- The basal pons, at all levels, contains scattered pontine nuclei; transverse pontocerebellar fibers; and perpendicularly coursing corticopontine, corticobulbar, and corticospinal fibers.
- Fascicles of the trigeminal nerve demarcate the basal pons medially from the middle cerebellar peduncle (MCP) laterally.

Clinical Correlations . . . .

The pontine arteries are "end" arteries; thus, the basal pons is a frequent site of hemorrhagic infarction.

Color the following structures red: MLF, TST, RST, SCP, CBT, and CST. Color blue the VSCT, MN, MT, DTT, VTT, ML, STHT, STET, PC, and MCP. Color the DLF and LC orange, the LL yellow, and the rootlets of V green. Use blue and red diagonal marks to color the CTT.

The greatest thing in family life is to take a hint when a hint is intended—
and not to take a hint when a hint isn't intended. – Robert Frost

78

Rostral Pons at Level of Locus Ceruleus

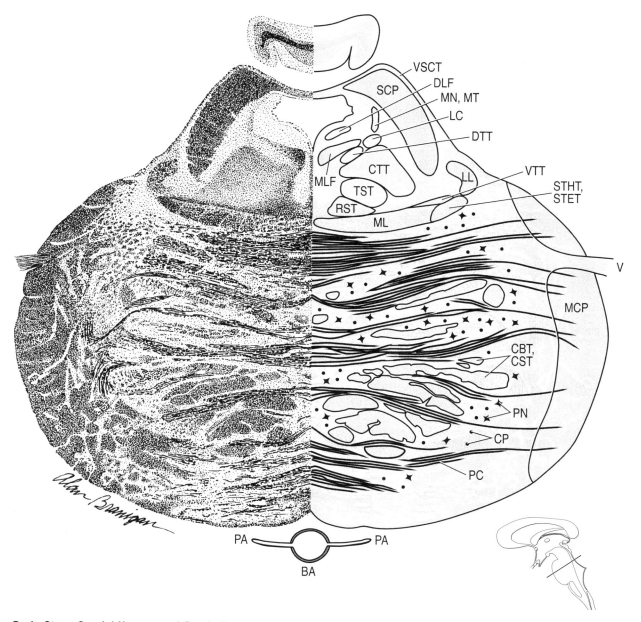

Structures Related to Afferent Input

MN, MT	Mesencephalic nucleus and tract of V
ML	Medial lemniscus
STHT	Spinothalamic tract
STET	Spinotectal tract
LL	Lateral lemniscus
VSCT	Ventral spinocerebellar tract
SCP, MCP	Superior and middle cerebellar peduncles
DTT	Dorsal trigeminothalamic tract
VTT	Ventral trigeminothalamic tract
V	Rootlets of V

Structures Related to Efferent Outflow

RST	Rubrospinal tract
MLF	Medial longitudinal fasciculus
TST	Tectospinal tract
SCP	Superior cerebellar peduncle
CBT, CST	Corticobulbar and corticospinal tracts
V	Rootlets of V

Arteries and Integrative Structures

BA	Basilar artery
CTT	Central tegmental tract
CP	Corticopontine fibers
PN	Pontine nuclei
PC	Pontocerebellar fibers
MCP	Middle cerebellar peduncle
DLF	Dorsal longitudinal fasciculus
LC	Locus ceruleus
PA	Pontine arteries

Pons at Level of Isthmus

Characteristics of the Pons at the Level of the Isthmus
- The fourth ventricle narrows and is continuous with the cerebral aqueduct.
- Decussating trochlear nerves are in the roof plate.
- The dorsal longitudinal fasciculus (DLF) contains ascending and descending fibers that influence the autonomic nervous system. The DLF is located in the ventral part of the periaqueductal gray and in the floor of the fourth ventricle just dorsal to the hypoglossal nucleus. It is composed of fibers mainly from the hypothalamus and dorsal tegmental nucleus (some are from the habenula), with endings in all cranial preganglionic parasympathetic nuclei and brain stem motor nuclei other than those innervating the ocular muscles.
- The locus ceruleus, mesencephalic nucleus, and tract of the trigeminal are in close proximity to the fourth ventricle.
- Decussating fibers are within the superior cerebellar peduncle (SCP).
- A well-demarcated lateral lemniscus and nucleus are lateral to the SCP.
- The dorsal and ventral tegmental nuclei are separated by the medial longitudinal fasciculus.
- The position of the medial lemniscus and the spinothalamic tract define the tegmentum from the basal pons.

- The base of the pons contains the nuclei and fibers previously identified at caudal levels, i.e., pontine nuclei and corticopontine, pontocerebellar, corticobulbar, and corticospinal fibers.

Clinical Correlations . . . .

The pons rests on the clivus in the posterior fossa. Midline tumors in the posterior fossa may block CSF flow and cause hydrocephalus, increased intracranial pressure, and nausea and vomiting.

Color the DLF, DTN, and VTN orange. Color the following structures red: rootlets of IV, MLF, TST, decussation of SCP, RST, CBT, and CST. Color blue the MN, MT, DTT, VTT, ML, STHT, STET, PC, and MCP. Color the LL yellow, and use red and blue diagonal marks to color the CTT.

Pons at Level of Isthmus

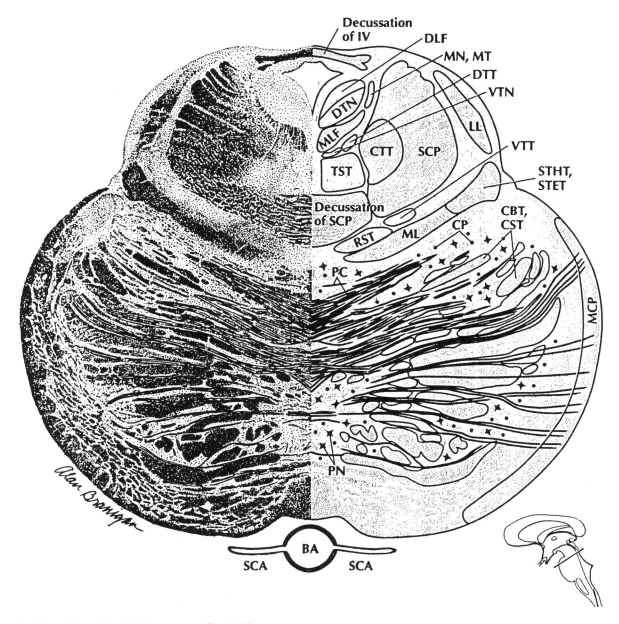

Decussation of IV

DLF

MN, MT

DTT

VTN

DTN

MLF

LL

CTT

SCP

VTT

TST

STHT, STET

Decussation of SCP

RST

ML

CP

CBT, CST

PC

PN

MCP

BA

SCA   SCA

Structures Related to Afferent Input

MN, MT	Mesencephalic nucleus and tract of V
ML	Medial lemniscus
STHT	Spinothalamic tract
STET	Spinotectal tract
LL	Lateral lemniscus
MCP	Middle cerebellar peduncle
SCP	Superior cerebellar peduncle
DTT	Dorsal trigeminothalamic tract
VTT	Ventral trigeminothalamic tract

Structures Related to Efferent Outflow

IV	Trochlear fibers
RST	Rubrospinal tract
MLF	Medial longitudinal fasciculus
TST	Tectospinal tract
SCP	Superior cerebellar peduncle
CBT, CST	Corticobulbar and corticospinal tracts

Arteries and Integrative Structures

BA	Basilar artery
SCA	Superior cerebellar artery
CTT	Central tegmental tract
CP	Corticopontine fibers
PN	Pontine nuclei
PC	Pontocerebellar fibers
MCP	Middle cerebellar peduncle
DLF	Dorsal longitudinal fasciculus
DTN, VTN	Dorsal and ventral tegmental nuclei

Mesencephalon at Level of Inferior Colliculus

Characteristics of the Mesencephalon at the Level of the Inferior Colliculus

- The oval-shaped inferior colliculi are dorsolateral in the tectum and receive fibers from the ascending lateral lemnisci. They are connected through the commissure of the inferior colliculus (CIC). The inferior colliculus has reciprocal connections with the medial geniculate nucleus of the thalamus via the inferior brachium. The inferior colliculus projects to the superior colliculus, establishing reflexes for turning the head and eyes toward or away from auditory stimuli.
- The massive decussation of the superior cerebellar peduncles (SCP) occurs in the tegmentum. These fibers originate in the intracerebellar nuclei and terminate predominantly in the red nucleus (cerebellorubral) and thalamus (cerebellothalamic).
- The trochlear nuclei and medial longitudinal fasciculi (MLF) are distinct features ventral to the cerebral aqueduct.
- The central tegmental tract (CTT) is prominent lateral to the MLF. It traverses the brain stem and terminates mainly on the surface of the inferior olivary nucleus. It contains fibers from the red nucleus and the periaqueductal gray matter and relays signals from the cerebral cortex, basal ganglia, and cerebellum. It also includes fibers that end on reticular neurons, the nucleus ambiguus, and, to some extent, the spinal cord.
- The cerebral aqueduct, surrounded by lightly stained periaqueductal gray, is characteristic of all levels of the mesencephalon. The periaqueductal gray is important in pain transmission and in somatic and autonomic responses in affective behavior, including the defense reaction.

- The substantial nigra, a large nucleus of melanin-containing cells, is present at caudal and rostral levels as are the fibers traversing the base of the cerebral peduncle. The homunculus (stick figure) shows the somatotopic organization of the corticobulbar and corticospinal fibers medial to lateral, respectively. The substantia nigra consists of a pars reticulata of scattered cells among fiber strands; a pars compacta of larger, more closely packed cells; and a small pars lateralis.
- The ventral tegmental area (VTA) lies between the substantia nigrae and the interpeduncular nucleus. It contains dopaminergic neurons that project to the nucleus accumbens in the mesolimbic pathway.
- The interpeduncular nucleus receives afferents from the habenular nucleus and medial mamillary nucleus, and projects to tegmental nuclei associated with the limbic system.

Clinical Correlations . . . .

The **dopaminergic neurons** in the pars compacta of the **substantia nigra degenerate** in **Parkinson's disease.**

Color blue the MN, MT, VTT, DTT, ML, STHT, and STET. Color red the IV, MLF, TST, decussation of SCP, RST, CBT, and CST. Color IC, LL, and BIC yellow. Use red and blue to draw diagonal lines through CTT. Draw red diagonal lines through FP and P-O-T. Color IPN and VTA orange.

Young man, the secret of my success is that at an early age I discovered I was not God. – Oliver Wendell Holmes, Jr.

82

Mesencephalon at Level of Inferior Colliculus

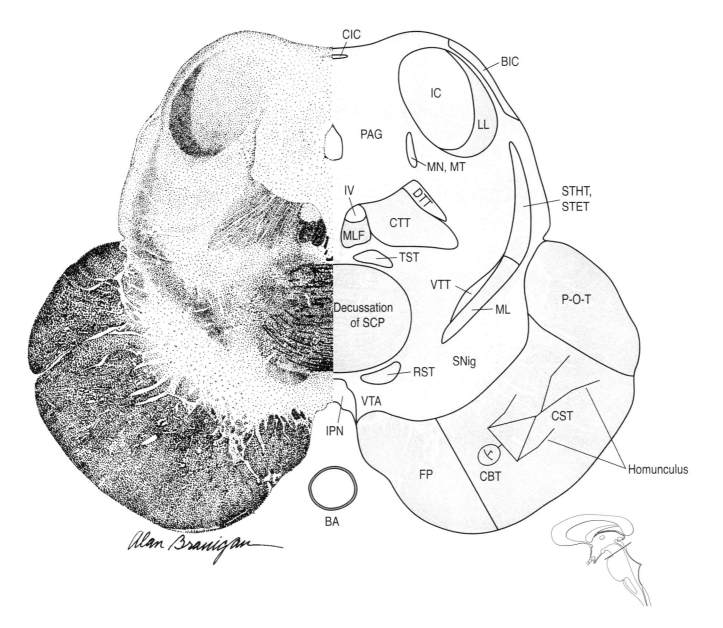

Structures Related to Afferent Input

MN, MT	Mesencephalic nucleus and tract of V
ML	Medial lemniscus
STHT	Spinothalamic tract
STET	Spinotectal tract
LL	Lateral lemniscus
DTT	Dorsal trigeminothalamic tract
VTT	Ventral trigeminothalamic tract
IC	Nucleus of inferior colliculus
BIC	Brachium of inferior colliculus
CIC	Commissure of inferior colliculus

Structures Related to Efferent Outflow

IV	Trochlear nucleus
MLF	Medial longitudinal fasciculus
TST	Tectospinal tract
CBT, CST	Corticobulbar and corticospinal tracts
Dec SCP	Decussation of superior cerebellar peduncles
RST	Rubrospinal tract
SNig	Substantia nigra

Arteries and Integrative Structures

BA	Basilar artery
CTT	Central tegmental tract
FP	Frontopontine fibers
P-O-T	Parieto-occipito-temporopontine fibers
IPN	Interpeduncular nucleus
PAG	Periaqueductal gray
VTA	Ventral tegmental area

Mesencephalon at Level of Superior Colliculus

Characteristics of the Mesencephalon at the Level of the Superior Colliculus

- The superior colliculi are dorsal to the cerebral aqueduct and are connected through the commissure of the superior colliculi (CSC). These nuclei receive projections from the cerebral cortex, retina, inferior colliculus, and spinal cord (spinotectal tract). The superior colliculus contains six cellular layers and has a laminated appearance. Cells in the deep layers give rise to tectospinal and tectobulbar fibers that mediate cranial nerve and cervical spinal nerve reflex response to visual, auditory, and cutaneous stimuli.
- The general somatic efferent nucleus and the general visceral efferent nucleus (Edinger-Westphal [E-W]) of the oculomotor nerve form a "V" in the midline of the tegmentum. The nucleus of Darkschewitsch and the interstitial nucleus of Cajal receive afferents from the globus pallidus and from the medial longitudinal fasciculus (MLF); efferent connections enter the MLF for discharge to motor nuclei of the brain stem.
- The prominent oval-shaped red nucleus is a feature in the tegmentum. It is named for its pink color in a fresh specimen, which is attributed to the richness of its vascularity in contrast to the surrounding tissue. It receives input from the cerebellum, cerebral cortex, globus pallidus, ventral thalamus, and superior colliculus. Its efferent connections include rubrospinal and reticulospinal connections and numerous fibers that reach the inferior olivary nucleus via the central tegmental tract.

- The medial lemniscus, spinothalamic, and spinotectal tracts lie dorsal to the substantia nigra.
- The medial geniculate nucleus (MGN) of the thalamus lies dorsal to the cerebral peduncle and medial to the lateral geniculate nucleus (LGN) of the thalamus. The MGN relays auditory impulses to the primary auditory cortex.
- The LGN relays visual impulses received from the retina to the primary visual cortex.
- The optic tract and pulvinar are apparent.

Clinical Correlations . . . .

A description of the mediobasal mesencephalic syndrome (of Weber) is on pages 122 and 123.

Color yellow the CSC, SC, BIC, MGN, BSC, LGN, and OT. Color red the III, MLF, TST, RN, RST, CR, CT, CBT, and CST. Color DLF, E-W, HPT, IPN, and VTA orange. Use red and blue to draw diagonal lines through CTT. Draw red lines through F-P and P-O-T.

Mesencephalon at Level of Superior Colliculus

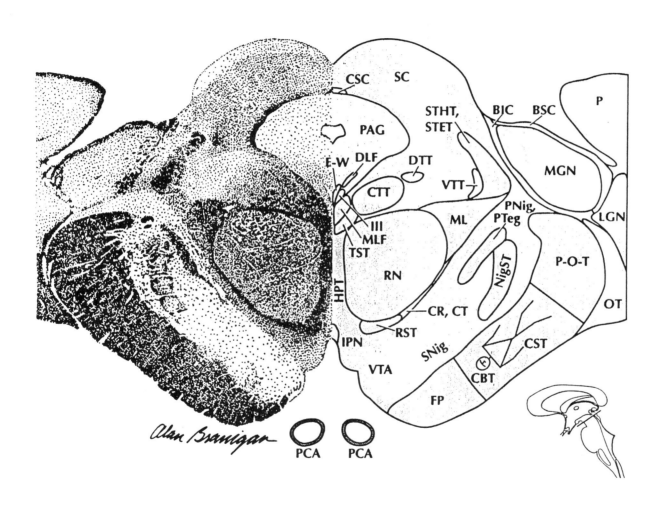

Structures Related to Afferent Input

ML	Medial lemniscus
STHT	Spinothalamic tract
STET	Spinotectal tract
DTT	Dorsal trigeminothalamic tract
VTT	Ventral trigeminothalamic tract
MGN	Medial geniculate nucleus
OT	Optic tract
LGN	Lateral geniculate nucleus
BIC	Brachium of inferior colliculus

Structures Related to Efferent Outflow

III	Oculomotor nucleus
E-W	Edinger-Westphal nucleus
MLF	Medial longitudinal fasciculus
TST	Tectospinal tract
CBT, CST	Corticobulbar and corticospinal tracts
RN, RST	Red nucleus, rubrospinal tract
SNig	Substantia nigra
NigST	Nigrostriatal tract
CR, CT	Cerebellorubral and cerebellothalamic fibers
PNig, PTeg	Pallidonigral and pallidotegmental tracts

Arteries and Integrative Structures

PCA	Posterior cerebral artery
CTT	Central tegmental tract
FP	Frontopontine fibers
P-O-T	Parieto-occipito-temporopontine fibers
PAG	Periaqueductal gray
IPN	Interpeduncular nucleus
HPT	Habenulopeduncular tract
DLF	Dorsal longitudinal fasciculus
SC	Superior colliculus
CSC, BSC	Commissure, brachium of SC
P	Pulvinar of thalamus
VTA	Ventral tegmental area

Cranial Nerve Summary

Table 3–1. Cranial Nerve Summary[a]

Roman Numeral	Nerve	Components	Function
I	Olfactory	SVA	Olfaction
II	Optic	SSA	Vision
III	Oculomotor	GSE, GVE	Moves eye medially, superiorly, inferiorly, and up and out (GSE); constricts pupil and accommodates eye (GVE)
IV	Trochlear	GSE	Moves eye down and out
V	Trigeminal: V1 ophthalmic V2 maxillary V3 mandibular	 GSA GSA GSA, SVE	Proprioception: Mesencephalic nucleus (GSA) Touch: chief sensory nucleus (GSA) Pain and temperature: spinal trigeminal nucleus (GSA) Moves jaw (SVE) and innervates tensor tympani, tensor palatini, mylohyoid and anterior belly of digastric
VI	Abducens	GSE	Moves eye laterally
VII	Facial	GSA, GVA, SVA, GVE, SVE	Facial expression, taste, salivation, lacrimation
VIII	Vestibulocochlear VIIIc VIIIv	SSA	 Audition Equilibrium
IX	Glossopharyngeal	GSA, GVA, SVA, GVE, SVE	Taste, salivation, swallowing, (carotid body and carotid sinus [GVA] monitor [O_2] and blood pressure, respectively)
X	Vagus	GSA, GVA, SVA, GVE, SVE	Taste, swallowing, lifts palate, talking (carotid body, monitors [O_2]) (parasympathetic of viscera)
XI	Accessory	SVE	Turns head, lifts shoulders
XII	Hypoglossal	GSE	Moves tongue

[a]Sensory: I, II, VIII (I, II are tracts of the brain); motor: III, IV, VI, XI, XII; mixed: V, VII, IX, X

Observe that motor nuclei lie medial to the sulcus limitans and that sensory nuclei are lateral to it. Medial to lateral, the motor nuclei are GSE, GVE, and SVE. Color brown the rostral part of the nucleus of the solitary tract (SVA) and color purple the caudal part (GVA). Color yellow the cochlear and vestibular nuclei (SSA). Color blue the mesencephalic, chief sensory, and spinal trigeminal nuclei (GSA). Color the GSE nuclei red, the GVE nuclei orange, and the SVE nuclei green (see summary at top of page 87). Finally, use the indicated colors to color the columns listing the components.

Cranial Nerve Nuclei and Components

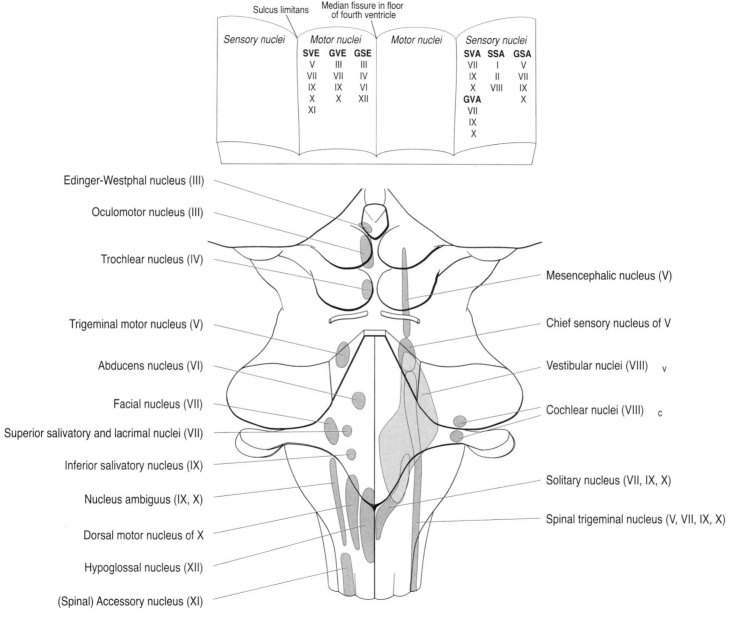

Sulcus limitans

Median fissure in floor
of fourth ventricle

Sensory nuclei	Motor nuclei			Motor nuclei	Sensory nuclei		
	SVE	**GVE**	**GSE**		**SVA**	**SSA**	**GSA**
	V	III	III		VII	I	V
	VII	VII	IV		IX	II	VII
	IX	IX	VI		X	VIII	IX
	X	X	XII		**GVA**		X
	XI				VII		
					IX		
					X		

Edinger-Westphal nucleus (III)

Oculomotor nucleus (III)

Trochlear nucleus (IV)

Mesencephalic nucleus (V)

Trigeminal motor nucleus (V)

Chief sensory nucleus of V

Abducens nucleus (VI)

Vestibular nuclei (VIII)   v

Facial nucleus (VII)

Cochlear nuclei (VIII)   c

Superior salivatory and lacrimal nuclei (VII)

Inferior salivatory nucleus (IX)

Solitary nucleus (VII, IX, X)

Nucleus ambiguus (IX, X)

Dorsal motor nucleus of X

Spinal trigeminal nucleus (V, VII, IX, X)

Hypoglossal nucleus (XII)

(Spinal) Accessory nucleus (XI)

Cranial Nerve I, Olfactory

Definitions

The **olfactory nerve** is composed of unmyelinated axons of receptor cells located in the olfactory mucosa in the nasal cavity. Taste and smell are intimately related; both are involved in **visceral functions** and are classified as SVA. Olfaction is unique in that (1) it is the only sensation that is transmitted directly to the cerebral cortex without first relaying through the **thalamus**, and (2) olfactory receptor cells are regularly replaced from precursor cells. The **primary olfactory cortex** (piriform cortex) is in the temporal and frontal lobes. The **amygdaloid body**, a subcortical structure, is located in the temporal lobe anterior to the hippocampus and the temporal horn of the lateral ventricle.

Structural and Functional Features

The first order neuron in the olfactory pathway is also the sensory receptor. Bipolar neurons with ciliated dendrites are located in the **olfactory mucosa** in the upper part of the nasal cavity. Secretions from supporting cells and glands (Bowman's) lubricate the epithelium. Particles in the air pass into solution, thus, the effective stimulus is **chemical.** The transduction mechanism is unclear but it is believed that odorants bind to receptor proteins on the cilia.

Axons of the receptor cells pass through **foramina** in the **cribriform plate** of the ethmoid bone to constitute about 20 olfactory fila on each side. Most of the axons terminate on **mitral cells** in the **olfactory bulb.** Within the olfactory bulb, the central process of the bipolar receptor cells forms brush-like synapses in specialized structures called **glomeruli.** Axons of numerous receptor cells converge onto mitral cells whose function is to relay the olfactory stimuli to the brain. Through collateral branches from mitral cells, and inhibitory neurons (granule and periglomerular cells), complex information processing occurs in the olfactory bulb. The relay from the mitral cells makes up the olfactory tract; therefore, this projection is, in reality, a tract of the brain, specifically of the telencephalon. The **anterior olfactory nucleus** is composed of loosely arranged neurons within the olfactory tract. Projections from the anterior olfactory nucleus through the **anterior commissure** contribute to the contralateral olfactory pathway.

The **olfactory tract** expands into the **olfactory trigone** at the **anterior perforated substance**. Most of the fibers in the tract follow the lateral olfactory stria to reach the primary olfactory cortex, which includes parts of the orbital surface of the frontal lobe, as well as the uncus, entorhinal area, and medial amygdaloid nucleus of the temporal lobe.

Caudal olfactory connections reach numerous structures including the hippocampal formation. Ultimately, olfactory input is likely to reach regions in the reticular formation including salivatory nuclei and the dorsal motor nucleus of the vagus nerve, the mediodorsal thalamic nucleus, and the medial amygdaloid nucleus (which in turn is related to the medial preoptic–hypothalamic region). Through these complex interconnections, the sense of smell influences **visceral functions (salivation, gastric secretions, peristalsis), social interaction**, and **reproductive behavior**.

Some of the pathways involved in transmitting olfaction include the medial forebrain bundle (to hypothalamus), stria medullaris thalami (to mediodorsal thalamus), stria terminalis (from amygdala to medial preoptic–anterior hypothalamus), and the dorsal longitudinal fasciculus (from hypothalamus to brain stem centers involved in visceral function).

Clinical Correlations . . . .

Fractures of the floor of the anterior cranial fossa involving the cribriform plate, avulsion of the delicate olfactory nerves, and tumors along the olfactory tract may interrupt olfactory pathways. Anterior cranial fossa fractures may also cause leakage of CSF from the subarachnoid space into the nasal cavity (**CSF rhinorrhea**). The significance of such fractures is that they provide a potential route whereby infectious agents can invade the meninges and brain.

Loss of the sense of smell is termed "anosmia." Disagreeable imaginary odors termed "olfactory hallucinations" sometimes precede seizure activity involving temporal lobe structures (**uncinate fits**). The olfactory nerve is tested by instructing the patient to close both eyes and to close one nostril. The patient is then asked to identify the smell of a familiar aromatic compound (coffee, cloves, etc.) presented to the open nostril.

Color the bipolar receptor cells, mitral cells, and their axons brown. Observe that the bipolar axons and mitral cell dendrites form synaptic contacts in the glomerulus. Note that the axons of the mitral cells, via the lateral olfactory stria terminate mainly in the uncus and amygdala.

Cranial Nerve I, Olfactory

Component: SVA

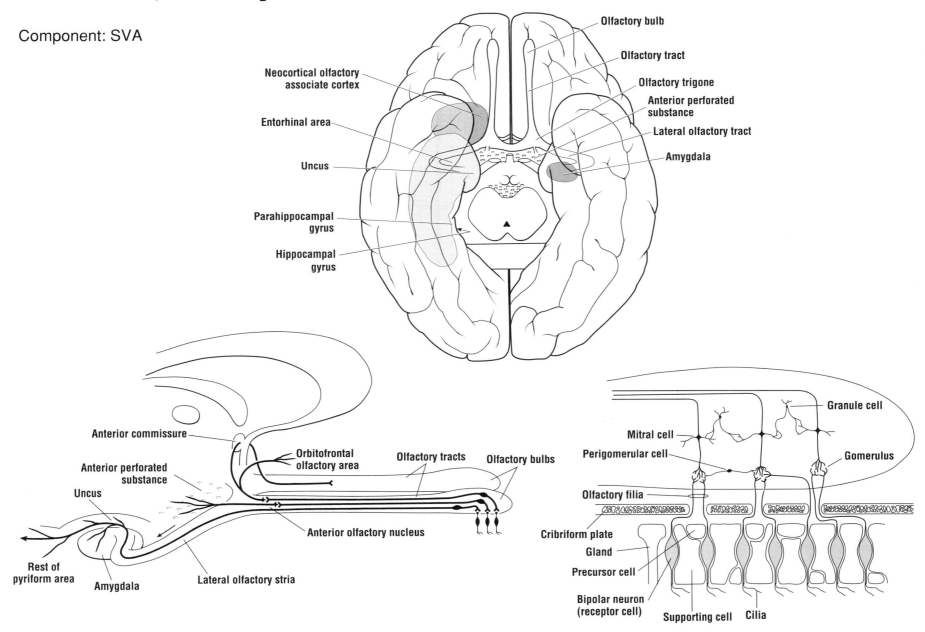

Olfactory bulb

Olfactory tract

Neocortical olfactory associate cortex

Olfactory trigone

Anterior perforated substance

Entorhinal area

Lateral olfactory tract

Uncus

Amygdala

Parahippocampal gyrus

Hippocampal gyrus

Anterior commissure

Granule cell

Mitral cell

Orbitofrontal olfactory area

Olfactory tracts

Olfactory bulbs

Perigomerular cell

Gomerulus

Anterior perforated substance

Uncus

Olfactory filia

Anterior olfactory nucleus

Cribriform plate

Gland

Rest of pyriform area

Precursor cell

Amygdala

Lateral olfactory stria

Bipolar neuron (receptor cell)

Supporting cell

Cilia

Cranial Nerve II, Optic

Definitions
Although the optic nerve actually forms a CNS tract at the level of the diencephalon, it continues to be called a "nerve." Vision is classified as SSA.

Structural and Functional Features
The receptor cells for vision are rods and cones. Integrative neurons in the retina (bipolar, amacrine, and horizontal) are interposed between the rods and cones and the ganglionic neurons, whose axons make up the optic nerve. **Rods** have a low threshold of excitability and are responsible for **night vision**. **Cones** have a high threshold of excitability and are responsible for **visual acuity** and **color discrimination**. Cones are densely packed in the fovea centralis region of the retina; rods are peripherally located. Ganglion cell axons exit the globe at the **optic disc** as the **optic nerve**.

Ganglion cell axons from the ipsilateral eye form the optic nerves, which traverse the optic canals and converge at the optic chiasm. Ganglion cell axons from the temporal retina continue in the ipsilateral optic tract, whereas ganglion cell axons in the nasal retina cross in the chiasm to the contralateral optic tract. A small population of axons leaves the optic tract to either (1) terminate in the pretectal area and provide the afferent stimulus for the pupillary light reflex or (2) terminate in the superior colliculus to provide afferent input that is integrated for reflex response via the tectospinal tract. The majority of optic tract axons terminate retinotopically in the lateral geniculate nuclei (LGN) of the thalami in distinct laminae within this six-layered structure. Geniculocalcarine fibers (optic radiation) project to the calcarine sulcus in the occipital lobe (primary visual cortex, area 17).

Clinical Correlations . . . .

Retinotopic organization is faithfully maintained throughout the visual system so that images received from the left visual hemifield terminate in the right occipital lobe. Images projected on the inferior region of the retina are relayed to the inferior bank of the calcarine sulcus (lingual gyrus), and those from the superior retina terminate in the gyrus along the superior bank (cuneus). Because one cerebral hemisphere subserves only a visual hemifield, it follows that quadrants of the visual field are represented inferiorly and superiorly along the calcarine sulcus, which is the **primary** (1°) visual cortex (area 17). It is surrounded by **visual association cortex, areas 18, 19**. Color, form, and movement are highly integrative aspects of the visual phenomenon that are functions of the association areas of the occipital lobe and of occipitotemporal and occipitoparietal interconnections.

The intactness of the visual pathway gives an anterior-to-posterior assessment of the cerebrum from the frontal to the occipital lobes. Because the visual system extends from the eyeball to the occipital pole and is retinotopically organized, lesions in the various locations cause predictable visual field deficits. Likewise, the nature of the deficits suggests the site of the lesion. The external world is projected onto the retina in an up–down (inverted) and right–left (reversed) fashion. Fibers in the nasal half of each retina (temporal field vision) decussate in the optic chiasm, whereas fibers in the temporal half of each retina

(nasal field vision) continue in the optic tract of the ipsilateral eye. It is essential to understand that visual deficits refer to the visual field loss and not to retinal areas.

Diseases of the eye per se are more common than are neurologic defects involving the pathways. **Cataract** (loss of transparency of the lens) and **glaucoma** (excessive intraocular pressure) are common causes of impaired vision. The central artery enters the eye at the optic disk and ramifies into several retinal branches. Swelling at the optic papilla, i.e., choked disk, can be observed in an ophthalmoscopic examination of the fundus. Increased intracranial pressure is one of the causes of **papilledema**. A cursory evaluation of the visual system can be obtained by the confrontation method in which the examiner moves an object into the patient's field of vision and the patient reports when it becomes visible.

The following discussion refers to lesions involving the **right visual pathway**. The circles below represent left and right visual fields, with the darkened areas depicting the **visual field** loss. Disease processes seldom result in clear-cut defects; however, depicting complete quadrant and hemifield involvement serves a didactic purpose. Complete lesions of the optic nerve cause blindness in the ipsilateral eye (monocular blindness, A). Most internal carotid aneurysms that affect vision arise at the junction of the internal carotid and ophthalmic arteries and compress the ipsilateral optic nerve, causing ipsilateral vision loss initially. A lesion of temporal retinal fibers relaying nasal field vision causes right nasal hemianopsia (B). Pituitary tumors grow upward into the chiasm and typically affect the temporal visual fields, causing bitemporal hemianopsia (C). A lesion of the optic tract near the LGN results in homonymous hemianopsia (D). Reflex response to light is maintained, however, because the lesion is posterior to the point at which axons diverge to the superior colliculus and pretectal nuclei.

The fibers in Meyer's loop relay stimuli from the lower retina to the inferior bank of the calcarine sulcus, mirroring upper field vision. **Interruption of Meyer's loop** causes a **contralateral superior quadrantanopsia** (E). An occlusion of a branch of the middle cerebral artery could selectively lesion Meyer's loop. Aneurysms of the anterior cerebral or the anterior communicating artery tend to involve the lower quadrant (inferior bitemporal quadrantanopsia, not shown).

Tumors and **intracerebral bleeding** cause defects of the **contralateral hemifield** (homonymous hemianopsia, F) if the encroachment is in the optic radiations as they traverse the temporal or parietal lobes en route to the primary visual area. Observe that a lesion of the optic tract (D) and a lesion of the optic radiation (F) both result in contralateral homonymous hemianopsia.

Color yellow the right temporal and the left nasal axons (SSA component). Observe that this is a ventral view; therefore, the right eye is on the left of the diagram. Color Meyer's loop fibers yellow; they terminate inferiorly along area 17. Color the other optic radiations yellow; they terminate superiorly along area 17.

Cranial Nerve II, Optic

Component: SSA

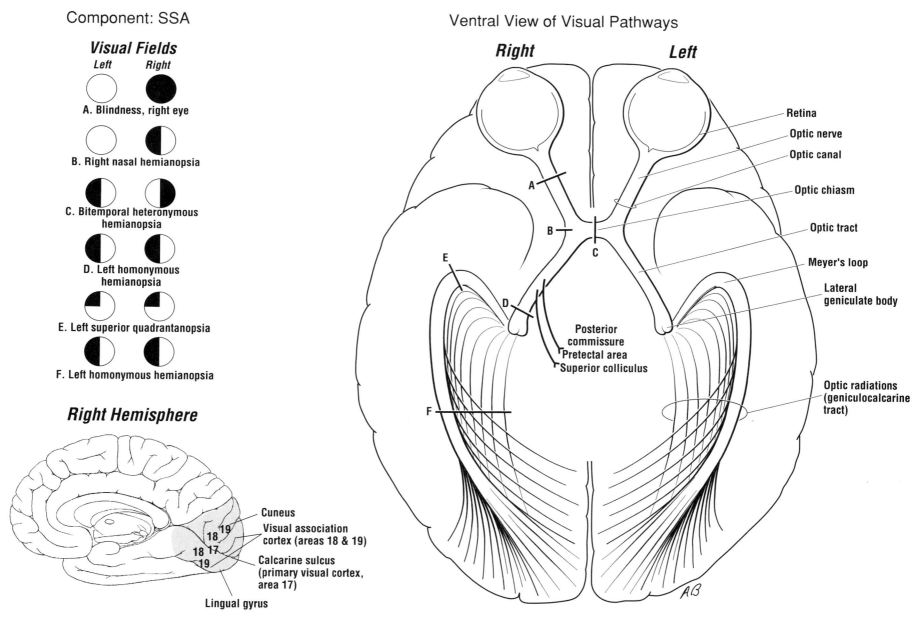

Visual Fields

Left   Right

A. Blindness, right eye

B. Right nasal hemianopsia

C. Bitemporal heteronymous hemianopsia

D. Left homonymous hemianopsia

E. Left superior quadrantanopsia

F. Left homonymous hemianopsia

Right Hemisphere

Cuneus

Visual association cortex (areas 18 & 19)

18 19
18 17
19

Calcarine sulcus (primary visual cortex, area 17)

Lingual gyrus

Ventral View of Visual Pathways

Right   Left

Retina

Optic nerve

Optic canal

Optic chiasm

Optic tract

Meyer's loop

Lateral geniculate body

Posterior commissure

Pretectal area

Superior colliculus

Optic radiations (geniculocalcarine tract)

AB

Cranial Nerve III, Oculomotor

Definitions

The oculomotor, trochlear, and abducens nerves supply the motor innervation (GSE) to the extraocular muscles, which control voluntary movement of the eyes (page 98). The trochlear and abducens nerves contain only the GSE component. In addition to the GSE component, the oculomotor nerve includes the GVE component of preganglionic parasympathetic fibers that arise from the Edinger-Westphal nucleus.

Structural and Functional Features

The **oculomotor nucleus** is actually a complex of several subnuclei that lies ventral to the cerebral aqueduct in the periaqueductal gray of the midbrain at the level of the superior colliculus. It is V-shaped and is located just rostral to the medial longitudinal fasciculus. The nucleus in cross section consists of multipolar motor neurons whose axons curve ventrally in the tegmentum and pass through the red nucleus. These fibers innervate the **inferior oblique**, the **superior, medial,** and **inferior recti muscles** and the **striated fibers** of the **levator palpebrae muscle** (smooth muscle fibers in the levator palpebrae are supplied by postganglionic sympathetic fibers).

The **Edinger-Westphal nucleus** contains small preganglionic parasympathetic cells whose axons accompany other oculomotor fibers into the orbit and terminate in the ciliary ganglion. Axons of the ganglion cells (postganglionic fibers) pass through the short ciliary nerves to supply the **sphincter pupillae** of the iris and the **ciliary muscle.** The GSE and GVE components together form the oculomotor nerve, which emerges from the midbrain in the interpeduncular fossa and passes between the superior cerebellar and the posterior cerebral arteries. The nerve pierces the dura, enters the cavernous sinus, runs along the lateral wall, passes through the superior orbital fissure, and splits into superior and inferior divisions (page 93) to reach four of the six extrinsic muscles and the intrinsic ocular muscles.

A group of nuclei at the rostral end of the oculomotor complex at the junction of the midbrain and diencephalon are involved in eye movements; are referred to as accessory oculomotor nuclei; and include the nucleus of Darkschewitsch, the interstitial nucleus of Cajal, the nucleus of the posterior commissure, and the rostral interstitial nucleus of the medial longitudinal fasciculus (MLF). The interstitial nucleus of Cajal consists of cells intermingled with the fibers of the posterior commissure. The nucleus of the posterior commissure consists, as the name implies, of cells associated with fibers of the posterior commissure. The rostral interstitial nucleus of the MLF is involved in vertical eye movements. These nuclei, as a group, are rather poorly understood. The **pretectal region** rostral to the superior colliculus is clinically significant. Pretectal neurons receive afferents from the optic tract, the visual cortex, and the lateral geniculate body. Some of the fibers from the accessory oculomotor nuclei and the pretectal region cross in the posterior commissure, which is situated caudal to the pineal gland at the point of transition between the cerebral aqueduct and the third ventricle. The **bilateralism** of the **pupillary reflexes** is mediated from **pretectal neurons** via the **posterior commissure.** Both pupils constrict when light is shown on the retina of one eye. The response of the ipsilateral eye is the **direct pupillary light reflex**; that of the contralateral eye is the **consensual reflex.** This pathway involves (1) retinal ganglion cell axons that reach the pretectal area via the optic nerve, optic tract, and brachium of the superior colliculus; (2) axons of pretectal neurons that terminate bilaterally in the Edinger-Westphal or accessory oculomotor nuclei; (3) preganglionic fibers in the CN III that synapse in the ciliary ganglion; and (4) postganglionic fibers that innervate the sphincter of the iris. Stated briefly, the afferent arc of the pupillary light reflex is **CN II** and the efferent arc is the **E-W nucleus** of **CN III.**

Visual fixation on a near object results in **ocular convergence** accompanied by **accommodation** of the lens. Impulses from the occipital cortex relayed to the E-W nucleus through the superior colliculus seem to initiate the **accommodation reflex.** Contraction of the ciliary muscle increases the thickness of the lens, thereby increasing refractive focusing on a near object. The sphincter pupillae muscle contracts at the same time.

Clinical Correlations . . . .

Examination of eye movements and the size, position, equality, and reaction of the pupils is important. Lesions of either the oculomotor nucleus or nerve (lower motor neuron lesions) are easily detected because of the objective signs present. These include **ptosis, dilation** of the **pupil,** a **downward, abducted eye position,** and **strabismus** (inability to direct both eyes toward the same object). **Diplopia** or double vision (a consequence of strabismus) and **paralysis of accommodation** are more difficult to evaluate. **Ptosis** is caused by paralysis of the levator palpebrae superioris and the unopposed action of the orbicularis oculi. The **downward, abducted eye position** results from the unopposed action of the superior oblique and lateral rectus muscles.

Interruption of the parasympathetic innervation results in **mydriasis** (dilated pupil), **loss of the pupillary light reflex,** and **loss of accommodation.** Because the preganglionic parasympathetic fibers are superficial in the nerve, they are readily affected by external pressure; therefore, slowness of the pupillary response to light is an early sign of oculomotor nerve compression.

The oculomotor nerve is vulnerable to compression from aneurysms (of either the superior cerebellar or the posterior cerebral artery) and to supratentorial herniations (discussion of medial longitudinal fasciculus and supranuclear control of eye movements, page 98).

Color the oculomotor nucleus and fibers red. Follow the superior and inferior divisions of the oculomotor nerve to their target muscles. Color the E-W nucleus orange. Color the preganglionic fibers orange, observing the synapse in the ciliary ganglion. Color the postganglionic fibers orange; note that they innervate muscles intrinsic to the globe.

Cranial Nerve III, Oculomotor

Components: GSE, GVE

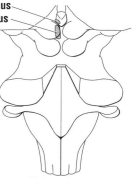

Edinger-Westphal nucleus
Oculomotor nucleus

Motor *Sensory*
nuclei *nuclei*

Left Eye

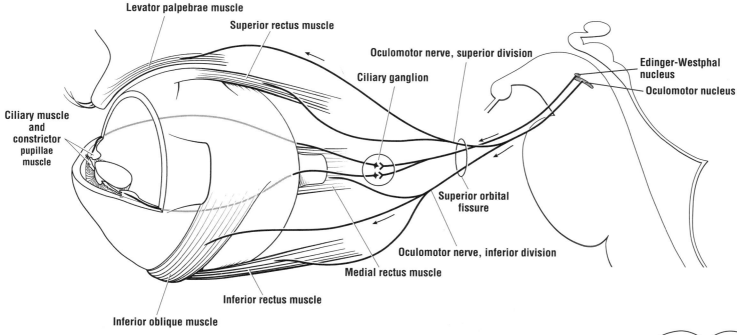

Levator palpebrae muscle

Superior rectus muscle

Oculomotor nerve, superior division

Ciliary ganglion

Edinger-Westphal nucleus

Oculomotor nucleus

Ciliary muscle and constrictor pupillae muscle

Superior orbital fissure

Oculomotor nerve, inferior division

Medial rectus muscle

Inferior rectus muscle

Inferior oblique muscle

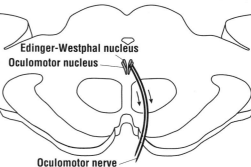

Edinger-Westphal nucleus
Oculomotor nucleus

Oculomotor nerve

Cranial Nerve IV, Trochlear

Definitions

The trochlear (pulley) nerve contains one functional component (GSE) and innervates only one muscle, the superior oblique.

Structural and Functional Features

The **trochlear nucleus** is located ventral to the cerebral aqueduct at the level of the inferior colliculus of the midbrain. The axons course dorsally around the aqueduct, decussate, and exit on the dorsal surface caudal to the colliculus. The nerve circles around the cerebral peduncle and passes ventrally with the oculomotor nerve between the posterior cerebral and superior cerebellar arteries. The nerve then runs along the lateral wall of the cavernous sinus and enters the orbit through the **superior orbital fissure.** It runs in the roof of the orbit across the levator palpebrae and superior rectus muscles to reach the superior oblique muscle. Contractions of the superior oblique muscle result in **inward rotation** and **downward and lateral movement** of the eye.

Clinical Correlations . . . .

Pathologic lesions in the cavernous sinus, aneurysms of either the posterior cerebral arteries or superior cerebellar arteries, or inflammatory disease may injure the trochlear nerve. Injury results in outward rotation of the affected eye and diplopia that is most pronounced when a patient is descending stairs. Tilting the head to the unaffected side minimizes diplopia.

Color the trochlear nucleus red, noting its position near the midline in the tegmentum. As you color the nerve, observe its decussation, dorsal exit, and entrance into the orbit via the superior orbital fissure.

The genius—in his works, in his deeds—is necessarily a prodigal:
his greatness lies in the fact that he expends himself. – Nietzsche

94

Cranial Nerve IV, Trochlear

Component: GSE

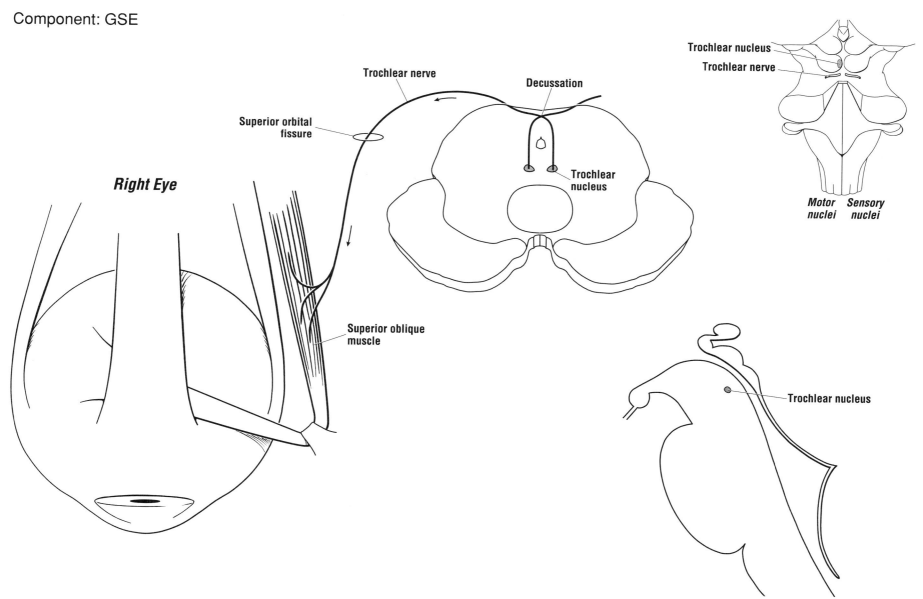

Right Eye

Trochlear nerve

Superior orbital fissure

Superior oblique muscle

Decussation

Trochlear nucleus

Trochlear nucleus

Trochlear nerve

Motor nuclei   Sensory nuclei

Trochlear nucleus

Cranial Nerve V, Trigeminal

Definitions

The trigeminal sensory nuclei transmit all GSA sensations (proprioception, pain, temperature, pressure, vibration, and discriminative touch) from the head and face. Cranial nerves VII, IX, and X mediate minimal GSA input to the spinal trigeminal nucleus; however, the trigeminal nerve is the main sensory nerve of the face and head. Additionally, CN V contains SVE motor fibers to striated muscles derived from mesenchyme of the first branchial arch.

Structural and Functional Features

The trigeminal (Gasserian, semilunar) ganglion rests in a depression in the middle cranial fossa. The dural recess that contains the roots of cranial nerve V and the ganglion are referred to as the trigeminal (or Meckel's) cave. The ganglion is composed of pseudounipolar neurons whose central processes enter the lateral surface of the pons and terminate either in the chief sensory or the spinal trigeminal nucleus. The peripheral processes leave the ganglion and exit the skull in one of three major divisions: the **ophthalmic (V1), maxillary (V2),** or **mandibular (V3) nerves.** Each of these divisions branches extensively after exiting the cranial cavity through the **superior orbital fissure (V1), foramen rotundum (V2),** or **foramen ovale (V3).** The **motor root** travels exclusively in the **mandibular division.** All GSA sensations from the face, excluding proprioception and small areas of skin around the external ear, are mediated by trigeminal ganglion cells. Proprioceptive impulses from the head and face are transmitted by the mesencephalic nucleus of CN V, whose peripheral processes travel in the V1 division. The cell bodies of pseudounipolar neurons located in the mesencephalic nucleus of CN V are the only sensory neurons within the CNS whose peripheral processes reach somatic structures (all others are in spinal or cranial nerve ganglia). These GSA "aberrant" neurons selectively mediate proprioception from the extraocular and the masticatory muscles. Collaterals from mesencephalic sensory axons terminate in the trigeminal motor nucleus, providing the afferent arc for the monosynaptic jaw (masseter) reflex.

The spinal trigeminal nucleus is a long column of cells extending from midpons to the spinal cord, where it merges with the dorsal gray matter. The spinal trigeminal tract and second order neurons of the spinal trigeminal nucleus are somatotopically arranged with V1 fibers ventral, V2 fibers intermediate, and V3 fibers dorsal. This nucleus processes pain, temperature, and tactile input with the **caudal area receiving** many **pain** and **temperature impulses.** The **chief sensory nucleus,** located in the pons near the point of entry of the nerve, comprises second order neurons concerned primarily with **discriminative touch sensation** from the face. Impulses originating in free and encapsulated endings in various tissues are processed in the chief sensory and spinal trigeminal nuclei. Axons from secondary sensory neurons ascend in either the uncrossed dorsal trigeminothalamic tract or the crossed ventral trigeminothalamic tract and synapse in the ventral posteromedial (VPM) nucleus of the thalamus. Axons from third order neurons in VPM ascend in the posterior limb of the internal capsule to terminate in the postcentral gyrus of the parietal lobe, the primary somatosensory cortex (areas 3,1,2). The central projections of the mesen-

cephalic nucleus mediating proprioception are less well understood. Nonetheless, proprioceptive input is essential for the precision required for conjugate eye movement and for chewing.

The SVE motor nucleus is medial to, and much smaller than, the chief sensory nucleus. Axons from these multipolar neurons join the mandibular nerve distal to the foramen ovale. Fibers in the anterior division of the mandibular branch supply the medial pterygoid, temporalis, masseter, and lateral pterygoid muscles. A small population of fibers passes through the otic ganglion (without synapsing) to innervate the tensor tympani and tensor veli palatini muscles. The inferior alveolar nerve (from the posterior branch of the mandibular) supplies the anterior belly of the digastric and the mylohyoid muscle.

Corticobulbar projections from the face area of the cerebral cortex provide **voluntary control of chewing.** Sensory branches of the trigeminal nerve and other CN input are integrated at pontine level for reflex responses, e.g., proprioceptive feedback via the mesencephalic nucleus for the stretch (jaw jerk) reflex and CN VIII input for tensor tympani response to sound intensity.

Clinical Correlations . . . .

Clinical testing for sensation should be done near the midline where the nerve supply is most consistent. The GSA component is tested by stroking the skin of the face in the dermatomes supplied by V1, V2, and V3 divisions. The **blink reflex** is checked by touching the cornea with a wisp of cotton and observing closure of the eye in response to the stimulus. In addition to the ophthalmic branch of CNV (afferent arc) and CN VII (efferent arc), the corneal blink reflex also involves CN III because it innervates the levator palpebrae muscle, which reopens the eye. The **jaw reflex** is tested by tapping the patient's chin with a percussion hammer. The **motor component of V3** is assessed by directing the patient to clench the teeth while the examiner palpates the masticatory muscles (page 130). (**Trigeminal neuralgia (tic douloureux)** is described on page 130.) Many disorders affect trigeminal pathways due to the wide distribution of the nuclei and nerve branches extending from the mesencephalon to the cervical spinal cord. Fractures of the facial bones or cranium, aneurysms of the internal carotid artery, tumors, and the lateral medullary vascular syndrome (pages 122 and 123) may disrupt sensory or motor functions or both. A hallmark of a lesion in the **lateral medulla** or upper cervical spinal cord is the interruption of **pain** and **temperature** sensation of the **face,** ipsilaterally, and of the **body, contralaterally.**

Color blue the GSA nuclei—mesencephalic, chief sensory, and spinal trigeminal. Beginning from the periphery, color fibers in V1, V2, and V3 blue; note their particular termination. Color the SVE motor nucleus and the motor fibers in V3 green.

Cranial Nerve V, Trigeminal

Components: GSA, SVE

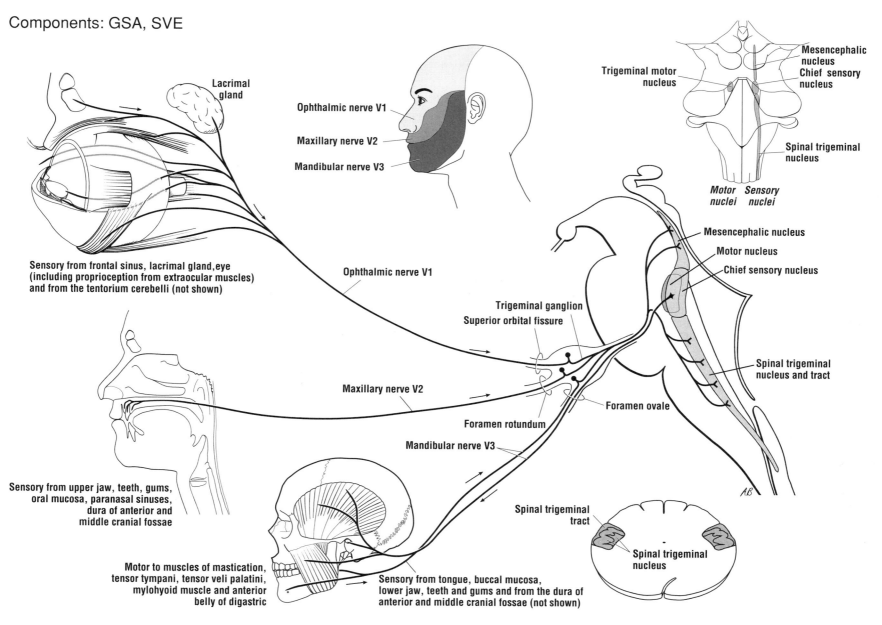

Lacrimal gland

Ophthalmic nerve V1

Maxillary nerve V2

Mandibular nerve V3

Trigeminal motor nucleus

Mesencephalic nucleus

Chief sensory nucleus

Spinal trigeminal nucleus

Motor nuclei   Sensory nuclei

Sensory from frontal sinus, lacrimal gland, eye (including proprioception from extraocular muscles) and from the tentorium cerebelli (not shown)

Ophthalmic nerve V1

Mesencephalic nucleus

Motor nucleus

Chief sensory nucleus

Trigeminal ganglion

Superior orbital fissure

Maxillary nerve V2

Spinal trigeminal nucleus and tract

Foramen ovale

Foramen rotundum

Mandibular nerve V3

Sensory from upper jaw, teeth, gums, oral mucosa, paranasal sinuses, dura of anterior and middle cranial fossae

Spinal trigeminal tract

Spinal trigeminal nucleus

Motor to muscles of mastication, tensor tympani, tensor veli palatini, mylohyoid muscle and anterior belly of digastric

Sensory from tongue, buccal mucosa, lower jaw, teeth and gums and from the dura of anterior and middle cranial fossae (not shown)

Cranial Nerve VI, Abducens

Definitions
The **abducens nerve** contains only one functional component (GSE) and innervates only one muscle, the **lateral rectus**. Ocular movements are described as conjugate when both eyes move in the same direction.

Structural and Functional Features
Like other GSE nuclei, the abducens nucleus is near the midline in the tegmentum. It is located in the pons just ventral to the fourth ventricle. The **internal genu** of the CN VII is a loop around the abducens nucleus that creates a bulge in the floor of the fourth ventricle (the facial colliculus). Axons from the abducens nucleus course through the tegmentum and emerge ventrally at the junction of the pons and the pyramid of the medulla. The nerve runs anteriorly in the subarachnoid space to reach the cavernous sinus, where it lies lateral to the internal carotid artery. The nerve enters the orbit through the **superior orbital fissure** to reach and supply the lateral rectus muscle. Contraction of this muscle results in abduction of the eye.

Both eyes must move together with a high degree of precision in order to maintain fixation on a moving object. The exquisite coordination of the extraocular muscles is possible due to several factors: (1) small motor units of the eye muscles; (2) proprioceptive input via the ophthalmic division of the trigeminal nerve; (3) complex subnuclear organization of the oculomotor nuclear complex; and (4) control of cranial nerves III, IV, and VI as a group by higher centers in the cortex and brain stem.

The **paramedian pontine reticular formation (PPRF)** located near the abducens nucleus serves as a **gaze center** for horizontal eye movements. PPRF projections through the medial longitudinal fasciculus (MFL) coordinate movements of the lateral rectus on one side with the medial rectus on the opposite side. The PPRF also receives afferent fibers from the vestibular nuclei and connects with the vertical gaze center in the periaqueductal gray matter of the midbrain at the level of the superior colliculus.

Clinical Correlations . . . .

Lesions of the abducens nerve result in (1) paresis or paralysis of the lateral rectus muscle, (2) inability to abduct the eye beyond the midline of gaze, (3) strabismus, and (4) diplopia. To some extent one can compensate for the strabismus by moving the head so that the affected eye is in line with the object of interest and the normal eye then fixates on the same object. Because the abducens runs a long course on the ventral surface of the pons, which rests on the clivus, it is particularly vulnerable to increased intracranial pressure. Its dysfunction, therefore, has no localizing value relative to etiology. In other words, involvement of cranial nerve VI, especially when bilateral, does not necessarily suggest a pontine lesion. Testing the **intactness** of the **MLF** is an important consideration when evaluating possible brain stem lesions. The MLF receives extensive input from vestibular and cerebellar nuclei as well as from supranuclear pathways. In lowered states of consciousness, the oculocephalic reflex (doll's eye phenomenon) is tested by holding the eyes open and passively moving the head rapidly from side to side. The reflex is intact if the eyes move in the direction opposite to that in which the head is moved. Absence of movement to one side suggests paralysis of conjugate gaze to that side and may be due to a cerebral or brain stem lesion. Pineal tumors may cause paralysis of upward gaze (sunset eyes).

The supranuclear pathway controlling **voluntary horizontal eye movement** originates in the frontal **eye field (area 8)** in the **contralateral middle frontal gyrus. Irritative lesions**, e.g., epileptic seizures, drive the eyes to the **contralateral side**, whereas **destructive lesions** of area 8 result in **looking at the lesion** due to the unopposed action of the opposite frontal eye field.

Another cortical center concerned with ocular movements lies in the visual cortex in the occipital lobe; however, this pathway is concerned with involuntary tracking movements of the eyes as in reading.

Color the abducens nucleus and fibers red. Note the intraaxial path and the long course of the nerve on the ventral surface of the pons en route to the cavernous sinus, superior orbital fissure, and, finally, the lateral rectus muscle.

internuclear opthalmoplegia
What are the 2 nuclei involved?

Cranial Nerve VI, Abducens

Component: GSE

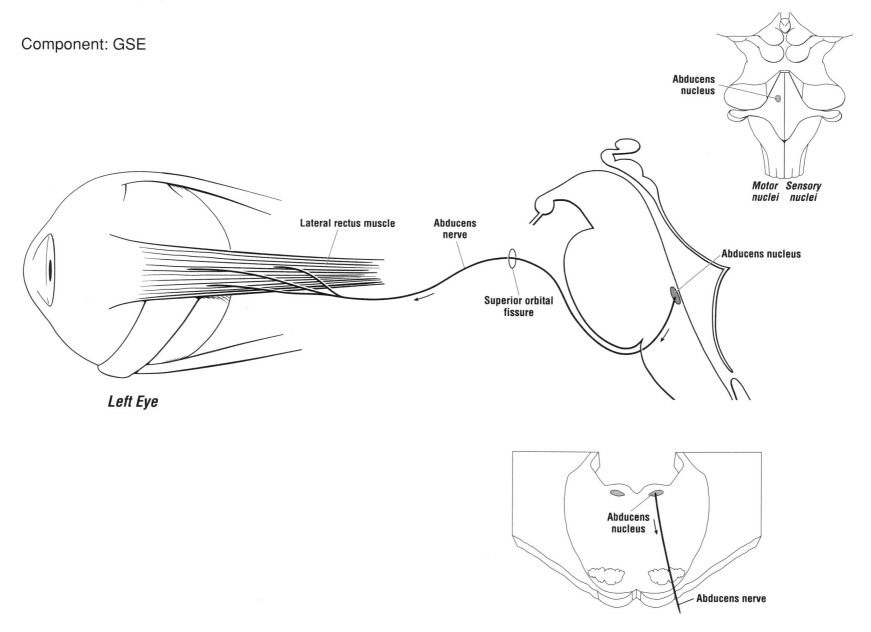

Abducens nucleus

Motor nuclei Sensory nuclei

Lateral rectus muscle

Abducens nerve

Abducens nucleus

Superior orbital fissure

Left Eye

Abducens nucleus

Abducens nerve

Cranial Nerve VII, Facial

Definitions

The facial nerve has a motor (**SVE**) component that innervates muscles derived from mesenchyme of the **second branchial arch** and forms the largest part of the facial nerve. The sensory components including GSA, GVA, and SVA are bound in a separate fascial sheath called the **intermediate nerve** (between the SVE component of VII and CN VIII in the cerebellopontine angle). **GVE components** are also located in the intermediate nerve.

Structural and Functional Features

SVE axons arise from multipolar neurons in the facial motor nucleus located in the pontine tegmentum. The axons course dorsomedially and encircle the abducens nucleus, creating the **internal genu** of the facial nerve. The fibers emerge from the ventrolateral pons and, in company with CN VIII, enter the internal auditory meatus. A "hairpin turn" within the facial canal creates the external genu of the facial nerve. A small twig innervates the **stapedius muscle** within the facial canal, then the nerve exits the canal via the **stylomastoid foramen.**

SVE fibers in the posterior auricular branch supply the occipitalis and muscles of the external ear. Other fibers form the nerves to the stylohyoid and posterior belly of the digastric. The main SVE component turns forward into the parotid gland and branches into temporal, zygomatic, buccal, mandibular, and cervical branches. These supply the **muscles** of **facial expression**: orbicularis oculi and oris, buccinator, zygomaticus major and minor, platysma, and frontalis.

The parasympathetic preganglionic (GVE) neurons are located in the **superior salivatory** and **lacrimal nuclei** in the pons. After the preganglionic axons from these neurons exit the brain stem in the intermediate nerve, they divide into two branches, the greater petrosal nerve and the chorda tympani nerve. Preganglionic axons in the greater petrosal nerve synapse on neurons in the **pterygopalatine ganglion** whose postganglionic axons in turn innervate the lacrimal gland and glandular tissue in the nasal and oral cavities. Preganglionic axons in the second branch, the **chorda tympani**, travel with the lingual nerve to synapse on postganglionic neurons in the **submandibular ganglion.** Neurons in the ganglion supply postganglionic innervation to the submandibular and sublingual glands.

All sensory components carried in the facial nerve (SVA, GVA, and GSA) are mediated by pseudounipolar neurons in the **geniculate ganglion** located at the external genu within the petrous portion of the temporal bone. Central processes of GVA ganglion cells terminate on neurons in the caudal part of the solitary nucleus. GVA information is integrated into medullary reticular circuits for regulation of ANS activity; the visceral input is integrated at an unconscious level.

The SVA component of CN VII is composed of fibers that mediate **taste** from the **anterior two thirds of the tongue** and travel with the **chorda tympani branch** of CN VII. The central processes of SVA ganglion cells terminate on neurons in the **rostral part of the solitary nucleus,** and second order neurons relay the input to the thalamus. Third order neurons in the thalamus relay taste information to the parietal operculum and the adjacent parainsular cortex (area 43). Gustatory (taste) representation is adjacent to the somesthetic area for the tongue.

The GSA component of CN VII mediates sensation from the skin posterior to the ear and from the external auditory meatus. Central processes from perikarya located in the geniculate ganglion mediating pain, temperature, and nondiscriminative touch join the spinal trigeminal tract and synapse on second order neurons in the spinal trigeminal nucleus. Second order neurons project via the dorsal and ventral trigeminothalamic tracts to the VPM of the thalamus, which, in turn, projects to the primary somatosensory cortex (areas 3,1,2) in the parietal lobe.

Clinical Correlations . . . .

Taste (SVA) on the anterior two thirds of the tongue is tested by placing a familiar compound on the tip of the tongue and asking the patient to identify it. The muscles of facial expression (SVE) are tested by asking the patient to smile, wrinkle the forehead, purse the lips, close the eyes, etc. Closure of the eye, the efferent arc of the blink reflex mediated by VII was discussed with CN V (page 96).

By knowing the components carried in the peripheral branches of CN VII, one can correlate the deficit with the site of the lesion. An isolated lesion of the greater petrosal nerve, e.g., would interrupt only GVE and GVA function to the lacrimal gland and to glands of the oral and nasal cavities.

It is clinically important to understand the difference between lower motor neuron lesions involving the facial nucleus or nerve (**Bell's palsy**) in contrast to upper motor neuron lesions. Bell's palsy is an **ipsilateral paralysis** of all of the **muscles of facial expression**. Conversely, a unilateral stroke (cerebrovascular accident) typically interrupts corticobulbar projections in the posterior limb of the internal capsule, resulting in an upper motor neuron lesion that spares the muscles in the upper quadrant of the face contralateral to the lesion. Bell's palsy is a condition of unknown etiology. Edema within the stylomastoid foramen is often postulated as a cause. Many cases show spontaneous recovery within about six weeks.

Color the facial motor nucleus and its SVE fibers green. Color the superior salivatory and lacrimal nuclei and the GVE fibers in the greater petrosal and chorda tympani branches orange. Color the fibers mediating taste and the rostral solitary nucleus brown. Color the sensory component from the ear and the GSA spinal trigeminal nucleus blue. Color the GVA components via the greater petrosal and chorda tympani and the caudal solitary nucleus purple.

Heavy thoughts bring on physical maladies;
when the soul is oppressed, so is the body. – Martin Luther

Cranial Nerve VII, Facial

Components: GSA, GVA, SVA, GVE, SVE

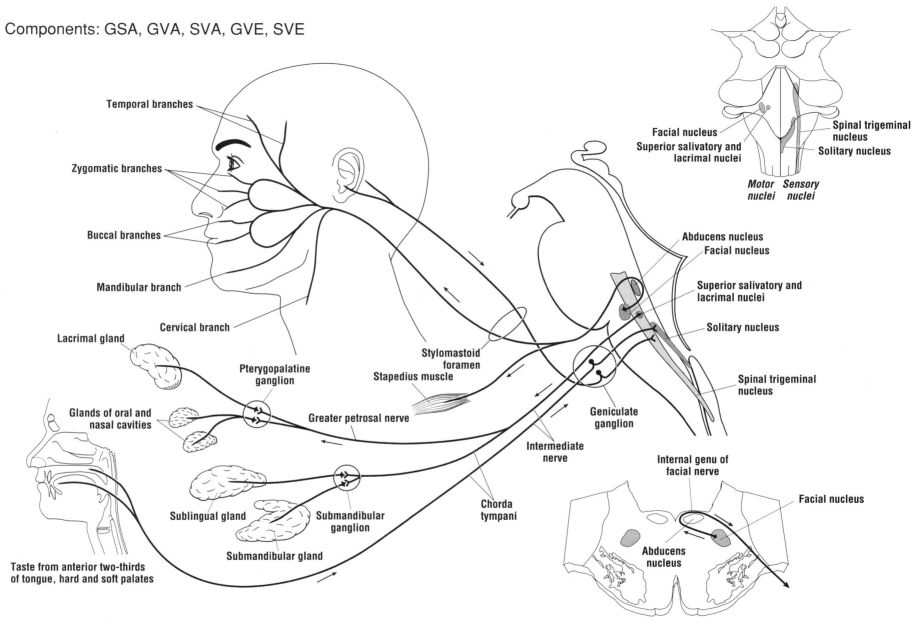

Temporal branches

Zygomatic branches

Buccal branches

Mandibular branch

Cervical branch

Lacrimal gland

Pterygopalatine ganglion

Glands of oral and nasal cavities

Sublingual gland

Submandibular gland

Submandibular ganglion

Taste from anterior two-thirds of tongue, hard and soft palates

Stylomastoid foramen

Stapedius muscle

Greater petrosal nerve

Chorda tympani

Intermediate nerve

Geniculate ganglion

Facial nucleus
Superior salivatory and lacrimal nuclei

Spinal trigeminal nucleus
Solitary nucleus

Motor nuclei   Sensory nuclei

Abducens nucleus
Facial nucleus

Superior salivatory and lacrimal nuclei

Solitary nucleus

Spinal trigeminal nucleus

Internal genu of facial nerve

Facial nucleus

Abducens nucleus

Cranial Nerve VIII, Vestibulocochlear

Definitions

The vestibulocochlear nerve serves two functions and actually is two nerves. The component carried in each of the nerves, the **vestibular (VIIIv)** and the **cochlear (VIIIc)**, is classified as **special somatic afferent (SSA).** VIIIv subserves **posture** and **equilibrium;** VIIIc transmits **sound frequencies.** The sensory receptors for both divisions are hair cells in the semicircular canals or in the cochlea located in the inner ear.

Structural and Functional Features

The vestibular ganglion contains **bipolar neurons** and lies in the petrous portion of the temporal bone. The peripheral processes of these bipolar cells terminate on hair cells in the crista ampullaris of the **semicircular canals** and maculae of the **utricle** and **saccule.** The central processes of the vestibular division enter the brain stem in the **cerebellopontine angle.** Most of the vestibular fibers terminate on second order neurons in four vestibular nuclei located in the rostral medulla and caudal pons. A minor number of first order vestibular fibers terminate in the flocculonodular lobe of the cerebellum.

The saccule and the utricle are referred to as the **static labyrinth** because their function is to detect the position of the head relative to gravity. The sensory receptors (macula; ciliated hair cells) are covered by a gelatinous mass. The otoliths are crystals of calcium carbonate embedded in the gel. The receptors are stimulated when the cilia of the hair cells bend in different directions in response to changes in position or rate of movement.

The semicircular canals are referred to as the **kinetic labyrinth** because they perceive angular movement of the head in space. Endolymph within the canals moves when the head is moved. The hair cells of the canals are located in the ampulla. Movement of endolymph causes the hair cells to bend, thereby eliciting an appropriate electrical stimulus that is transmitted to the vestibular nerve. Secondary sensory neurons in the vestibular nuclei send axons to the cerebellum, brain stem, and spinal cord to influence lower motor neurons controlling postural muscles. The lateral vestibulospinal tract originates in the lateral vestibular (Deiters') nucleus. This pathway facilitates the action of anterior motor horn cells that innervate antigravity muscles.

Reciprocal connections between the medial and inferior vestibular nuclei and the cerebellum provide coordinated movement.

The peripheral processes of bipolar neurons located in the spiral ganglion terminate on hair cells in the organ of Corti. The central processes of the bipolar neurons course through the internal auditory meatus, enter the brain stem in the cerebellopontine angle, and terminate in the **dorsal** and **ventral cochlear nuclei**.

CNS connections involving the superior olivary nucleus (SON), nuclei in the lateral lemniscus, inferior colliculus, and medial geniculate nucleus of the thalamus ultimately terminate in the transverse temporal gyri (Heschl's convolutions). These gyri, located in the floor of the lateral sulcus within the superior temporal gyrus, contain the **primary auditory cortex (areas 41,42).**

The **lateral lemniscus** in the brain stem tegmentum is the pathway between the cochlear nuclei and the inferior colliculus. Fibers from the ventral cochlear nuclei en route to the SON cross in the pontine tegmentum and form the **trapezoid body.**

CNS auditory pathways are characterized by tonotopic localization of pitch at all levels. The bilateralism of auditory projections is such that lesions within the CNS may diminish hearing but do not produce deafness.

Clinical Correlations . . . .

Lesions of the vestibular nerve result in disturbances in **equilibrium, nystagmus, nausea, and vomiting**. The most common cause of damage is an acoustic neuroma (Schwann cell tumor) that usually arises from the vestibular portion of CN VIII and expands into the cerebellopontine angle. The integrity of the vestibular apparatus is tested by irrigation of the external auditory meatus with cold and warm water. Normally, irrigation with cold water produces nystagmus to the opposite side. Irrigation with warm water results in nystagmus to the same side.

Skull fractures and **infections (otitis media)** may damage the auditory apparatus or the cochlear nerve and result in a decrease or loss of hearing in the affected ear. An acoustic neuroma may damage the nerve within the internal auditory meatus. **Conduction deafness** refers to the inability of sound waves to pass through the external ear (obstruction) or middle ear (otosclerosis), whereas **sensorineural deafness** results from lesions of the cochlea, cochlear nerve, or CNS pathways. Wax in the ear may obstruct the flow of sound waves. **Otosclerosis** is defined as a new formation of spongy bone about the stapes and oval window, resulting in progressively increasing deafness without signs of disease in the Eustachian tube or tympanic membrane. Whispering to a patient or performing simple tuning fork tests can be informative relative to whether or not there is a loss of hearing. Auditory acuity must be clinically evaluated to determine the nature of the problem, i.e., whether there is a conduction or neural deficit.

Color the afferent fibers from the vestibular ganglion and the vestibular nuclei yellow. Color the afferent fibers from the spiral ganglion and the cochlear nuclei yellow. In the cross section of the medulla, color the VIIIv and VIIIc branches yellow; note their different routes relative to the inferior cerebellar peduncle.

Only one absolute certainty is possible to man,
namely that at any given moment the feeling which he has exists. – T.H. Huxley

102

Cranial Nerve VIII, Vestibulocochlear

Component: SSA

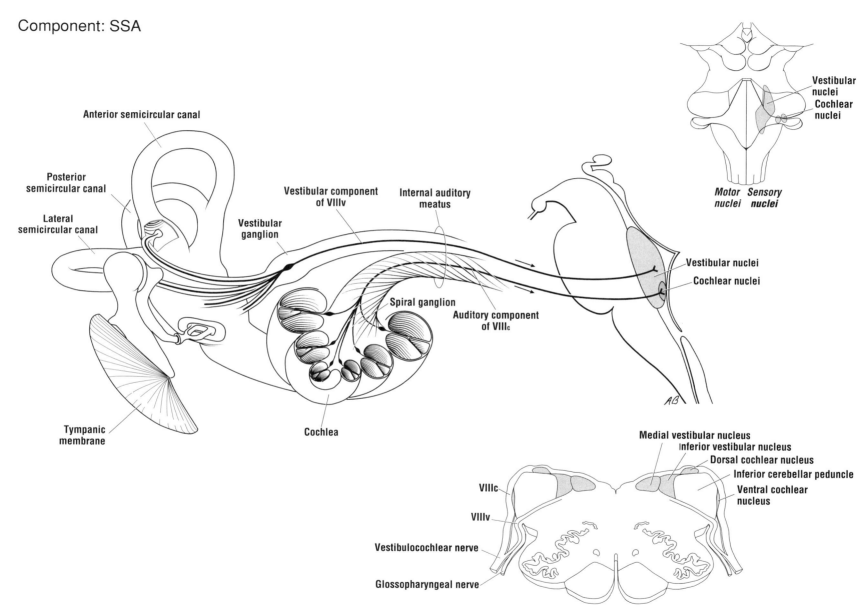

Anterior semicircular canal

Posterior semicircular canal

Lateral semicircular canal

Vestibular ganglion

Vestibular component of VIIIv

Internal auditory meatus

Spiral ganglion

Auditory component of VIIIc

Tympanic membrane

Cochlea

Vestibular nuclei

Cochlear nuclei

Motor nuclei   Sensory nuclei

Vestibular nuclei

Cochlear nuclei

Medial vestibular nucleus
Inferior vestibular nucleus
Dorsal cochlear nucleus
Inferior cerebellar peduncle
Ventral cochlear nucleus

VIIIc

VIIIv

Vestibulocochlear nerve

Glossopharyngeal nerve

Cranial Nerve IX, Glossopharyngeal

Definitions

The glossopharyngeal nerve contains SVE fibers that innervate the striated **stylopharyngeus muscle** that develops from **third branchial arch mesenchyme**. The nerve also has a **parasympathetic component (GVE)** as well as **GVA, SVA,** and **GSA** components. Unipolar neurons in the **superior** and **inferior** (petrosal) **ganglia**, located on the nerve near the jugular foramen, mediate the somatic functions (GSA) and visceral sensory functions (GVA, SVA), respectively.

Structural and Functional Features

SVE neurons in the **nucleus ambiguus** give rise to the motor fibers in CN IX that emerge in the postolivary sulcus (rostral to the rootlets of CN X) to supply the stylopharyngeus muscle. The preganglionic parasympathetic axons arise from the **inferior salivatory nucleus,** emerge in CN IX, pass through the jugular foramen, and ultimately reach the otic ganglion via the lesser petrosal nerve. Postganglionic axons from the otic ganglion innervate the **parotid gland** via the auriculotemporal nerve, a branch of the mandibular division of CN V.

GSA fibers innervate the mucosa of the pharynx providing the **afferent limb** of the **gag reflex**. The **carotid sinus** (GVA) monitors **arterial blood pressure** via baroreceptors (stretch receptors) at the bifurcation of the carotid artery; the carotid body monitors oxygen. Central processes of inferior ganglion cells mediate this input to the **solitary nucleus** (caudal part). This information is integrated into reflex responses involving the reticular formation and hypothalamus, which affect respiration, blood pressure, and cardiac output.

SVA fibers traveling in CN IX mediate **taste** sensation from the **posterior one third** of the **tongue** to the **solitary nucleus** (rostral part). Taste information is used reflexly but also reaches the cortex via the thalamus.

GSA sensation from the external auditory meatus and from the skin posterior to the ear is also transmitted by CN IX. Cells in the superior ganglion mediate pain, temperature, and nondiscriminative touch to the spinal trigeminal nucleus. The information reaches the cortex via the thalamus.

Clinical Correlations . . . .

Lower motor neuron damage to the glossopharyngeal nerve results in the **absence** of a **gag reflex** after stroking the palatine tonsils or tonsilar fossa with a tongue depressor. Taste on the posterior one third of the tongue would also be impaired. **Glossopharyngeal neuralgia** defines sudden sharp attacks of pain in the throat, side of the neck, front of the ear, and back of the lower jaw. The onset may occur with swallowing or protrusion of the tongue; the cause is unknown. (The involvement of CN IX in the lateral medullary syndrome is described on page 122).

Color the nucleus ambiguus (SVE) and fibers to the stylopharyngeus green. Color the inferior salivatory nucleus (GVE) and fibers from it orange. Color purple the solitary nucleus (caudal part) and the GVA fibers that terminate there. Color brown the SVA taste fibers from the tongue and the solitary nucleus (rostral part). Color blue the GSA fibers from the tonsils and pharynx and the spinal trigeminal nucleus.

Cranial Nerve IX, Glossopharyngeal

Components: GSA, GVA, SVA, GVE, SVE

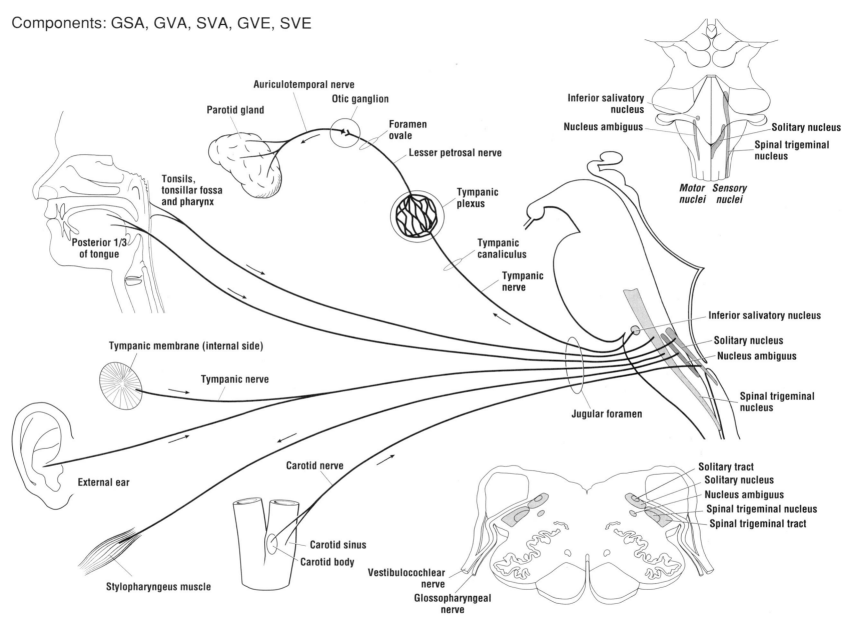

Auriculotemporal nerve

Otic ganglion

Parotid gland

Foramen ovale

Tonsils, tonsillar fossa and pharynx

Lesser petrosal nerve

Tympanic plexus

Posterior 1/3 of tongue

Tympanic canaliculus

Tympanic nerve

Tympanic membrane (internal side)

Tympanic nerve

External ear

Carotid nerve

Stylopharyngeus muscle

Carotid sinus

Carotid body

Vestibulocochlear nerve

Glossopharyngeal nerve

Inferior salivatory nucleus

Nucleus ambiguus

Solitary nucleus

Spinal trigeminal nucleus

Motor nuclei   Sensory nuclei

Inferior salivatory nucleus

Solitary nucleus

Nucleus ambiguus

Spinal trigeminal nucleus

Jugular foramen

Solitary tract

Solitary nucleus

Nucleus ambiguus

Spinal trigeminal nucleus

Spinal trigeminal tract

Cranial Nerve X, Vagus

Definitions

The vagus nerve (1) supplies striated muscles that develop from mesenchyme in the fourth and sixth branchial arches (SVE), (2) has extensive secretomotor preganglionic parasympathetic fibers (GVE), (3) provides important GVA feedback from visceral sensory structures, and (4) contains minimal GSA and SVA components. Superior (jugular) and inferior (nodose) ganglia mediate the somatic (GSA) and visceral sensory functions (GVA and SVA) respectively. These five components subserve functions in the head, neck, and body cavities. In the neck, the vagus descends between the internal jugular vein and the internal carotid artery within the carotid sheath.

Structural and Functional Features

The SVE fibers arise from the **nucleus ambiguus** and the GVE fibers from the dorsal motor nucleus of the vagus. The fibers emerge along the **postolivary sulcus** in the medulla as a series of rootlets that converge, travel briefly with CN XI, and exit the skull through the **jugular foramen**.

The **SVE** component supplies the **pharyngeal constrictor muscles** and the **intrinsic muscles** of the **larynx**. The pharyngeal branches, via the pharyngeal plexus, supply superior, middle, and inferior constrictors of the pharynx and all muscles of the soft palate except the stylopharyngeus (IX) and tensor veli palati (V3)—levator palati, salpingopharyngeus, palatopharyngeus, and one muscle of the tongue, the palatoglossus. The cricothyroid muscle is supplied by the superior laryngeal nerve.

The **right** and **left recurrent laryngeal nerves** take different paths; the former arises from the right vagus nerve anterior to the subclavian artery, hooks under the artery, and ascends in a groove between the trachea and the esophagus; the latter arises from the left vagus on the aortic arch, hooks under the arch, and ascends to the left side to reach the groove. The right and left recurrent laryngeal nerves supply the **intrinsic muscles** of the **larynx** (except the cricothyroid). An aortic aneurysm may press on the left recurrent laryngeal nerve.

Corticobulbar fibers descend from premotor and motor cortical areas to provide voluntary control over the **nucleus ambiguus.** The nucleus ambiguus also receives sensory signals used in reflex responses, e.g., coughing and vomiting.

GVE preganglionic parasympathetic cells located in the **dorsal motor nucleus** of the **vagus** supply the secretomotor fibers in the vagus. The dorsal motor nucleus of the vagus receives input from the nearby solitary nucleus, the olfactory system, the hypothalamus, and the reticular formation. **Preganglionic fibers** join plexuses around blood vessels to the lungs and heart and synapse on neurons located within the walls of the organs. In the gut, postganglionic parasympathetic fibers emerge from myenteric (Auerbach) and submucosal (Meissner) plexuses.

The **GVA** component of the vagus nerve is **anatomically massive** and is important for **homeostasis.** Visceral afferent neurons in the inferior ganglion relay unconscious sensory information from structures in the body cavities and from the **carotid body** (**monitors oxygen** tension). The central processes terminate in the caudal part of the **solitary nucleus,** which projects to reticular neurons in the medulla that influence reflex visceral function.

The SVA pathway mediating taste from the epiglottis and root of the tongue (a minor component) follows the one described above with the exception that the central processes terminate in the rostral rather than the caudal part of the solitary nucleus. Taste information is used reflexly but also reaches the cortex via the thalamus.

The **GSA** component of the vagus (also minor) is mediated via cells in the superior ganglion whose central processes terminate in the spinal trigeminal nucleus. The modalities mediated are pain, temperature, and nondiscriminative touch from the tympanic membrane, external auditory meatus, and the skin posterior to the ear.

Clinical Correlations

Unilateral lesions of the SVE component of the vagus nerve cause **hoarseness and difficulty in swallowing.** The function is tested by having the patient swallow and by observing the uvula while the patient says "aaahhh." On examination, the **soft palate droops** and the **uvula deviates away from the lesioned side**.

Hypersecretion of acidic gastric fluids can be treated by severing the right and left gastric nerves, if conservative measures are ineffective. The GVA input can be stimulated to increase parasympathetic tone to the heart. **Massaging the neck** at the **carotid bifurcation stimulates** the **carotid body** (CN IX and X) and **sinus** (CN IX), thus **reducing heart rate**.

Color the nucleus ambiguus (SVE) and axons from it green. Color the dorsal motor nucleus of X (GVE) and axons from it orange. Color purple the solitary nucleus (caudal part) and the GVA fibers that terminate there. Color brown the SVA fibers and solitary nucleus (rostral part). Color the GSA fibers and spinal trigeminal nucleus blue.

Cranial Nerve X, Vagus

Components: GSA, GVA, SVA, GVE, SVE

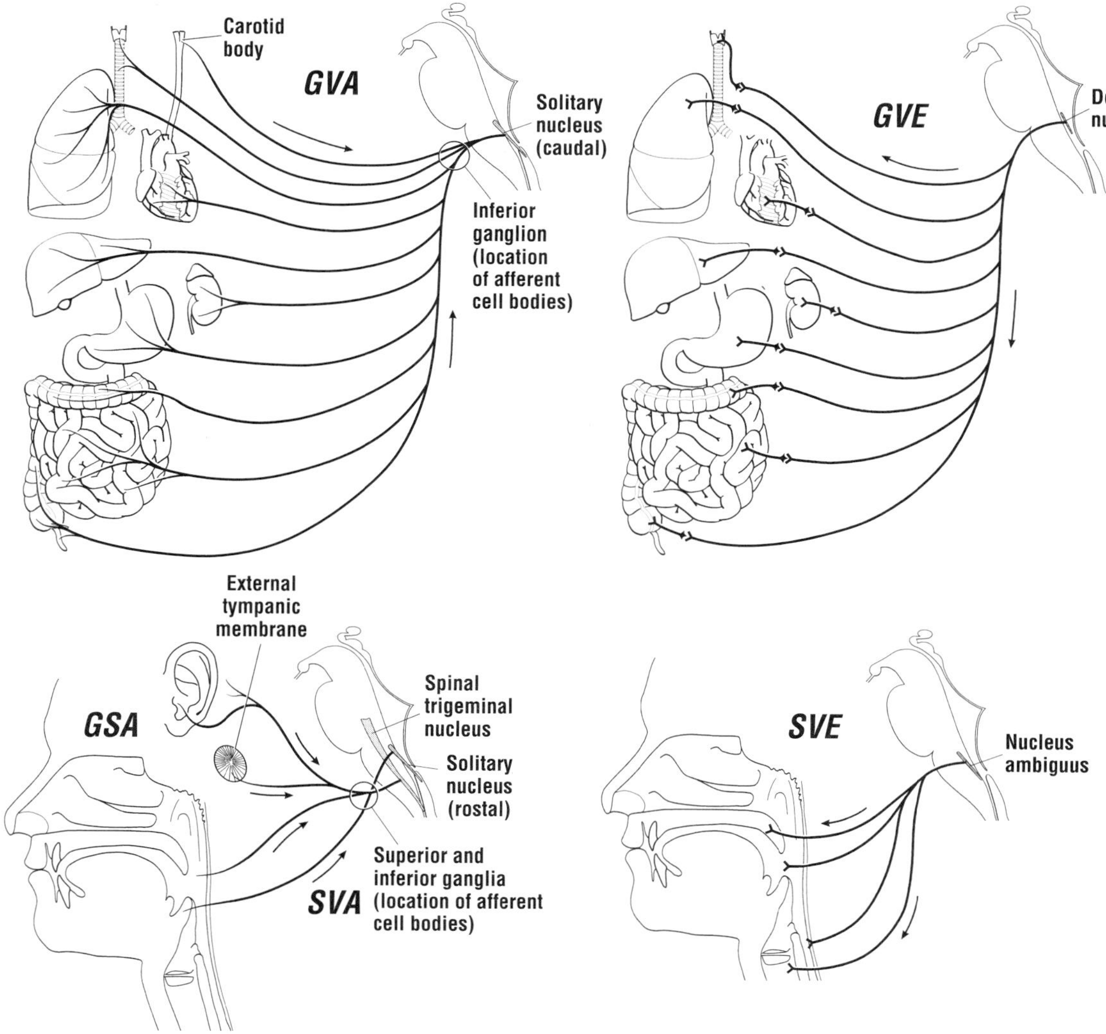

Carotid body

GVA

Solitary nucleus (caudal)

Inferior ganglion (location of afferent cell bodies)

GVE

Dorsal motor nucleus of X

Nucleus ambiguus

Dorsal motor nucleus of X

Motor nuclei   *Sensory nuclei*

Solitary nucleus

Spinal trigeminal nucleus

External tympanic membrane

GSA

Spinal trigeminal nucleus

Solitary nucleus (rostal)

Superior and inferior ganglia (location of afferent cell bodies)

SVA

SVE

Nucleus ambiguus

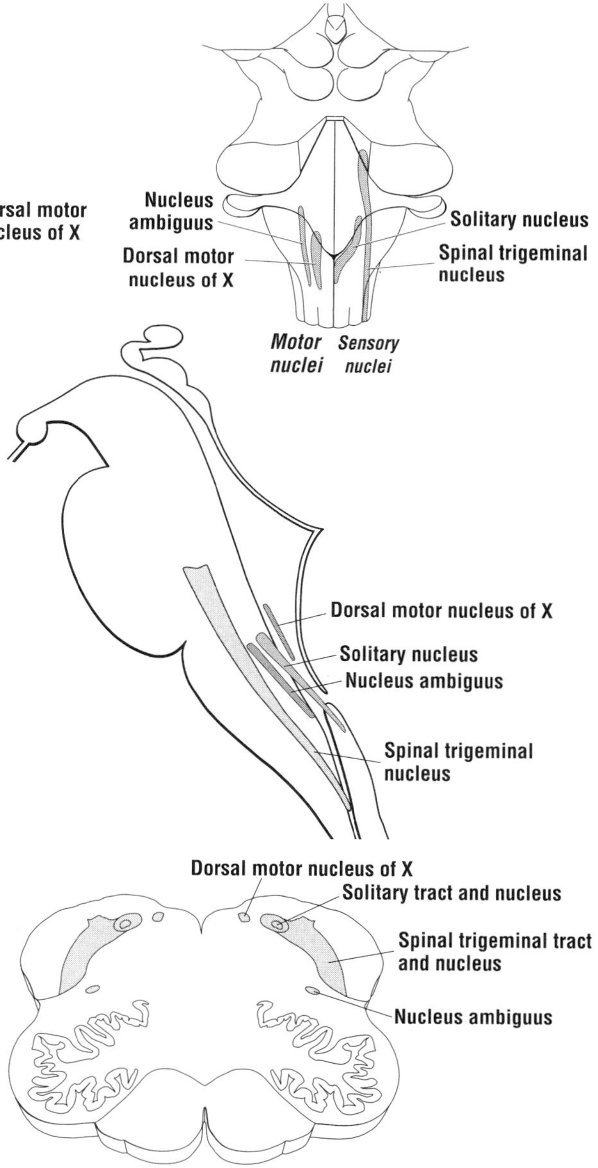

Dorsal motor nucleus of X

Solitary nucleus

Nucleus ambiguus

Spinal trigeminal nucleus

Dorsal motor nucleus of X

Solitary tract and nucleus

Spinal trigeminal tract and nucleus

Nucleus ambiguus

Modified from Demarest

Cranial Nerve XI, Accessory

Definitions
The SVE accessory nerve originates from the accessory nucleus, which consists of anterior motor horn cells located in cervical spinal cord segments C1-C5. Accessory axons innervate the ipsilateral sternocleidomastoid and trapezius muscles of branchiomeric origin.

Structural and Functional Features
The accessory nucleus is laterally located in the cervical spinal cord. Rootlets from these neurons emerge between the dorsal and ventral roots in line with other SVE components. The rootlets ascend to the cranium dorsal to the denticulate ligament. The nerve enters through the **foramen magnum** and exits through the **jugular foramen**. Within the cranium, the accessory nerve runs with the vagus nerve but separates from it after its emergence from the jugular foramen. Therefore, the cranial axons that arise from the nucleus ambiguus are often considered to be part of the vagus nerve.

Clinical Correlations . . . .

Damage to the accessory nucleus or nerve results in a lower motor neuron lesion in which there is a downward and lateral rotation of the scapula and drooping of the shoulder due to the denervated trapezius. The strength of the trapezius is tested by asking the patient to shrug the shoulder against the resistance of the examiner's hand placed on the shoulder.

Contraction of the sternocleidomastoid rotates the head to the opposite side and tilts the chin upward. It is tested by placing resistance with the hand on the mandible and asking the patient to turn the head to the side opposite the lesion. Always test bilaterally for comparison.

Supranuclear lesions (lesions of upper motor neurons or their axons) can result in spastic paresis of the contralateral sternocleidomastoid and trapezius muscles.

Space-occupying lesions (glomus tumors, Schwannomas, meningiomas, and other tumors), vascular occlusions, syringomyelia, and torticollis may involve the accessory nerve or nucleus. Intracranial lesions of CN XI usually involve CN IX, X, and XII as well because these four nerves are all in the medulla. **Radical neck surgery** of laryngeal carcinomas requires **vigilant attention** to the **accessory nerve** because of its proximity to superficial cervical lymph nodes.

Color the accessory nucleus, the rootlets, and the nerve green. Note the ascent of the nerve through the foramen magnum and its exit from the cranium via the jugular foramen.

Hypocrite—the man who murdered both his parents
and then pleaded for mercy on the grounds that he was an orphan. – Abraham Lincoln

108

Cranial Nerve XI, Accessory

Component: SVE

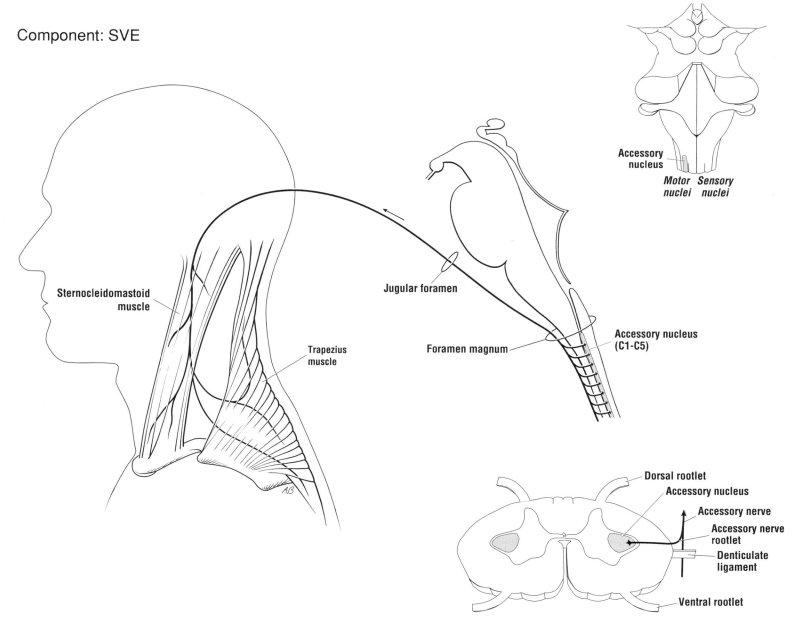

Accessory nucleus

Motor   Sensory
nuclei   nuclei

Jugular foramen

Sternocleidomastoid
muscle

Trapezius
muscle

Foramen magnum

Accessory nucleus
(C1-C5)

Dorsal rootlet

Accessory nucleus

Accessory nerve

Accessory nerve
rootlet

Denticulate
ligament

Ventral rootlet

Cranial Nerve XII, Hypoglossal

Definitions

The hypoglossal nerve arises from a long GSE cell column near the midline in the tegmentum of the medulla. The hypoglossal nerve supplies all of the intrinsic and the extrinsic muscles of the tongue (except the palatoglossus, which is supplied by the vagus nerve).

Structural and Functional Features

Axons from the hypoglossal nucleus emerge from the medulla as a series of rootlets between the pyramid and the olive (preolivary sulcus). The rootlets form the hypoglossal nerve, which exits the skull through the hypoglossal canal. The corticobulbar projections to the nucleus are said to be exclusively from the contralateral hemisphere. (Most cranial nerves receive a minor projection from the ipsilateral hemisphere as well.)

Clinical Correlations . . . .

To test the hypoglossal nerve, the patient is asked to protrude the tongue. The paired genioglossus muscles protrude the tongue. In a **lower motor neuron lesion** of the hypoglossal nerve, the unopposed action of the intact genioglossus pushes the **tongue toward** the **side** of the **lesion**. Additionally there is **flaccid paralysis, fasciculation**, and **atrophy** of the **tongue** on the **affected side**.

An **upper motor neuron lesion** of the corticobulbar projection to the hypoglossal nucleus results in **deviation** of the **tongue** to the **side opposite** the **lesion.** For example, a left capsular insult results in right hemiplegia and the tongue deviates to the right.

The **medial medullary syndrome** (due to vascular lesions of the anterior spinal artery or of a medullary branch of the vertebral artery) produces a combined upper and lower motor neuron deficit due to involvement of the medullary pyramid and the hypoglossal nerve. This syndrome is termed "alternating hemiplegia" and is characterized by **ipsilateral paralysis** of the **tongue** (lower motor neuron) and **contralateral hemiplegia** (upper motor neuron). An intramedullary lesion of the hypoglossal nucleus may result in unilateral involvement of the tongue; however, bilateral involvement is more probable due to the proximity of the nuclei to the midline.

Color the hypoglossal nucleus and nerve red. Note the course of the axons between the pyramid and inferior olivary nucleus as well as the longitudinal extent of the nucleus.

That best portion of a good man's life, his little,
nameless unremembered acts of kindness and of love. – William Wordsworth

110

Cranial Nerve XII, Hypoglossal

Component: GSE

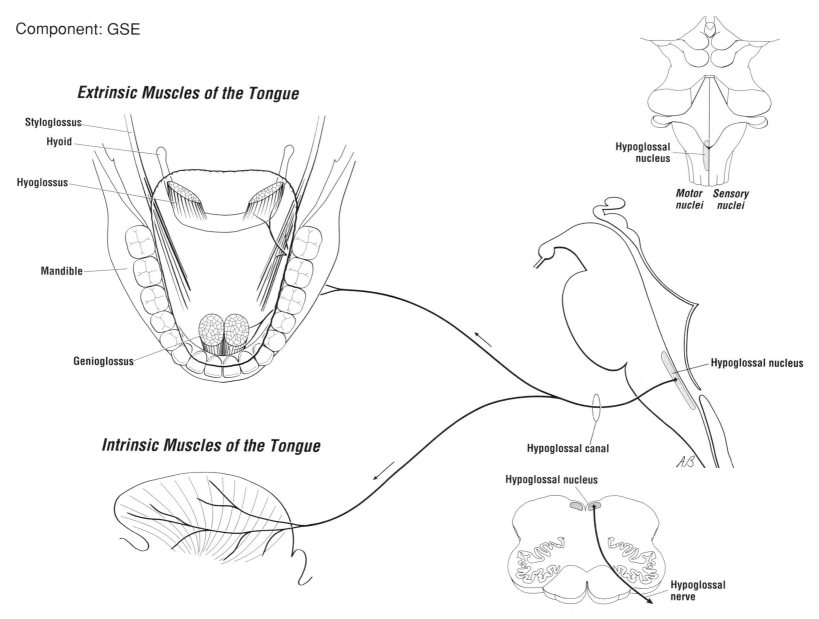

Extrinsic Muscles of the Tongue

Styloglossus

Hyoid

Hyoglossus

Mandible

Genioglossus

Hypoglossal nucleus

Motor nuclei   Sensory nuclei

Hypoglossal nucleus

Hypoglossal canal

Intrinsic Muscles of the Tongue

Hypoglossal nucleus

Hypoglossal nerve

Intramedullary Course of the Cranial Nerves

Definitions
Some cranial nerves exit from the ventral surface of the brain stem, some from the ventrolateral surface, and one—the trochlear—is unique in that it exits dorsally.

Structural and Functional Features
The infratentorial cranial nerves (CN III–XII) are depicted in a brain stem "shell," showing their nuclei of origin, intramedullary course, and exit or, in the case of sensory fibers, their entrance into the CNS. To fully appreciate the compactness of brain stem structures longitudinally, one needs to superimpose the schematic on page 63 of other brain stem nuclei and to visualize sensory pathways ascending and motor tracts descending through this part of the neuraxis. The topography of the spinal cord is simple in comparison. This view of the intramedullary course of cranial nerves is critical to understanding the plethora of signs and symptoms of the classical vascular syndromes depicted on page 123.

Corticobulbar (supranuclear) projections to the brain stem arise from the **face area** of the cerebral cortex, traverse the region of the genu in the internal capsule, and descend in the base of the brain stem. At their level of destination, they pass through the tegmentum and **terminate** either on **cranial nerve motor nuclei**, on **reticular neurons**, or on **sensory nuclei**. The motor nucleus of the trigeminal, the upper part of the facial motor nucleus, and the hypoglossal nucleus receive direct fibers. All cranial nerve nuclei, including V, VII, and XII, receive indirect projections via reticular neurons.

Sensory nuclei that receive **corticobulbar projections** include the **gracile** and **cuneate, sensory trigeminal nuclei**, and the **solitary nucleus**. The influence of cortical input on sensory impulses at the second neuronal level may be either excitatory or inhibitory. This is a mechanism (discussed relative to the dorsal horn of the spinal cord) whereby the ongoing activity of the cerebral cortex influences incoming stimuli.

Clinical Correlations

The causes of **brain stem lesions** include, among others, **vascular occlusion** or **hemorrhage, tumors, trauma**, and **herniations** through the tentorial incisure or through the foramen magnum, or both. Bilateral lesions involving corticobulbar fibers result in **pseudobulbar palsy**. Weakness of the muscles involved in **swallowing, chewing, breathing**, and **speaking** may occur with relatively little involvement of the limbs. Labile emotions, e.g., inappropriate laughing and crying, are a part of this syndrome.

Brain stem mechanisms through the **reticular formation** are important in **maintaining alertness**; therefore, **lesions** of the tegmentum, especially in the pons and midbrain, may **cause coma**. Conversely, bilateral lesions of the ventral pons may disrupt the corticobulbar and corticospinal tracts. In this case, the patient is quadriplegic, unable to speak and with facial paralysis. This resembles coma because of the inability to communicate either verbally or through gestures other than movement of the eyelids or eyes. The patient **perceives stimuli** ascending through the tegmentum; therefore, **consciousness** is **unimpaired**, but the patient is completely **immobile**. This is referred to as a **locked-in syndrome**.

Color blue the GSA cell column: mesencephalic, chief sensory, and spinal trigeminal nuclei. (The solitary nucleus for SVA and GVA input is not shown.) Color red the GSE cell column: III, IV, VI, and XII. Color green the SVE cell column: V and VII; IX and X (nucleus ambiguus), and XI (spinal) accessory. Color orange the GVE nuclei: Edinger-Westphal, salivatory (one structure represents superior, lacrimal, and inferior nuclei), and dorsal motor nucleus of X.

In each case use the same color as the nuclei to trace the intramedullary course of the fibers beginning at the periphery for incoming sensory and at the nucleus of origin for outgoing motor fibers.

Intramedullary Course of the Cranial Nerves

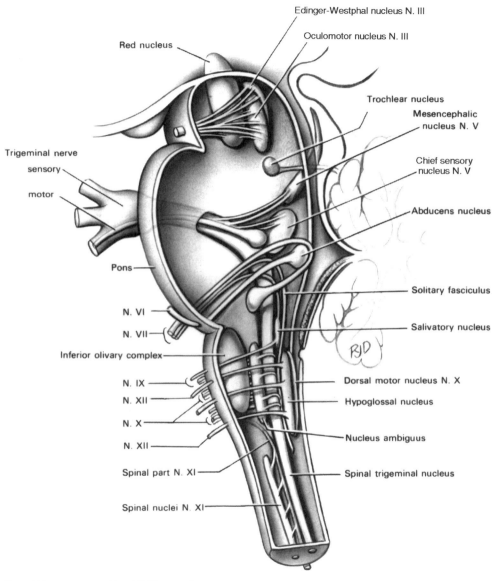

(Reprinted with permission from Carpenter MB. Core Text of Neuroanatomy. 4th ed. Williams & Wilkins, 1991:139.)

Basal View of the Diencephalon, Brain Stem, and Cerebellum

Definitions

In the posterior cranial fossa, the **clivus** is a downward **sloping surface** from the dorsum sellae to the foramen magnum, formed by parts of the sphenoid and occipital bones, on which the brain stem and cerebellum rest.

The large size of the cerebellum in the human brain is attributed to the need for synergy of muscles in maintaining the upright posture and in performing activities that require exquisite hand movements. The cerebellar cortex is composed of many narrow, transversely oriented laminae known as folia, which are separated by fissures. Two of these, the **primary fissure** (not apparent in this view) and the **posterolateral fissure** (8), are significant because they divide the cerebellum transversely into **anterior, posterior**, and **flocculonodular lobes**. The latter lobe lies at the rostral edge of the inferior surface and essentially makes up the **vestibulocerebellum**. The anterior lobe makes up the **spinocerebellum,** and the posterior lobe makes up the **pontocerebellum (neocerebellum)**.

Structural and Functional Features

The cerebellum and brain stem fill the posterior cranial fossa and are covered by the tentorium cerebelli, which attaches along the superior margin of the petrous temporal bone and to the anterior and posterior clinoid processes. The **optic chiasm** (27) lies above the diaphragma sellae. The **infundibulum** (2) connects the hypophysis to the tuber cinereum and hypothalamus through an opening in the diaphragma sellae. The relation of the diencephalon to the hypophysial fossa and the basal surface of the brain stem to the clivus of the occipital bone can be seen on pages 117 and 119. The **optic tract** (26) is located posterior to the optic chiasm and circles around the midbrain to reach the lateral geniculate nucleus. The **anterior perforated substance** (1) is lateral to the optic chiasm.

Mamillary bodies (3) are nuclei in the posterior region of the hypothalamus. The **oculomotor nerves** (25) exit ventrally in the interpeduncular fossa, at the level of the superior colliculus of the midbrain. The oculomotor is therefore the most rostrally located cranial nerve of the brain stem because the olfactory nerve is an outgrowth from the telencephalon, and the **optic nerve** (28) originates from the diencephalon. The trochlear nerve is not visible here. It exits posteriorly, caudal to the inferior colliculus. The **trigeminal nerve** (24) exits at the junction of the pons and the middle cerebellar peduncle (MCP). The **abducens nerves** (23) emerge lateral to the **pyramids** (5) at the junction of the medulla and pons and begin their long route to enter the superior orbital fissure.

Laterally, at the junction of the medulla and **pons** (4), one sees the **facial** (21) and **vestibulo-cochlear nerves** (20), where the pons, medulla, and cerebellum meet to form the cerebellopontine angle. Rootlets of the **vagus** (19) and **glossopharyngeal** (18) nerves exit lateral to the **inferior olivary nucleus** (17). Rootlets of the **hypoglossal nerve** (22) exit lateral to the pyramid.

The cerebellum consists of a midline **vermis** (11) and the **hemispheres** (15), which are separated by the **posterior notch** (12). The **cerebellar flocculi** (7) lie laterally in the cerebellopontine angle. The **tonsils** (10) lie superior to the foramen magnum. All cranial nerve nuclei are located in the **tegmentum** (16) of the brain stem, which is labeled here in the cross section of the medulla. Throughout the brain stem, the **sulcus limitans** (14) is a landmark for a medial–lateral delineation of cranial nerve motor versus sensory nuclei, respectively. The **fourth ventricle** (13) lies dorsal to the brain stem and ventral to the cerebellum. Tufts of **choroid plexuses** (6) poke through the foramina of Luschka through which CSF flows from the fourth ventricle into the pontine cistern. Vermis means "worm" and describes the mid-portion of the cerebellum. The nodule of the **vermis** (9) is labeled separately and, together with the flocculi, forms the **flocculonodular lobe,** which is separated from the **posterior (middle) lobe** by the **posterolateral fissure** (8).

Clinical Correlations . . . .

Lesions of the cerebellum cause **disturbances of motor function** without voluntary paralysis. The flocculonodular lobe (vestibulocerebellum) has extensive reciprocal connections with the vestibular nuclei and functions to maintain equilibrium and posture. Pathology that affects the **vermis** and **flocculonodular lobe,** e.g., medulloblastoma in children or chronic alcoholism in adults, produces an unsteady, staggering, **ataxic gait.** Cerebellar ataxia can be differentiated from dorsal column lesions (sensory ataxia) by the fact that **visual clues improve sensory**, but **not cerebellar ataxia**. Lesions of the anterior lobe (**spinocerebellum**) affect **trunk** and **proximal limb** muscles. The cerebellar hemispheres (**pontocerebellum**) control the ipsilateral limbs; therefore, cerebellar lesions produce ipsilateral disturbances. The **pontocerebellar syndrome** is characterized by **dysmetria, past pointing, adiadochokinesia** (difficulty with rapidly alternating movements), **asynergy**, and **intention tremor** (occurs during movement). **Lesions** of the **intracerebellar nuclei** and of the **superior cerebellar peduncle** produce more **severe pathology** than do cerebellar cortical lesions. In fact, **cortical lesions** improve markedly with time, especially in children.

The anatomy and **position** of the **cerebellar tonsils is** clinically significant. A shift of a supratentorial mass into the posterior fossa may cause herniation of the cerebellar tonsils and the medulla through the foramen magnum. Death could be imminent due to pressure on vital centers in the reticular formation controlling respiration and heart rate, as has already been mentioned.

 Color the cranial nerves yellow, the flocculi and nodule green, and the tuft of choroid plexus and tonsils orange.

Basal View of the Diencephalon, Brain Stem, and Cerebellum

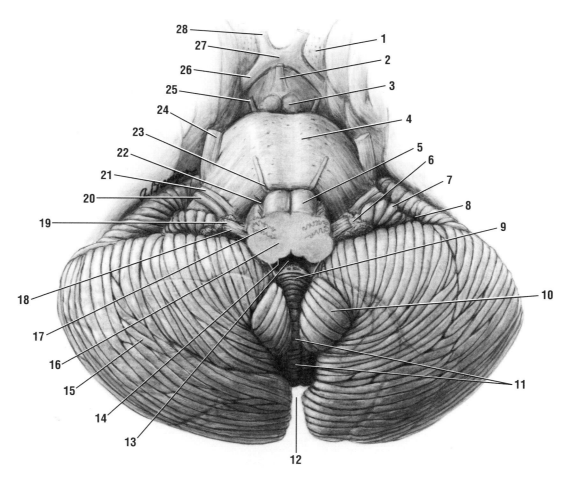

1. Anterior perforated substance
2. Tuber cinereum and infundibulum
3. Mamillary body
4. Pons (base of)
5. Pyramid of medulla
6. Tuft of choroid plexus
7. Flocculus
8. Posterolateral fissure
9. Nodule of vermis
10. Tonsil
11. Vermis
12. Posterior cerebellar notch
13. Fourth ventricle
14. Sulcus limitans
15. Cerebellar hemisphere
16. Tegmentum of medulla
17. Inferior olivary nucleus
18. Vagus nerve
19. Glossopharyngeal nerve
20. Vestibulocochlear nerve
21. Facial nerve
22. Hypoglossal nerve
23. Abducens nerve
24. Trigeminal nerve
25. Oculomotor nerve
26. Optic tract
27. Optic chiasm
28. Optic nerve

Base of the Skull, Calvaria Removed, Internal Aspect

Definitions

The **crista galli** is the vertical part of the ethmoid bone. On either side of the crista galli lies the cribriform plate that houses the olfactory bulbs. The **foramen cecum** (2) occasionally transmits an emissary vein from the nose to the superior sagittal sinus. The **foramina rotundum, ovale,** and **spinosum** transmit structures in the middle cranial fossa (see below). The **foramen lacerum** is an irregular aperture in the middle cranial fossa; however, no structures pass through it.

Structural and Functional Features

The shape of the internal surface of the skull conforms to that of the brain. The three cranial fossae are separated by prominent ridges. The **anterior cranial fossa** (28) houses the frontal lobe and the **middle cranial fossa** (24) contains the temporal lobe. The middle cranial fossa is elevated medially where the **hypophysial fossa** (8) is located, and the superior margin of the petrous temporal bone forms its posteromedial border. The medulla, pons, and cerebellum fill the **posterior cranial fossa** (17), which is covered by the tentorium cerebelli. The occipital lobes rest on the tentorium cerebelli. The **lesser** wing of the **sphenoid bone** (26) ends in the anterior clinoid process, which serves as attachment for the free border of the tentorium cerebelli. This dural partition attaches along the **superior margin** of the **petrous temporal bone** (11) and helps to define two supratentorial spaces above and a single infratentorial space below. Bone density varies in the skull and is an important factor in head trauma. In the anterior cranial fossa, the **orbital plate** (5) of the frontal bone fractures easily where there are thin regions. The delicate olfactory nerves pass through orifices in the **cribriform plate** (4). The falx cerebri, housed within the longitudinal fissure, attaches to the tentorium cerebelli posteriorly and to the **frontal crest** (1) and **crista galli** (3) anteriorly. The falx cerebri separates the anterior cerebral arteries, which nourish medially located structures including the paracentral lobule, the somatomotor area of the leg. The **planum (jugum) sphenoidale** (27) is a flat area of the sphenoid bone just anterior to the **chiasmatic sulcus** (6).

There are a number of foramina in the middle cranial fossa. The **optic canal** (7) transmits the optic nerve and the ophthalmic artery. The superior orbital fissure transmits all of the following to the the orbit: oculomotor, trochlear, ophthalmic, and abducens nerves and superior ophthalmic vein. The fissure is not visible in this view but is inferior to the lesser wing of the sphenoid bone. The maxillary nerve traverses the **foramen rotundum** (25), whereas the **foramen ovale** (23) transmits the mandibular nerve, the lesser petrosal nerve (occasionally), and the accessory meningeal artery. The **foramen spinosum** (22) transmits the meningeal branch of the mandibular nerve and the middle meningeal artery and vein. An irregular aperture, the **foramen lacerum** (21) marks the entry of the internal carotid artery into the cavernous sinus. Lateral to the foramen lacerum is a shallow depression for the trigeminal ganglion.

In the posterior fossa, the pons and medulla rest on the thick, **sloping clivus** (10), which is composed of the **dorsum sellae** (9) and the basilar part of the occipital bone. This deep fossa is pierced by several foramina. It also contains grooves for the **transverse** (16) and **sigmoid** (12) venous sinuses. The confluence of sinuses is located at the **internal occipital protuberance** (15). The attachment of the falx cerebelli and the course of the occipital sinus are in line with the **internal occipital crest** (14). The largest opening is the **foramen magnum** (13), which permits continuity of the medulla oblongata and spinal cord along with their surrounding meninges. Also, the vertebral arteries and the (spinal) accessory nerves ascend through this foramen. The inferior petrosal and sigmoid sinuses pass through the **jugular foramen** (19) as do the glossopharyngeal, vagus, and (descending spinal) accessory nerves. Details of the **hypoglossal canal** (18) and the **internal acoustic meatus** (20) are on page 118.

Clinical Correlations . . . .

Epidural hematomas or brain tumors may crowd the supratentorial compartment and result in herniation of tissue through the tentorial notch (page 16). Tumors of neuronal origin occur infrequently because mature neurons do not undergo mitosis. Tumors within the cranium arise predominantly from the glia or meninges. Focal meningiomas of the falx encroaching on the medial surface of the hemisphere cause leg symptoms unilaterally or bilaterally, depending on the size and rate of growth. In the anterior cranial fossa, **meningiomas** tend to occur in the area of the **planum sphenoidale**. Pituitary tumors expand upwardly, press on the optic chiasm, and result in bitemporal hemianopsia. The position of the temporal lobe in the middle fossa renders it vulnerable to accelerating injuries of the head from behind. A rapid force thrusts the temporal pole into the greater wing of the sphenoid bone. Trauma to **mesiotemporal structures**, especially if the injury is bilateral, may result in **memory impairment**. Trigeminal tic douloureux is often attributed to the fact that only the meninges separates the trigeminal ganglion from bone, rendering it vulnerable to intermittent vascular pressure.

Base of the Skull, Calvaria Removed, Internal Aspect

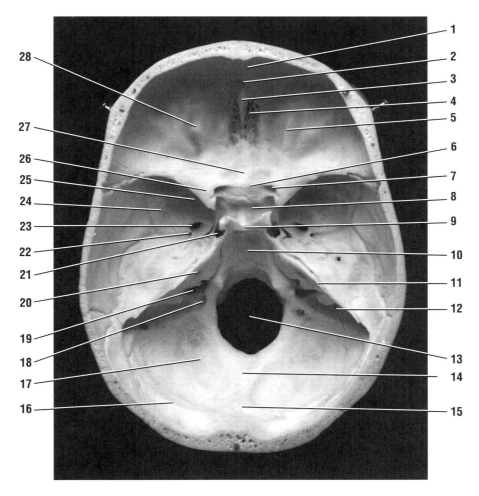

1. Frontal crest
2. Foramen cecum
3. Crista galli
4. Cribriform plate of ethmoid bone
5. Ridged orbital plate
6. Chiasmatic sulcus
7. Optic canal
8. Hypophysial fossa (sella turcica)

9. Dorsum sellae
10. Clivus
11. Superior margin of the petrous temporal bone
12. Groove for sigmoid sinus
13. Foramen magnum
14. Internal occipital crest
15. Internal occipital protuberance

16. Groove for transverse sinus
17. Posterior cranial fossa
18. Hypoglossal canal
19. Jugular foramen
20. Internal acoustic meatus
21. Foramen lacerum
22. Foramen spinosum
23. Foramen ovale

24. Middle cranial fossa
25. Foramen rotundum
26. Lesser wing of sphenoid
27. Planum sphenoidale
28. Anterior cranial fossa

Median Section Through the Skull, Internal Aspect of the Left Basal Portion

Definitions

The **occipital condyles** (5) are the weight-bearing surfaces of the skull that rest on the superior articular facets of the axis.

Structural and Functional Features

This view shows the increase in depth of the cranial fossae from shallow in the **anterior** (1), to intermediate in the **middle** (10), to deep in the **posterior** (9). Branches of the **middle meningeal artery** create numerous **grooves** (2) within the middle cranial fossa. These vessels lie between the dura mater and bone in a potential epidural space. The **hypophysial fossa** (4) and **dorsum sellae** (3) are features of the body of the sphenoid bone in the middle cranial fossa.

In the posterior fossa, the hypoglossal nerve exits the skull via the **hypoglossal canal** (6). The **internal acoustic meatus** (8) tunnels into the petrous part of the temporal bone. Fascicles of the facial and vestibulocochlear nerves travel about 1 cm in this tunnel and pierce apertures in a thin bony plate lateral to the internal ear. The groove for the **sigmoid sinus** (7) is readily apparent. At the jugular foramen, the sigmoid sinus becomes continuous with the internal jugular vein.

Clinical Correlations

Trauma to the dorsolateral surface of the head may tear the meningeal arteries and result in spurting arterial bleeding with rapid accumulation of blood between the dura and skull (epidural hematoma). If diagnosed, the hematoma can easily be evacuated; if untreated, the serious sequelae to tentorial herniation may occur.

Median Section Through the Skull, Internal Aspect of the Left Basal Portion

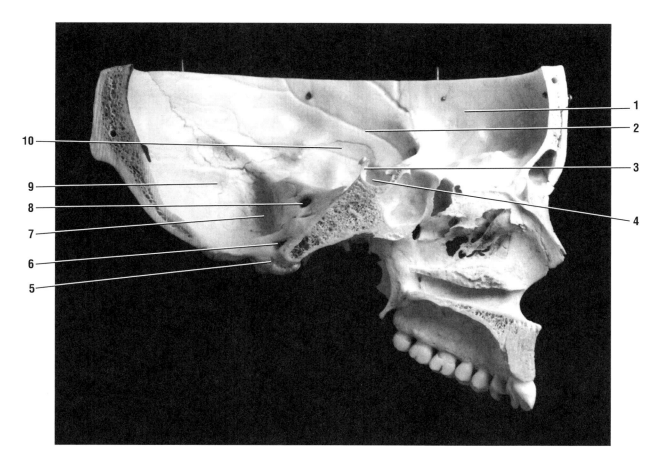

1. Anterior cranial fossa
2. Groove for middle meningeal artery
3. Dorsum sellae
4. Hypophysial fossa (sella turcica)
5. Occipital condyle
6. Hypoglossal canal
7. Groove for sigmoid sinus
8. Internal acoustic meatus
9. Posterior cranial fossa
10. Middle cranial fossa

Dorsal and Ventral Spinocerebellar and Cuneocerebellar Tracts: Proprioceptive Input

Definitions

The **cerebellum** (little brain) is essentially a **motor** part of the brain that functions indirectly in providing synergy of movements and the maintenance of posture. The cerebellum contains a cortex of gray matter and a core of white matter (medullary center) in which four pairs of **intracerebellar nuclei** (intrinsic, central, deep) are embedded. The histology of the cortex is uniform throughout. The intracerebellar nuclei are similar histologically but vary in respect to their topographical relation to the cortex. From medial to lateral, the nuclei are: **fastigial, globose, emboliform**, and **dentate**. The cortex of the midline vermis projects to the fastigial nucleus, the paravermal zone of the hemisphere projects to the globose and emboliform nuclei, and the remainder of the hemisphere projects to the dentate nucleus. Therefore, the cerebellum has a **longitudinal histological organization** and a **transverse division** into **lobes** (page 114). Three pairs of **inferior** (ICP), **middle** (MCP), and **superior** (SCP) **cerebellar peduncles** composed of fibers connect the cerebellum with the brain stem.

Structural and Functional Features

The cerebellar cortex consists of **five types** of **neurons** organized into **three cortical layers.** From the surface, these are the molecular layer, the Purkinje cell layer, and the granule cell layer. The granule cell uses the **excitatory** transmitter glutamate and the stellate, basket, Golgi, and Purkinje cells all release the **inhibitory** transmitter, gamma-aminobutyric acid. The afferent fibers are classified as **mossy, climbing**, or **aminergic. Climbing fibers** from the **inferior olivary nucleus (ION)** activate Purkinje cells and the intracerebellar nuclei. Aminergic fibers originate in reticular nuclei whose projections are **serotonergic** (raphe) or **noradrenergic** (locus ceruleus). All other input is of the "mossy" fiber type, which includes input from the spinal cord, vestibular nuclei, reticular formation, and pontine nuclei that is **excitatory** to granule cells and to the intracerebellar nuclei. Mossy fibers terminate in a synaptic formation (glomerulus) in the granular layer. Axons of the granule cells ascend to the molecular layer, bifurcate, and run as parallel fibers to make synaptic contact with the transversely oriented dendritic tree of numerous Purkinje cells. The Purkinje cell is **inhibitory** to the intracerebellar nuclei and is the **single output** source from the cortex. Output from the cerebellum per se, however, is **excitatory** via axons from the intracerebellar nuclei, which traverse the SCP to terminate in the contralateral red nucleus and ventral lateral nucleus of the thalamus. Of the three peduncles, the ICP and MCP are predominantly afferent. The ICP links the cerebellum to the spinal cord and medulla, and the MCP links the cerebellum with the cerebral cortex. The SCP contains some afferent fibers but is mainly an efferent route that is part of the corticopontocerebellar-thalamocortical circuit. This circuit provides a pathway for the control of synchronous, highly skilled motor function.

First order neurons of the **dorsal spinocerebellar tract (DSCT)** are located in dorsal root ganglia (DRG) at spinal levels C8 and below. Second order neurons originate in the dorsal nucleus of Clarke (Rexed's lamina VI) at levels C8-L3. The **DSCT** ascends ipsilaterally in the lateral funiculus of the spinal cord and enters the cerebellum via the ICP. The DSCT transmits proprioceptive and exteroceptive signals from the trunk and lower limb.

First order neurons of the **cuneocerebellar tract (CCT)** are located in DRG at C7 and above, and synapse in the accessory cuneate nucleus in the medulla. It is the brain stem counterpart of the dorsal nucleus of Clarke at spinal cord level. The **CCT** ascends **ipsilaterally** with the dorsal column fibers and, after relaying in the accessory cuneate nucleus, enters the cerebellum via the ICP. The CCT mediates proprioceptive stimuli from the upper limb and neck.

First order neurons of the **ventral spinocerebellar tract (VSCT)** are located in DRG, and second order fibers originate in neurons in the intermediate ventral gray matter. The **VSCT** ascends **contralaterally** in the lateral funiculus of the spinal cord and enters the cerebellum via the SCP. The VSCT transmits proprioceptive input from the leg and trunk. Some authors discuss a rostral counterpart of the VSCT for the arm and neck.

Both the **DSCT** and the **VSCT** are located in the lateral funiculus; however, the **VSCT** is more ventrally located. Both are in peripheral positions in the spinal cord and in the caudal medulla (pages 67 and 69). The DSCT, CCT, VSCT, and vestibular input to the cerebellum is mainly integrated at an **unconscious** level.

In summary, the cerebellum receives **sensory** information from numerous sources: muscles and joints (proprioceptive); visceral organs (interoceptive); the skin; and visual, auditory, and vestibular systems (exteroceptive). **Excitatory** input is conveyed to the cortex by fibers that give off collaterals that terminate on the intracerebellar nuclei. The cortical input summates onto the Purkinje cell. The Purkinje cells project inhibitory signals to the intracerebellar nuclei and to the lateral vestibular nucleus. Because the output from the cerebellum per se is via the intracerebellar nuclei, their output equals original input minus cortical output. Therefore, the term **comparator** is used to describe the cerebellum's regulation and control of movement—it transforms motor intention into motor execution, compares intention with performance, and compensates for errors.

Clinical Correlations . . . .

See page 114.

Color all the fibers blue, beginning peripheral to the DRG, and color the DSCT and CCT blue, noting that these pathways enter via the ICP and transmit proprioceptive signals ipsilaterally from the leg and trunk and from the arm and neck, respectively. Color the entry fibers and VSCT blue and note its contralateral ascent and entry via the SCP. On the right side of the cerebellum, color the vermis green, color yellow the paravermal zone (delineated by the broken line), and color blue the hemisphere (lateral to the broken line).

Dorsal and Ventral Spinocerebellar and Cuneocerebellar Tracts: Proprioceptive Input

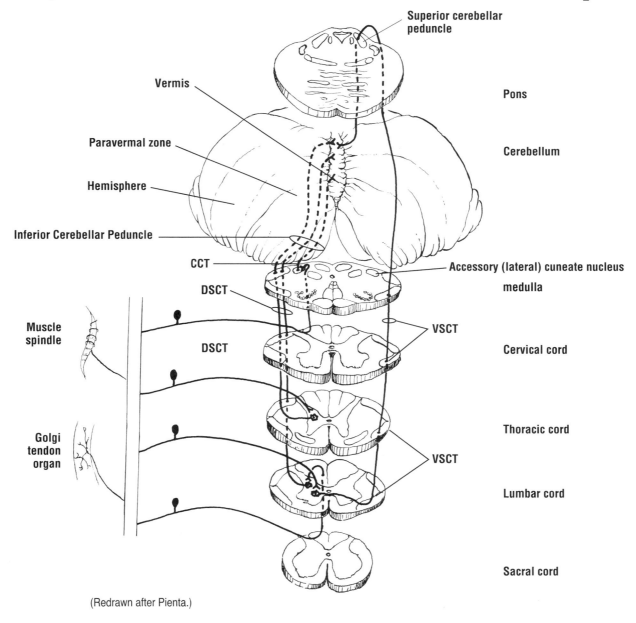

(Redrawn after Pienta.)

Table 3-2 Brain Stem Lesions and Syndromes

In addition to learning the function of the normal nervous system, the ultimate goal is to be able to predict disabilities resulting from a destructive lesion of an anatomic structure or to predict the site of the lesion if the disabilities are described. "Pure" syndromes rarely exist; however, delineation of these syndromes provides insight into the functional anatomy of the brain stem and illustrates how a detailed knowledge of brain stem anatomy facilitates solving clinical problems. The following examples show the correlation between neurologic signs and the location of the lesion. Of the various types of pathology, vascular lesions are among the more important. Hemorrhage into the brain stem usually has more serious consequences than does vascular occlusion.

Destruction of **cranial nerve nuclei** or **fibers** produces **lower motor neuron (LMN) deficits** whereas **interruption** of the **corticospinal tract** causes **upper motor neuron (UMN) signs.** Because of the compactness and functional importance of brain stem structures, a single lesion usually damages several structures and produces an assortment of clinical signs. Cranial nerves run perpendicular to the long axis; the tracts run parallel to the long axis. A discrete lesion may affect one or more cranial nerves; however, it may also interrupt a descending (motor) tract below the level of the lesion or interrupt ascending (sensory) tracts. By identifying the cranial nerve involved, it is possible to predict the level of lesion. **Alternating hemiplegia** is a term for **ipsilateral** motor involvement of a **cranial nerve** and **contralateral** motor involvement of the **body** with respect to the site of a lesion. This combination is a hallmark of brain stem insult. A cranial nerve listed under "Structures Affected" refers to either nucleus or fibers.

Medial Medullary Syndrome (of Dejerine)

Arteries Involved	Signs and Symptoms
Anterior spinal artery	
Vertebral artery (medullary branch)	

Structures Affected	
Hypoglossal	Atrophy, paresis and fasciculation of tongue (**ipsilateral**)
	Tongue deviates to the side of the lesion on protrusion
Medial lemniscus	Loss of discriminative touch and position sense (**contralateral**)
Pyramid (corticospinal fibers)	Paresis or paralysis of limbs (**contralateral**)

Basal Pontine Syndrome

Arteries Involved	Signs and Symptoms
Basilar artery (pontine branches)	

Structures Affected	
Abducens	Inward deviation of the eye (**ipsilateral**)
Facial	Paralysis of the face (**ipsilateral**)
Medial lemniscus	Loss of discriminative touch and position sense (**contralateral**)
Corticospinal fibers	Hemiparesis (**contralateral**)

Lateral Medullary Syndrome (of Wallenberg)

Arteries Involved	Signs and Symptoms
Vertebral, PICA, sometimes AICA	
Posterior inferior cerebellar artery (PICA)	
Anterior inferior cerebellar artery (AICA)	

Structures Affected	
Spinal trigeminal nucleus and tract	Loss of pain and temperature sense of the face (**ipsilateral**)
Spinothalamic tract	Loss of pain and temperature sense of the body (**contralateral**)
Nucleus ambiguus	Loss of gag reflex, dysphagia (difficulty in swallowing), dysarthria (difficulty articulating), dysphonia (hoarseness) (**ipsilateral**)
Inferior cerebellar peduncle	Ataxia (loss of coordination) of limbs (**ipsilateral**)
Vestibular nuclei	Nystagmus, nausea, vertigo (**ipsilateral**)
Descending sympathetic fibers	Horner's syndrome: miosis (small pupil), pseudoptosis (slight drooping of eyelid), anhidrosis (warm, dry skin of face) (**ipsilateral**)
Dorsal motor nucleus of X	Vomiting

Mediobasal Mesencephalic Syndrome (of Weber)

Arteries involved	Signs and Symptoms
Posterior part of Circle of Willis (aneurysm)	
Basilar artery (paramedian thalamo-perforating branches)	

Structures affected	
Oculomotor (Edinger-Westphal)	Outward deviation of eye (**ipsilateral**)
	Dilated pupil and absence of light reflex (**ipsilateral**)
Corticospinal tract	Hemiparesis (**contralateral**)
Red nucleus	Cerebellar ataxia (**contralateral**)

 Color the following red: CN III, VI, and XII; FP, CBT, CST, pyramid, and red nucleus. Color the following blue: ML, STT, STN, STHT, STET, and ICP. Color E-W and X nuclei orange and NA green. Color the vestibular nuclei yellow.

There are two times in a man's life when he should not speculate:
when he can't afford it, and when he can. – Mark Twain

122

Brain Stem Lesions and Syndromes

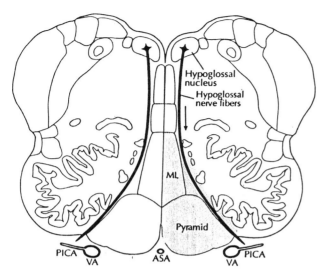

Medial Medullary Lesion

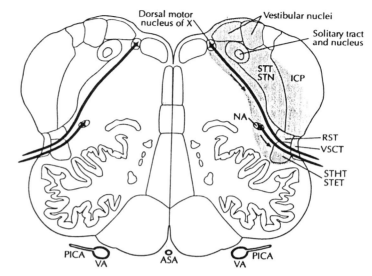

Lateral Medullary Lesion

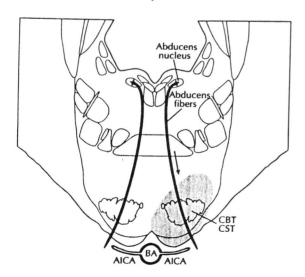

Basal Pontine Lesion

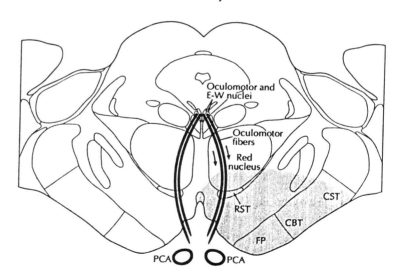

Mediobasal Mesencephalic Lesion

Chapter Three Study Questions

Questions 1–5
Directions: Each question below contains four or five suggested answers. Choose the **one best** response to each question.

1. **Which of the following is a mismatch of brain–ventricular relations?**
   (a) Rostral medulla–fourth ventricle
   (b) Diencephalon–cerebral aqueduct
   (c) Caudal medulla–central canal
   (d) Pons–fourth ventricle
   (e) Cerebral hemisphere–lateral ventricle

2. **The cranial nerve that emerges from the brain stem between the pyramid and the olive and is damaged in a medial medullary lesion is the**
   (a) Vagus
   (b) Hypoglossal
   (c) Glossopharyngeal
   (d) Vestibulocochlear
   (e) Facial

3. **Axons from which of the following cranial nerves terminate in the lateral geniculate nucleus of the thalamus?**
   (a) Olfactory
   (b) Cochlear division of CN VIII
   (c) Vestibular division of CN VIII
   (d) Vagus
   (e) Optic

4. **Which of the following is a mismatch of nuclei–brain stem location?**
   (a) Oculomotor: midbrain
   (b) Trigeminal: pons
   (c) Facial: medulla
   (d) Abducens: pons
   (e) Glossopharyngeal: medulla

5. **Projections from reticular midbrain raphe neurons to the dorsal horn of the spinal cord that actively suppress the conscious awareness of pain use the transmitter**
   (a) Serotonin
   (b) Norepinephrine
   (c) Acetylcholine
   (d) Dopamine
   (e) Glutamate

Questions 6–10: Match the lettered brain regions with the numbered items. Each lettered brain region may be used more than once or not at all.

   (a) Telencephalon
   (b) Diencephalon
   (c) Midbrain–pons junction
   (d) Rostral medulla–caudal pons
   (e) Rostral (open) medulla
   (f) Caudal (closed) medulla

6. **Decussation of the trochlear nerves**

7. **Decussation of the pyramidal tract**

8. **Location of the vestibular nuclei**

9. **Decussation of the dorsal column–medial lemniscal pathway**

10. **Primary auditory cortex**

Case History
Jill, a second year medical student, invited Jack, a first year medical student, to accompany her to observe an autopsy. The pathology resident performing the autopsy called their attention to a concave area surrounding the lateral sulcus in the left cerebral hemisphere. There was a diffuse loss of tissue involving the inferior frontal gyrus, the inferior portions of the precentral and postcentral gyri, and the superior temporal gyrus. Jack astutely observed that the arachnoid remained intact and bridged over the various sulci.

11. **Is it likely that the left hemisphere lesion was the cause of death? Why or why not?**

12. **Is it likely that the lesion involves gray matter? White matter?**

13. **Was motor deficit of the left side of the body likely? Why or why not?**

14. **Would you surmise that the patient had speech or language problems? Explain.**

15. **Why was Jack's observation regarding the arachnoid significant?**

16. **Where did Jack and Jill go after the autopsy?**

Answers and Explanations for Chapter Three Study Questions

1. **b** [page 64] The cerebral aqueduct in the midbrain connects the third ventricle, located in the diencephalon, to the fourth ventricle, which is dorsal to the pons and rostral medulla and ventral to the cerebellum.

2. **b** [pages 122 and 123] The hypoglossal nerve is composed of a series of rootlets that originates from a long column of cells located medially in the medulla. Damage to the nerve results in atrophy, paresis, and fasciculation of the tongue ipsilaterally. On protrusion, the tongue deviates to the side of the lesion. In a vascular lesion, which also destroys the medial lemniscus and pyramid, are contralateral loss of discriminative touch and position sense and paresis of the contralateral limbs (alternating hemiplegia). The vagus and glossopharyngeal nerves are dorsolaterally located in the medulla and are likely to be damaged due to a **lateral medullary lesion.** The vestibulocochlear nerve is in the cerebellopontine angle and the facial nerve originates in the pons and emerges medial to CN VIII.

3. **e** [pages 90 and 91] Axons from retinal ganglion cells traverse the optic nerve and tract to reach the lateral geniculate nucleus. Olfactory nerves terminate in the olfactory bulb, cochlear and vestibular axons terminate in the brain stem nuclei, and the central processes of afferent vagal fibers may end in the solitary or spinal trigeminal nuclei.

4. **c** [pages 64 and 65] The facial nerve emerges at the medullopontine junction; however, the nucleus per se is in the tegmentum of the pons.

5. **a** [page 62] Serotonergic terminals dampen pain transmission in the dorsal horn of the spinal cord. Norepinephrine is the principal neurotransmitter for postganglionic sympathetic neurons and in CNS pathways that originate in the locus ceruleus. Acetylcholine is the principal neurotransmitter at the neuromuscular junction, the peripheral ganglia of the ANS, many autonomic organs, and many of the synapses in the CNS. Dopamine pathways include the nigrostriatal from the substantia nigra to the caudate and putamen and connections from the ventral tegmental area of the midbrain to other limbic-related structures. Glutamate, an excitatory amino acid, is one of the principal neurotransmitters in the CNS.

6. **c** [pages 94 and 95] The trochlear nerve originates from a nucleus in the tegmentum of the midbrain, arches around the cerebral aqueduct, and crosses dorsally as it emerges from the dorsal surface of the midbrain below the inferior colliculus, i.e., at the midbrain–pons junction.

7. **f** [pages 66 and 67] The motor or pyramidal decussation occurs in the caudal medulla, caudal to the **medial lemniscal** (sensory) decussation.

8. **d** [pages 102 and 103] The vestibular nuclei are in the floor of the rhomboid fossa. They span a region in the rostral medulla and caudal pons.

9. **f** [pages 68 and 69] (Refer to number 7 above.)

10. **a** [pages 102 and 103] The primary auditory cortex is in the temporal lobe of the telencephalon.

Case History

11. **No.** The appearance of the left hemisphere is compatible with a long-standing (chronic) vascular lesion. Loss of tissue occurs over time. It is likely, however, that such an acute vascular lesion could result in death.

12. **Yes.** The cortex of neurons is 2 to 4 mm thick. Such a loss of brain mass probably would involve the underlying white matter as well as the cortical mantle of gray.

13. **No.** Fibers emanating from the left hemisphere essentially control the right sides of the lower face and body.

14. **Yes.** Understanding the semantics of speech and the delivery of speech (i.e., the motor component of speech) is localized to the left hemisphere in more than 95% of the population.

15. **The presence of an intact arachnoid suggests that the insult originated internally, rather than externally, to the brain. Likewise, it is a clue that a natural process (e.g., phagocytic activity) accounts for the loss of tissue.**

16. **An unfair question.** Joe, a former attorney and classmate of Jack's, eloquently articulated and proved beyond a reasonable doubt that this point was not discussed in class, nor could it be found in any of the course materials.

CHAPTER 4 Lateral View of Major Pathways in the Brain Stem

Ascending Pathways in the Tegmentum*

VSCT, SCP The **ventral spinocerebellar** tract (VSCT) enters the cerebellum via the **superior cerebellar peduncle** (SCP); however, most of the fibers in the SCP originate in the deep cerebellar nuclei.

DSCT, ICP The **dorsal spinocerebellar** (DSCT) tract enters the cerebellum via the **inferior cerebellar peduncle** (ICP).

LL The **lateral lemniscus** (LL) originates from auditory nuclei and terminates in the inferior colliculus (IC) of the midbrain and in the medial geniculate nucleus (MGN) of the thalamus.

ML The **medial lemniscus** (ML) relays in the ventral posterolateral nucleus of the thalamus (VPL).

GF, CF, DC The **gracile fasciculus** (GF) and **cuneate fasciculus** (CF) ascend ipsilaterally in the dorsal column (DC) of the spinal cord.

GN, CN, ML The GF and CF terminate ipsilaterally in the **gracile nucleus** (GN) and **cuneate nucleus** (CN) of the medulla. Second order fibers from these nuclei cross in the medulla (internal arcuate fibers) and form the **medial lemniscus** (ML) of the brain stem.

STHT The **spinothalamic tract** (STHT) originates mainly from neurons in Rexed's laminae I, IV, V of the dorsal horn of the spinal cord and relays in the thalamus (VPL).

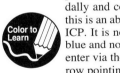

Blue represents GSA and yellow represents SSA pathways. Color the **ascending** pathways blue. Always color in the direction that impulses are flowing. Begin caudally and color the VSCT, which traverses the SCP. Be aware as you color that this is an aberrant route. It would be more direct if these fibers entered through the ICP. It is not known why the VSCT overshoots its destination. Color the DSCT blue and note its entry into the cerebellum via the ICP (many other pathways also enter via the ICP). Draw the LL in yellow from the pons to the IC and add an arrow pointing to the thalamus, where it relays in the MGN. Draw ascending fibers from the GF and the CF in the spinal cord to the GN and CN in the medulla, then indicate the crossing of the ML and its ascent through the tegmentum, ending with

an arrow to the VPL. The STHT crossed on entry at cord level so color it straight up through the tegmentum, ending with an arrow indicating that it relays in the VPL. Color yellow the optic tract, lateral geniculate nucleus (LGN), MGN, superior colliculus (SC), and IC.

Descending Pathways Ventrally Located

CB The **corticobulbar fibers** (CB) originate from cortical motor neurons and terminate on cranial nerve nuclei.

CS The **corticospinal fibers** (CS) originate from cortical neurons and terminate on spinal motor neurons.

CP, PC, MCP The **corticopontine** (CP) fibers originate from cortical motor neurons and terminate on nuclei in the ventral pons. The **pontocerebellar** (PC) fibers originate from pontine neurons and enter the cerebellum via the **middle cerebellar peduncle** (MCP).

LCST The **lateral corticospinal tract** (LCST) decussates in the caudal medulla and descends in the lateral funiculus of the spinal cord.

VCST The **ventral corticospinal tract** (VCST) descends in the ventral funiculus of the spinal cord without crossing.

All Other Descending Pathways Traverse the Tegmentum of the Brain Stem

*Recall that the tegmentum is defined as the portion of the brain stem dorsal to the base of the pons and of the cerebral peduncles and ventral to the cerebral aqueduct and fourth ventricle.

Color the **descending** pathways red. Begin rostrally and color the CB fibers, indicating their termination at all levels of the brain stem. Color the CS fibers and note their ventral position throughout the brain stem. Note the decussation of the LCST in the caudal medulla and the descent of the LCST and VCST in the spinal cord. Although the CP fibers are afferent to the cerebellum, color them red also to indicate their descent from the cerebral cortex. Include a synapse in the basal pons and show the entry of the PC fibers through the MCP. Color yellow the optic tract, LGN, MGN, SC, and IC.

Lateral View of Major Pathways in the Brain Stem

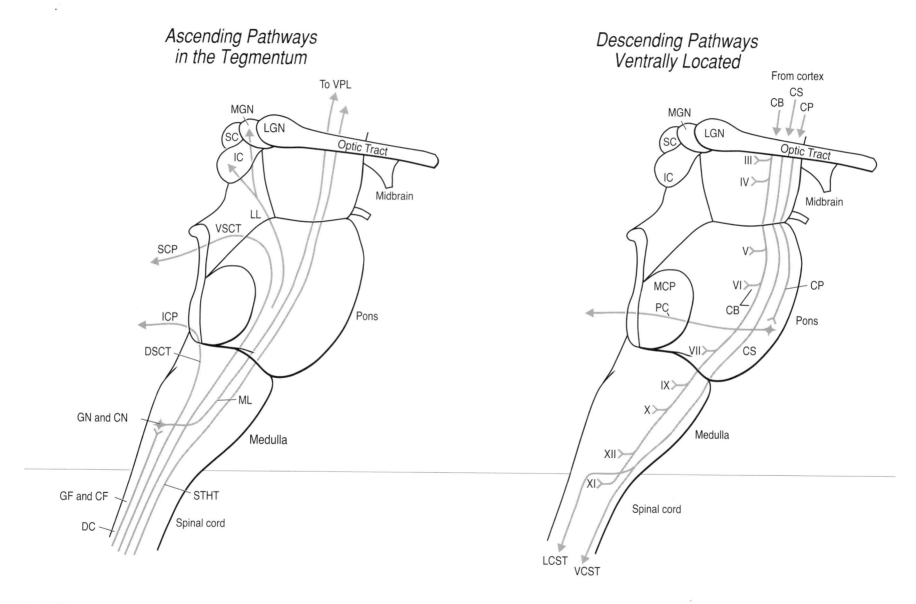

Ascending Pathways
in the Tegmentum

Descending Pathways
Ventrally Located

Ventrolateral System: Pain, Temperature, and Nondiscriminative Touch

Definitions

The ventrolateral system includes the spinothalamic tract that terminates in the postcentral gyrus (somatosensory cortex) of the parietal lobe. Mixed in among these fibers in the ventral and lateral funiculi of the spinal cord are **spinoreticular** fibers, which terminate in the reticular formation of the brain stem, and **spinotectal** fibers, which terminate in the tectum. Thus, the ventrolateral system (spinal lemniscus) subserves both conscious and unconscious appreciation of pain, temperature, and nondiscriminative touch.

Structural and Functional Features

The **spinothalamic tract** relays information from small, first order cell bodies in the dorsal root ganglia, which project to the **posteromarginal nucleus (lamina I)** or **nucleus proprius (laminae IV and V)** in the spinal cord. Additionally, second order neurons from the posteromarginal nucleus ascend or descend in **Lissauer's tract** and transmit pain impulses that are used unconsciously via intersegmental reflex responses. Axons of second order neurons from the posteromarginal nucleus and the nucleus proprius cross obliquely (usually within one spinal segment) and **ascend** in the **ventrolateral funiculus** on the **contralateral** side. Many fibers from second order neurons **relay** in the **ventral posterolateral nucleus** (VPL) of the thalamus; however, some terminals synapse in the posterior and intralaminar nuclei of the thalamus. The somatotopic arrangement in the spinal cord is such that fibers from the upper body are medial, and those from the lower body are lateral. The drawing shows this relative to the position and ascent of arm and leg fibers. Third order neurons terminating in the somatosensory cortex (areas 3,1,2) subserve conscious appreciation of pain, temperature, and nondiscriminative touch. These modalities are appreciated to some extent at the thalamic level of integration.

The **spinoreticular** tract contains crossed and uncrossed fibers that feed into the reticular formation of the brain stem and are involved in reflex activity. Other fibers reach the intralaminar and midline nuclei of the thalamus and project to diffuse cortical regions. This phenomenon is referred to as the **ascending reticular activating system** (ARAS), to distinguish it from the descending motor component of the reticular system. Fibers terminating in the periaqueductal gray, midbrain raphe, and tectum constitute the spinotectal tract, which is related to a pain-inhibiting system. Although information relayed over the spinothalamic, spinoreticular, and spinotectal tracts concerning pain, temperature, and nondiscriminative touch is integrated in the thalamus for an unconscious awareness, only the **spinothalamic tract**, with its relay in **VPL** and **termination** in the **somatosensory cortex** (areas 3,1,2) of the parietal lobe, contributes to the **conscious** appreciation of these modalities.

Clinical Correlations . . . .

Interruption of the **ventrolateral tract** produces **loss** of **pain** and **temperature** on the **opposite side** of the body, beginning about one segment below the level of the lesion. Additionally, there is a **segmental deficit** at the level of the lesion. The irritation of the **dorsal root** by a **bony spur** or a **slipped disk** can produce **pain** in a dermatome, as can herpes zoster (page 48). **Syringomyelia interrupts** the **pain** and **temperature fibers** as they **cross** in the ventral white commissure and produces a characteristic **yoke-like deficit** (page 56).

The **perception** of **pain** is a complex phenomenon as evidenced by **phantom pain** in an amputated limb or the overriding of pain by virtue of the stressful events of combat. In combat a wounded soldier may not experience pain until the crisis is over. **Stoicism**, the ignoring of discomfort, as opposed to a low threshold for pain, and as related to **cultural heritage**, also speaks to the behavioral complexity of pain.

Note the different receptors as you color them blue. Locate the small first order neuron in the dorsal root ganglion of the lines representing input via the leg and the arm (an interneuron in the dorsal horn is typical). Color blue in an ascending direction, noting the terminals that feed into the brain stem from the second order neuron. Also note that crossing occurs from this neuron. Observe that arm fibers are medial to leg fibers. Color the cross section of the tract blue; note its position at all levels. Finally, color the fibers from the third order neurons in the VPL to their cortical destination, i.e., **leg** fibers to the medial surface and **arm** fibers to the **dorsolateral** surface of the hemisphere.

Ventrolateral System: Pain, Temperature, and Nondiscriminative Touch

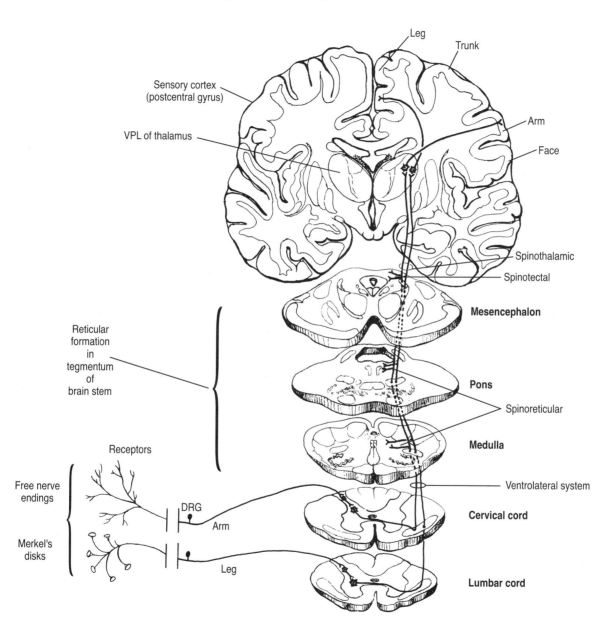

Trigeminal System: Pain, Temperature, Touch, Pressure, and Proprioception

Definitions

The **trigeminal** system serves the **face** and **head** in the way that the ventrolateral and **dorsal column–medial lemniscal pathways** serve the body. The trigeminal nerve (V) leaves the lateral surface of the pons and, peripheral to its ganglion, divides into three branches based on the regions of the face that it serves. These are the **ophthalmic** (V1), the **maxillary** (V2), and the **mandibular** (V3) divisions that leave the cranial cavity through different routes. Fibers from small first order neurons in the trigeminal (Gasserian, semilunar) ganglion descend and relay pain and temperature sensations from the face to the **spinal trigeminal nucleus** (STN). Fibers from second order neurons in the STN cross and ascend in the **ventral trigeminothalamic tract**; uncrossed fibers ascend in the **dorsal trigeminothalamic tract**; both tracts relay in the ventral posteromedial nucleus (VPM) of the thalamus. Third order neurons from VPM terminate in the somatosensory cortex (areas 3,1,2) for conscious recognition of pain, temperature, and touch from the face.

Fibers from large first order neurons in the trigeminal ganglion synapse in the **chief sensory (main) nucleus** of **CN V** and relay information concerning discriminative touch and pressure. Fibers from second order neurons in the chief sensory nucleus ascend to VPM in the trigeminothalamic tracts, and fibers from third order neurons in the VPM terminate in the face area of the somatosensory cortex (areas 3,1,2).

The **mesencephalic nucleus** of **CN V** is unique in that it contains the only unipolar cells within the CNS. Peripheral processes traveling in the mandibular branch (V3) relay proprioceptive input particularly from stretch receptors of the muscles of mastication, teeth, and gums. The central processes of these unipolar cells project to the motor nucleus of V, which then projects the efferent arc of the jaw reflex via V3. The ascending central connections of the **mesencephalic nucleus** of **V** are poorly understood. (The mesencephalic nucleus and **tract** are depicted at midbrain cross-sectional levels on pages 82 and 83. Their position has been indicated on the diagram on page 131.)

The **trigeminal** is the largest of the cranial nerves. It contains a large sensory component, **general somatic afferent** (GSA), and a much smaller motor component, **special visceral efferent** (SVE). SVE describes the innervation of muscles of **branchiomeric** origin. Motor fibers travel in the mandibular branch to innervate the muscles of mastication. The tensor tympani and the tensor veli palatini are also innervated by CN V3.

In addition to numerous trigeminal fibers that terminate in the spinal trigeminal nucleus, a few fibers from cranial nerves VII, IX, and X relay in this nucleus.

Clinical Correlations

A **peripheral lesion** of CN V3 results in **ipsilateral paralysis** or **paresis** of the muscles of mastication. When the jaw is clenched, it deviates toward the side of the lesion, and bite strength and muscle mass are diminished unilaterally. A **central** (UMN) **lesion** causes a **hyperactive jaw reflex.**

A lesion in the medulla or high cervical spinal cord may interrupt the descending tract of CN V and the ascending spinothalamic tract. This can result in an **ipsilateral loss** of pain and temperature of the **face** and a **contralateral loss** of pain and temperature of the body. This combination occurs only when a lesion is at these levels.

Trigeminal neuralgia (tic douloureux) is a recurrent lancinating pain that localizes to one side of the face in one or more branches of the trigeminal nerve, usually the maxillary or mandibular divisions. The disorder is of unknown etiology and is often triggered by a slight tactile stimulus. Vascular decompression of the trigeminal ganglion (recently made popular by Dr. Peter J. Jannetta) usually affords relief, if analgesics do not control the pain.

The trigeminal ganglion, like other sensory ganglia, may be infected by the herpes virus. Whereas **neuralgia** affects the **V2** and **V3** branches, **herpes zoster** affects the **V1** branch more often. (Herpes zoster in spinal nerves is discussed on page 48.)

Make the distinction between the motor nucleus of CN V (branchiomeric) in contrast to cranial nerves of somatic origin. Color the motor nucleus and fibers of CN V green to designate it as special visceral efferent (**SVE**); the motor fibers are in V3. General somatic efferent (GSE) cranial nerve nuclei include III, IV, VI, and XII. **SVE** as well as **GSE** fibers innervate striated skeletal muscle.

Color blue the spinal trigeminal and chief sensory nuclei and all sensory fibers. Observe the small DRG cell whose fiber transmits pain and temperature and descends to the spinal nucleus, whereas larger neurons subserve touch (chief sensory) and proprioception (mesencephalic nucleus). Note that the third order neuron is in the **VPM** and projects to the face area of the somatosensory cortex.

Trigeminal System: Pain, Temperature, Touch, Pressure, and Proprioception

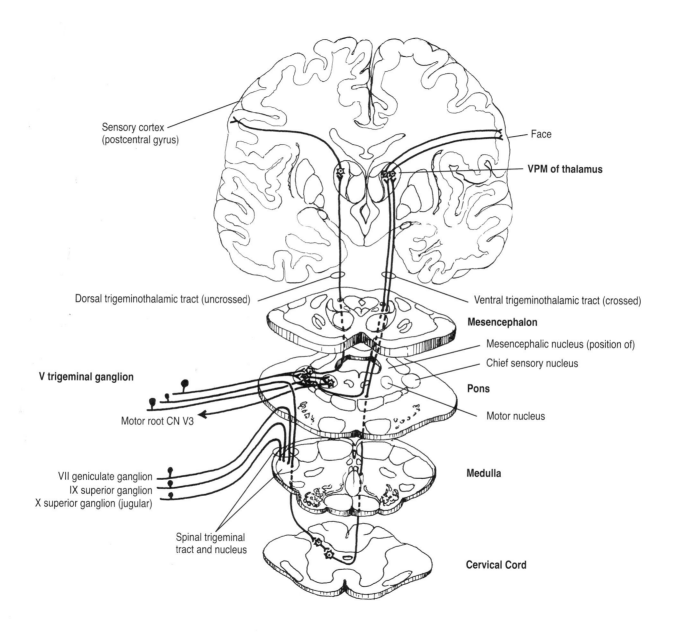

Sensory cortex (postcentral gyrus)

Face

VPM of thalamus

Dorsal trigeminothalamic tract (uncrossed)

Ventral trigeminothalamic tract (crossed)

Mesencephalon

Mesencephalic nucleus (position of)

Chief sensory nucleus

V trigeminal ganglion

Pons

Motor nucleus

Motor root CN V3

VII geniculate ganglion
IX superior ganglion
X superior ganglion (jugular)

Medulla

Spinal trigeminal tract and nucleus

Cervical Cord

Dorsal Column–Medial Lemniscal System: Proprioception, Vibration, Pressure, and Discriminative Touch

Definitions

The **dorsal column–medial lemniscal pathway** relays the modalities of **discriminative touch** via Meissner's corpuscles; **pressure** via deep receptors; **vibration** via Pacinian corpuscles; and **proprioception** via muscle spindles, Golgi tendon organs, and unencapsulated nerve endings. The impulses conveyed by this highly specific sensory pathway are concerned with either **touch pressure** or **kinesthesia** (sense of position or movement).

Structural and Functional Features

The first order neurons are large cell bodies located in the dorsal root ganglia. The axons are heavily myelinated and conduct impulses rapidly. The axons have ascending or descending collaterals in the spinal cord that form the afferent limb of reflex arcs. These may terminate on dorsal horn interneurons for local reflexes or, in the case of an afferent fiber from the muscle spindle, end directly on an anterior motor horn cell forming a monosynaptic reflex (stretch reflex). All other reflexes are polysynaptic and have one or more interneurons between the afferent and efferent components. Fibers entering at **T5** and **above** ascend ipsilaterally as the **cuneate fasciculus** and synapse in the cuneate nucleus. Fibers from **T6** and **below** ascend ipsilaterally as the **gracile fasciculus** and synapse in the gracile nucleus, which lies medial to the cuneate nucleus in the caudal medulla. Only about 25% of the fibers in the dorsal columns reach these nuclei.

Second order neurons in the **gracile** and **cuneate nuclei** give rise to **internal arcuate fibers,** which cross the midline and form the **medial lemniscus** in the medulla. Fibers arising in the medially located gracile nucleus swing ventral to those arising from the laterally located cuneate nucleus as they cross to the opposite side.

The **medial lemniscus rotates** as it ascends rostrally through the pons and midbrain to synapse in the **ventral posterolateral nucleus** (VPL) of the thalamus (arm medial, leg lateral). Axons from third order neurons in the thalamus traverse the **posterior limb** of the **internal capsule** and terminate in the somatosensory gyrus (areas 3,1,2) in a somatotopic manner.

Position sense includes the position of a limb in space (static) and kinesthesia (movement of a limb) and is dependent on proprioceptive receptors.

Many of the muscle spindle fibers and Golgi tendon organ afferent fibers that ascend in the dorsal column are destined to reach the cerebellum. Those from the lower limb ascend in the gracile fasciculus and project to the dorsal nucleus of Clarke. Those fibers from the upper limb that enter rostral to the dorsal nucleus of Clarke ascend in the cuneate fasciculus to reach the accessory (lateral) cuneate nucleus in the medulla. Both the dorsal nucleus of Clarke and the accessory cuneate nucleus project to the cerebellum via the ICP through the dorsal spinocerebellar and cuneocerebellar tracts, respectively (pages 120 and 121).

Clinical Correlations . . . .

Dorsal column–medial lemniscal (DC–ML) **lesions interfere** with **tactile** and **kinesthetic sense.** The pathway is **ipsilateral** (uncrossed) in the spinal cord and **contralateral** (crossed) in the brain stem; therefore, the **laterality** of the deficit depends on the level of the lesion. The loss of proprioceptive input **impairs coordination** resulting in **sensory ataxia,** which, if involving the legs, results in **disturbances** of **equilibrium, stance,** and **gait.** Sensory ataxia is improved by visual input; cerebellar ataxia is not. Difficulty maintaining balance with the eyes closed is a sign of impaired position sensibility (Romberg's sign). (Dorsal column lesions are discussed on page 54.)

Subacute combined degeneration involves the **dorsal columns** and the corticospinal tracts (page 52).

After coloring all the receptors blue, begin distal to the DRG and color blue in the ascending direction of the DC–ML pathway. Observe that the crossing occurs in the medulla. It is important to note where first, second, and third order neurons are located and in what cortical region the pathway terminates. Observe at every brain stem level the fiber lamination, i.e., relation of arm and leg fibers. Also color blue the sensory nuclei—cuneate and gracile. Color the fibers and nuclei in the inset blue.

Humanly speaking, let us define truth,
while waiting for a better definition as "a statement of the facts as they are." – Voltaire

132

Dorsal Column–Medial Lemniscal System: Proprioception, Vibration, Pressure, and Discriminative Touch

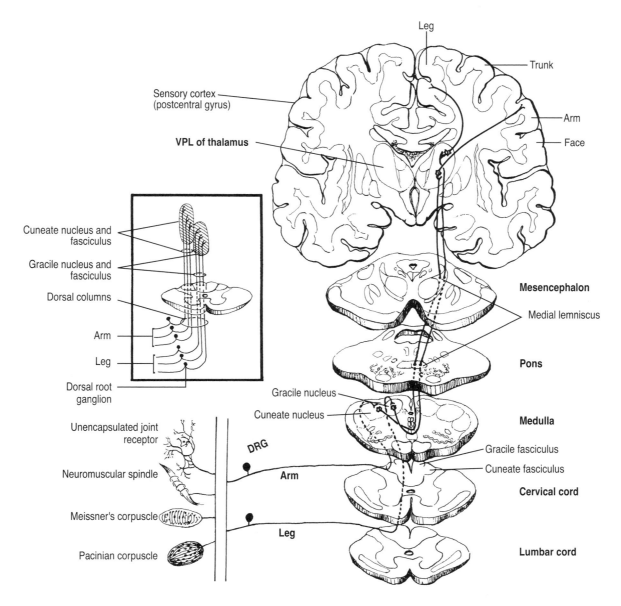

Leg

Trunk

Sensory cortex
(postcentral gyrus)

Arm

Face

VPL of thalamus

Cuneate nucleus and
fasciculus

Gracile nucleus and
fasciculus

Dorsal columns

Arm

Leg

Dorsal root
ganglion

Mesencephalon

Medial lemniscus

Pons

Gracile nucleus

Cuneate nucleus

Medulla

Gracile fasciculus

Cuneate fasciculus

Unencapsulated joint
receptor

DRG

Neuromuscular spindle

Arm

Cervical cord

Meissner's corpuscle

Leg

Pacinian corpuscle

Lumbar cord

Spinal Cord Ascending Pathways: Somatosensory Pathways (Limbs and Trunk)

Specific Input to the Primary Somatosensory Area of the Cerebral Cortex

Information consciously perceived arises predominantly from the contralateral face and body areas. Stimuli originating in peripheral sensory receptors are faithfully transmitted so that information is both place and modality specific, e.g., both the precise location and character of the stimuli are known. Two clinically important specific pathways are the **spinothalamic component** of the **ventrolateral system** and the **dorsal column–medial lemniscal system.** Both relay in the **ventral posterolateral nucleus** of the **thalamus** and terminate in the **postcentral gyrus** of the **parietal lobe.** The postcentral gyrus is synonymous with the **somatosensory area** and with **Brodmann's areas 3,1,2.**

Nonspecific Input to Diffuse Areas of the Cerebral Cortex

Stimuli transmitted in the **spinoreticulothalamic pathway** are of a nonspecific, general nature. This pathway transmits information that is not somatotopically organized, projects to widespread cortical areas, and functions to arouse and alert the cortex. It constitutes the **ascending reticular activating system** (ARAS).

Clinical Correlation . . . .

Interruption of the spinothalamic tract anywhere in the neuraxis results in **contralateral deficits** of pain and temperature caudal to the lesion. Interruption of the **dorsal column** results in **ipsilateral** loss of proprioception, vibration, pressure, and discriminative touch; however, these modalities are impaired **contralateral** to the lesion if the lesion is in the **medial lemniscus** at the brain stem level.

Begin with dorsal root fibers and color all of these sensory pathways blue. For the pathways that reach the postcentral gyrus, color with attention to the location of the first, second, and third order neurons. Observe the level of the crossing of the spinothalamic fibers in the spinal cord and the medial lemniscus in the brain stem. Also, take note of the cortical region receiving the impulses for conscious recognition of the modalities transmitted to the parietal lobe. Note that the ARAS may project terminals into all brain stem regions or may relay in intralaminar nuclei of the thalamus en route to widespread cortical regions.

Spinal Cord Ascending Pathways

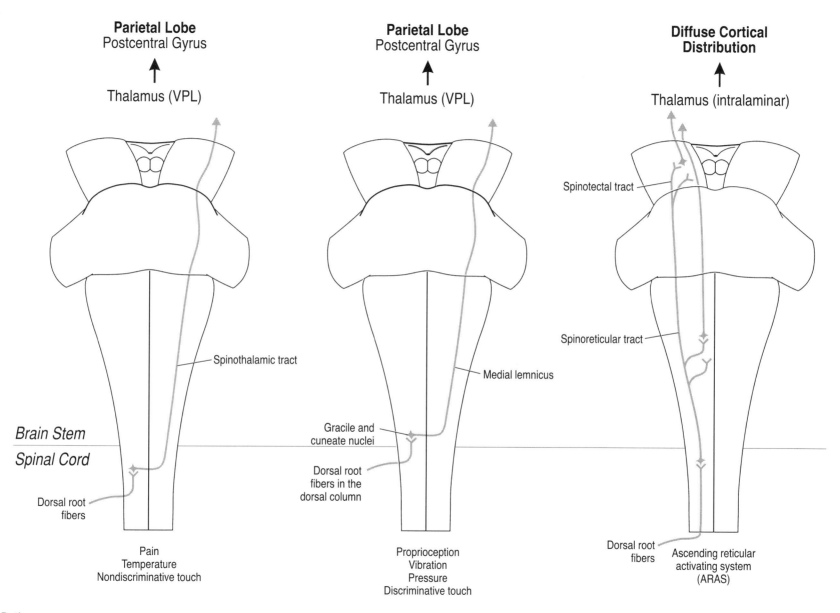

Parietal Lobe
Postcentral Gyrus

↑

Thalamus (VPL)

Parietal Lobe
Postcentral Gyrus

↑

Thalamus (VPL)

**Diffuse Cortical
Distribution**

↑

Thalamus (intralaminar)

Spinotectal tract

Spinoreticular tract

Spinothalamic tract

Medial lemnicus

Brain Stem

Spinal Cord

Gracile and
cuneate nuclei

Dorsal root
fibers in the
dorsal column

Dorsal root
fibers

Dorsal root
fibers

Pain
Temperature
Nondiscriminative touch

Proprioception
Vibration
Pressure
Discriminative touch

Ascending reticular
activating system
(ARAS)

Lateral and Ventral Corticospinal Tracts: Volitional Control of Limbs and Trunk

Definitions
Impulses from one **cerebral hemisphere control** the opposite side of the body via the **corticospinal tracts.** These fibers **descend ipsilaterally** from the **cortex** to the **caudal medulla.** At the junction of the medulla and spinal cord, the majority of fibers cross to the opposite side to exert voluntary control of limb musculature.

Structural and Functional Features
Of the one million fibers in each **corticospinal tract,** more than half originate from pyramidal cells in the precentral gyrus (area 4). The premotor cortex (areas 6,8), the primary somatosensory cortex (areas 3,1,2), and the superior parietal lobule (areas 5,7) also contribute fibers to the corticospinal tract. Fibers from giant cells of Betz in area 4 make up about 3% of the corticospinal tract and terminate directly on anterior motor horn cells of the spinal cord. Other fibers terminate on interneurons; many in lamina VIII. In the ventral medulla, about 85% of the corticospinal fibers **decussate** and descend in the lateral funiculus of the spinal cord as the **lateral corticospinal tract** (LCST). The 15% that do not cross, descend in the ventral funiculus of the spinal cord as the **ventral corticospinal tract** (VSCT). (An insignificant number of fibers that do not cross descend in the lateral funiculus.)

Like sensory fibers, motor fibers are somatotopically arranged. This efficient layering facilitates their termination at various levels, e.g., cervical (C) and thoracic (T) fibers are medially located, which facilitates their entry into the gray matter at rostral levels. At lower levels, only lumbar (L) and sacral (S) fibers make up the LCST. Note the position of the fibers of the face (F), arm (A), and leg (L) in the internal capsule and in the basis pedunculi of the midbrain.

As mentioned on page 138, there are fibers that descend from the cortex and from subcortical nuclei that travel with the motor fibers and function to modulate sensory activity. It is thought that the sensory modulation is mediated by fibers originating in the parietal lobe (areas 3,1,2,5,7). This modulation usually occurs at the second order neuron in the sensory pathway and generally, although not always, is inhibitory.

Clinical Correlations . . . .

Quadriplegia, paraplegia, and hemiplegia are defined on page 56. The characteristics of upper and lower motor neuron lesions are listed on page 138. **Interruption** of the corticospinal fibers **above** the **foramen magnum** results in a **contralateral motor deficit** caudal to the **lesion,** whereas a lesion in the **spinal cord** causes an **ipsilateral loss** of function. The deficit is most pronounced in the hands and feet.

Note in this diagram that the internal capsule is viewed from the front. Think about descent, lamination of fibers at various levels, and level of crossover as you color this pathway red. The final common pathway from the anterior motor horn cell to skeletal muscle in all spinal nerves is **general somatic efferent** (GSE). Color the cross-sectional LCST red. Also color the VSCT red and observe that fibers per se are not shown.

Lateral and Ventral Corticospinal Tracts: Volitional Control of Limbs and Trunk

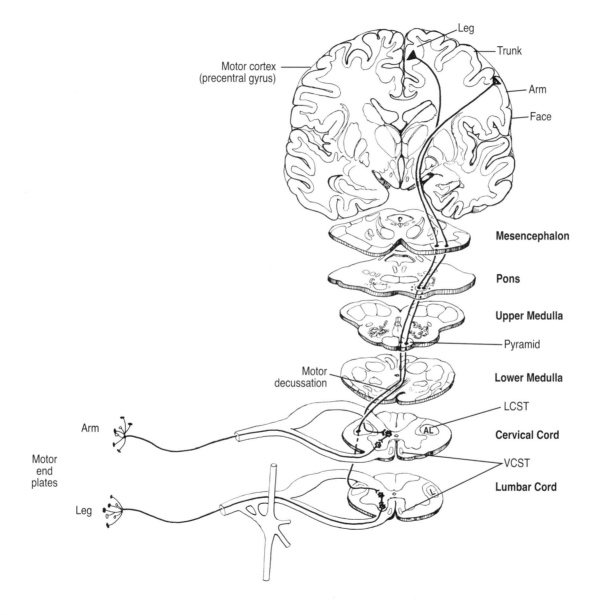

Leg

Trunk

Motor cortex
(precentral gyrus)

Arm

Face

Mesencephalon

Pons

Upper Medulla

Pyramid

Motor
decussation

Lower Medulla

LCST

Arm

AL

Cervical Cord

Motor
end
plates

VCST

Lumbar Cord

L

Leg

Descending Pathways Converge on Motor Neurons

1   **Cortical Motor Neurons** originate predominantly from Brodmann's areas 4,6,3,1,2,5,7 and descend to cranial nerve nuclei in the brain stem and to anterior motor horn cells in the spinal cord to exert volitional control over skeletal muscle.

Subcortical Pathways
Mesencephalon

2   The tectospinal and tectobulbar tracts from the superior colliculus of the tectum integrate reflex response to visual, auditory, and cutaneous stimuli.

3   The **medial longitudinal fasciculus** (MLF) contains ascending and descending fibers involved with reflexes of the vestibular system. MLF integrates movements of the eyes, head, and neck.

4   The **rubrospinal tract** originates from neurons of the red nucleus and descends in the tegmentum of the brain stem and in the lateral funiculus of the spinal cord; its most important function concerns control of tone in flexor muscle groups.

Pons

5   The **pontine (medial) reticulospinal tract** descends in the tegmentum of the brain stem and in the ventral funiculus of the spinal cord. It mediates excitatory input.

Medulla

6   The **(lateral) vestibulospinal tract** originates in the lateral vestibular nucleus and descends in the tegmentum of the brain stem and the ventral funiculus of the spinal cord. Its influence is facilitative.

7   The **medullary (lateral) reticulospinal tract** descends in the ventral part of the lateral funiculus. Stimulation of these fibers results in inhibitory effects.

8   **Interneurons (association neurons)** compose the majority of neurons throughout the CNS and serve an integrative function.

9   **Motor neurons** in the brain stem and in the ventral horn of the spinal cord receive corticobulbar or corticospinal fibers, respectively, as well as input from many subcortical nuclei. Volitional motor control of skeletal muscles supplied by cranial and spinal nerves results from synchronous interplay of multiple influences on the motor neuron, which is referred to as the final common pathway.

Clinical Correlations . . . .

Interruption of cortically or subcortically originating pathways results in an upper motor neuron (UMN) lesion, whereas death or injury of the motor neurons in the brain stem or spinal cord constitutes a lower motor neuron (LMN) lesion. Characteristics of each are as follows:

UMN Lesion
Spastic paralysis or paresis
No significant atrophy
Hyperreflexia; clonus
Babinski sign usually present
No fibrillation or fasciculation

LMN Lesion
Flaccid paralysis or paresis
Pronounced atrophy
Hyporeflexia or areflexia
No Babinski sign
Fibrillation and fasciculation

Clonus is a repetitive alternating contraction and relaxation of muscles. The Babinski sign consists of extension of the great toe in response to stroking the sole of the foot after injury to the corticospinal tract. The same response occurs normally in infants prior to medullation of the corticospinal fibers.

Color all of the lines red. Observe the spatial origin of pathways from various subcortical levels and note that only axons originating in the cortex terminate directly on the lower motor neurons. These axons reach their destination one synapse ahead of all the rest. As you color, consider the temporal summation of multiple impulses traveling different distances at different rates to exert inhibitory or excitatory influences on the lower motor neuron.

Descending Pathways Converge on Motor Neurons

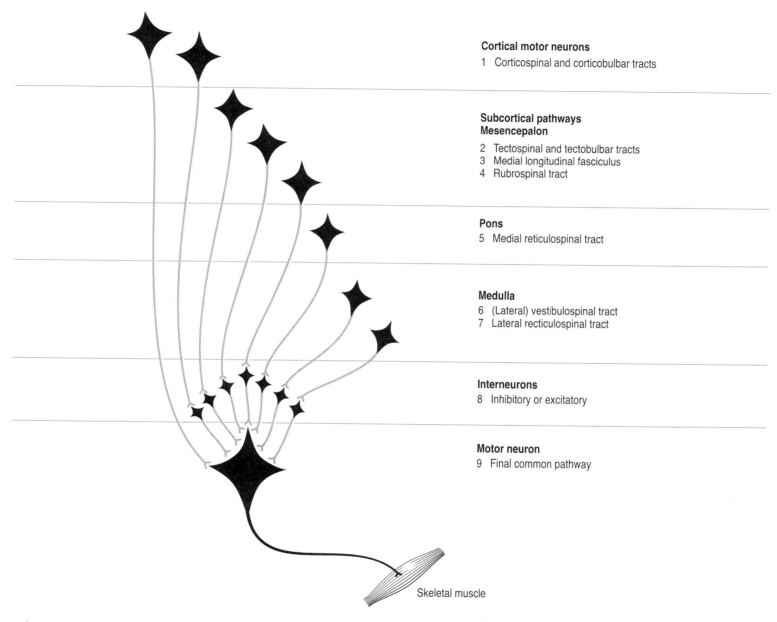

Cortical motor neurons

1 Corticospinal and corticobulbar tracts

Subcortical pathways
Mesencepalon

2 Tectospinal and tectobulbar tracts
3 Medial longitudinal fasciculus
4 Rubrospinal tract

Pons

5 Medial reticulospinal tract

Medulla

6 (Lateral) vestibulospinal tract
7 Lateral recticulospinal tract

Interneurons

8 Inhibitory or excitatory

Motor neuron

9 Final common pathway

Skeletal muscle

Corticobulbar Tract: Volitional Control of the Face and Head

Definitions

Corticobulbar fibers originate from the motor and somatosensory cortex and terminate on cranial nerve nuclei in the midbrain, pons, or medulla. These fibers are to cranial nerve nuclei what corticospinal fibers are to anterior motor horn cells at spinal levels.

Structural and Functional Features

Corticobulbar fibers take origin from pyramidal cells in Brodmann's areas 3,1,2,4,6 and **descend** with the **corticospinal fibers** through the internal capsule, base of the cerebral peduncle, basal region of the pons, and the ventral area of the medulla. Most fibers terminate on interneurons of the reticular formation; a few terminate directly on motor neurons in the brain stem subserving cranial nerve function.

Corticobulbar fibers exert **volitional control** over skeletal (GSE and SVE) muscles at cranial and, in the case of CN XI, the accessory nerve, at upper cervical levels. Cranial nerves that innervate muscles of **somatic** origin are **general somatic efferent** (GSE). Cortical projections relay through reticular formation neurons or terminate on cranial nerve nuclei, which then project GSE fibers; these nuclei include the oculomotor (III), the trochlear (IV), the abducens (VI), and the hypoglossal (XII). Cranial nerves that innervate muscles of **branchiomeric** (branchial arch) origin are **special visceral efferent** (SVE). Cranial nerve nuclei that are influenced by cortical projections and then project SVE fibers include the trigeminal motor nucleus (V), facial motor nucleus (VII), nucleus ambiguus (IX, X), and the accessory (spinal) nucleus (XI).

Corticobulbar pathways from the cortex to the brain stem are predominantly **crossed;** however, cortical **ipsilateral** projections are sufficient in number for the muscles of the **face** and **head** to function bilaterally (a notable exception is VII). **For visual simplicity, only the projections from the contralateral cortex are depicted.**

Mixed among the corticobulbar **motor** fibers are fibers that terminate in sensory relay nuclei (gracile, cuneate, sensory CN V, and the solitary nucleus) to modulate sensory activity.

Observe the internal capsule inset and the descent of corticobulbar fibers nearest the genu. The topographic arrangement of fibers in the posterior limb of the internal capsule is face (F), arm (A), trunk (T), and leg (L). This dorsal view of the brain stem shows cranial nerve nuclei in relation to the midline and to the floor of the rhomboid fossa.

Clinical Correlations . . . .

A **lesion** of the **corticobulbar projections** to the facial nucleus results in paresis or paralysis of the muscles of facial expression in the **lower quadrant** of the face **contralateral** to the lesion. A supranuclear lesion is often in the internal capsule and usually involves the contralateral limbs as well.

First, draw a dotted line through the midline of the brain stem to be cognizant that the corticobulbar fibers are **predominantly** contralateral. Color the fibers from the cortex to the cranial nerve nuclei red. These are efferent to the nuclei. The component designation refers to the brain stem motor nuclei that give rise to the fibers exerting volitional control over muscles of the face and head. Color the nuclei of III, IV, VI, and XII red for GSE. Color the nuclei of V, VII, IX, and X (nucleus ambiguus) and the accessory nucleus (SVE) green.

Every man feels instinctively that all the beautiful sentiments in the world weigh less than a single lovely action. – Rousseau

140

Corticobulbar Tract: Volitional Control of the Face and Head

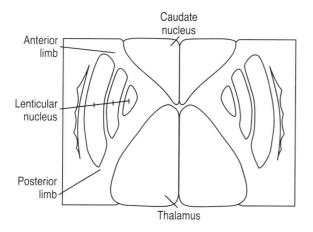

Horizontal (Axial) Section through the Internal Capsule

Caudate nucleus

Anterior limb

Lenticular nucleus

Posterior limb

Thalamus

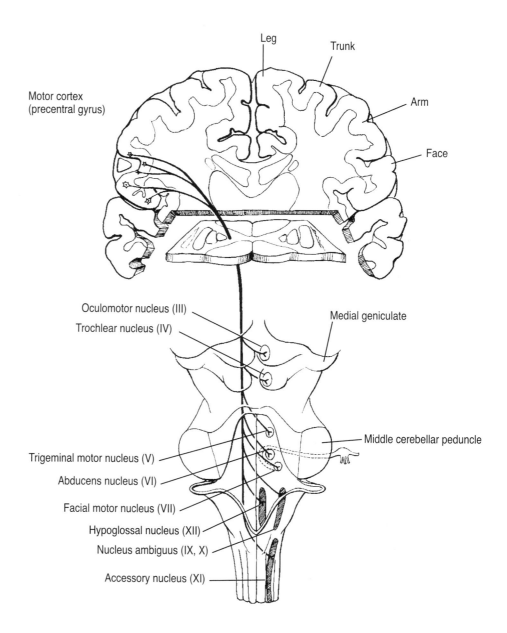

Leg

Trunk

Motor cortex (precentral gyrus)

Arm

Face

Oculomotor nucleus (III)

Trochlear nucleus (IV)

Medial geniculate

Trigeminal motor nucleus (V)

Abducens nucleus (VI)

Facial motor nucleus (VII)

Hypoglossal nucleus (XII)

Nucleus ambiguus (IX, X)

Accessory nucleus (XI)

Middle cerebellar peduncle

Corticobulbar and Corticospinal Summary

Definitions

The term pyramidal system (tract) originally referred to fibers in the medullary pyramids and was used to describe the corticospinal pathway under voluntary control. Extrapyramidal system (tract) referred to all other descending motor pathways. It seems preferable to use the terms corticobulbar, corticospinal, and subcortically originating pathways to name the parts of one unified motor system.

Structural and Functional Features

Axons from cortical pyramidal cells descend through the telencephalon as the **corona radiata.** They traverse the **internal capsule** (telencephalic–diencephalic area) and the basal region of the midbrain, the pons, and the medulla. Fibers destined for cranial nerve nuclei terminate throughout the brain stem. In the caudal medulla about 85% of the corticospinal fibers cross and descend in the lateral funiculus of the cord as the **lateral corticospinal tract. The ventral corticospinal tract** continues **uncrossed** in the ventral funiculus of the spinal cord. (A few **uncrossed** fibers descend in the lateral funiculus. For simplicity, ignore them.)

The majority (97%) of the corticospinal axons terminate on **interneurons** in Rexed's laminae V–VIII. A few (3%) terminate directly on anterior motor neurons in the medial and lateral cell columns in lamina IX. Axons from motor neurons (final common pathway) reach striated muscle via peripheral nerves.

The Roman numerals in the diagram represent the rostral to caudal location of cranial nerve motor nuclei in the brain stem. III and IV are at midbrain level; V, VI, and VII are in the pons; IX, X, and XII are in the medulla; and XI arises from neurons at upper cervical spinal cord levels. Cortical control of the cranial nerves is predominantly contralateral but a significant number of corticobulbar fibers are ipsilateral. Cranial nerves I, II, and VIII lack motor components. CN I,

the olfactory nerve, is in the telencephalon; CN II, the optic nerve, is in the diencephalon; and CN VIII, the vestibulocochlear nerve, is at the medullopontine junction.

There are also fibers descending from the cortex and from subcortical nuclei that travel with the motor fibers but function to modulate activity in the sensory pathways and in spinal reflexes; therefore, corticobulbar fibers are important for sensory modulation of cranial nerve input as well as motor control of voluntary and autonomic functions (pages 146 and 147) mediated through the cranial nerves.

Color the circles of the **general somatic efferent** (GSE) components red (cranial nerve nuclei III, IV, VI, and XII).

Color the circles of the **special visceral efferent** (SVE) components green (cranial nerve nuclei V, VII, IX, X, and XI).

Parasympathetic nuclei make up the **general visceral efferent** (GVE) component of cranial nerves III, VII, IX, and X (pages 146 and 147) and will be colored on page 147.

Color the corticobulbar and corticospinal projections red. Color the lateral and ventral corticospinal tracts red.

Color the caudate nucleus and the putamen green, the globus pallidus red, and the thalamus blue. Consider that the putamen and globus pallidus, which are lateral to the internal capsule, compose the lenticular (lens-shaped) nucleus. The caudate nucleus and thalamus are medial to the internal capsule.

Corticobulbar and Corticospinal Summary

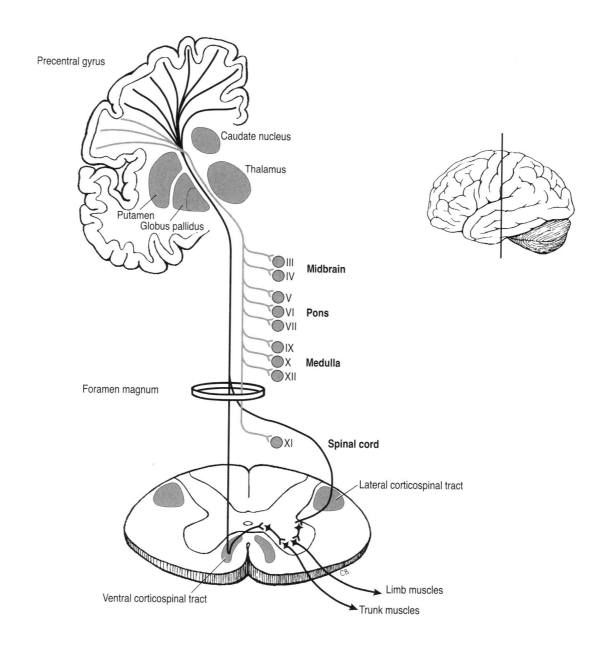

Precentral gyrus

Caudate nucleus

Thalamus

Putamen
Globus pallidus

III
IV **Midbrain**

V
VI **Pons**
VII

IX
X **Medulla**
XII

Foramen magnum

XI **Spinal cord**

Lateral corticospinal tract

Ventral corticospinal tract

Limb muscles

Trunk muscles

Sympathetic (Thoracolumbar) Division of the Autonomic Nervous System

Introduction of ANS

The efferent component of the autonomic motor system innervates visceral organs, glands, and the cardiovascular system through a two-neuron pathway. The **preganglionic neuron,** whose cell body is in the **CNS,** projects to a **peripheral ganglion** containing a **postganglionic neuron** whose axon terminates on the target organ. Sympathetic and parasympathetic divisions (pages 146 and 147) that are anatomically and neurochemically distinct make up the ANS. **Acetylcholine** (ACh) is the principal neurotransmitter of **all preganglionic neurons** in both divisions. Parasympathetic postganglionic neurons also use ACh as do postganglionic sympathetic neurons that innervate sweat glands. All other postganglionic sympathetic neurons use **norepinephrine.** Other transmitters such as peptides also occur in autonomic neurons.

The enteric nervous system, a third division of the ANS, consists of neuronal plexuses in the gastrointestinal tract and functions essentially autonomously. Many homeostatic functions are maintained through local circuits in peripheral ganglia, the spinal cord, or the brain stem. Complex functions are integrated through diencephalic structures (especially the hypothalamus) and basal forebrain structures. A prominent pathway is the **dorsal longitudinal fasciculus** with connections to and from the hypothalamus and preganglionic neurons in the brain stem and spinal cord.

Table 4-1. Sympathetic (Thoracolumbar) Division of the Autonomic Nervous System

Preganglionic Fibers		Postganglionic Fibers		
Cells of Origin	**Route**	**Cells of Origin**	**Route**	**Organs Innervated**
Intermediolateral cell column T1-L2	Ventral root and white communicating ramus to:	Chain (paravertebral) ganglion at level of entry	Gray communicating ramus and spinal nerve	Peripheral blood vessels Glands of skin Smooth muscle (arrector pili)
	Ascend or descend in sympathetic trunk	Chain ganglia above or below level of entry		
	Ventral root and white communicating ramus; ascend in thoracic sympathetic trunk	**Cervical ganglia** Superior	Carotid plexus along blood vessels	Head: blood vessels, glands, smooth muscles and glands of skin
		Middle Inferior	Cardiac nerves	Eye: smooth muscle of the lid and orbit, dilator pupillae Heart
	Ventral root and white communicating ramus	**Upper thoracic chain ganglia**		Bronchi and lungs
	Continue transversely through the sympathetic chain, still as preganglionics (splanchnic nerves)	**Prevertebral ganglia** Celiac		Liver, gallbladder, stomach, pancreas, and kidney
		Superior mesenteric		Small intestine and ascending colon
		Inferior mesenteric		Large intestine, rectum, urinary and reproductive tracts
			Adrenal gland	Paracrine/endocrine influence on organs by epinephrine and norepinephrine released into blood

Color orange the preganglionic fibers (solid lines) at T1-L2. Note that only these levels contain sympathetic neurons and white rami (unmyelinated fibers). At other levels, spinal nerves receive preganglionic sympathetic fibers that originate in upper or lower levels and ascend or descend in the sympathetic trunk. Postganglionic fibers are unmyelinated and compose the gray rami (broken lines) to all spinal nerves (represented to the left of the sympathetic trunk). Postganglionic fibers that innervate visceral structures are to the right. Color **all** postganglionic fibers orange. Certain preganglionic fibers to the abdominal and pelvic viscera are called splanchnic nerves; these as well as those to the head and thorax usually reach their destination via arteries.

Sympathetic (Thoracolumbar) Division of the Autonomic Nervous System

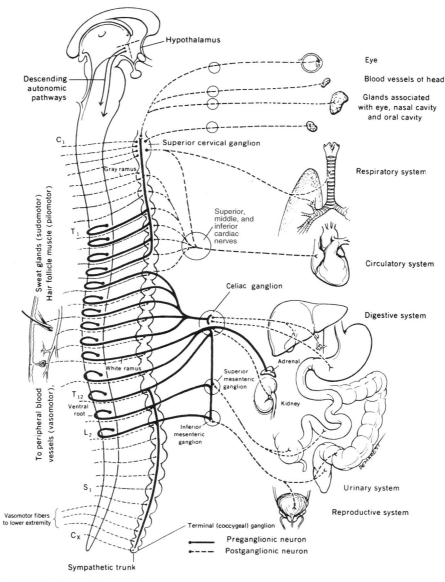

(Reprinted with permission from Noback CR, Strominger RL, Demarest RJ. **The Human Nervous System.** Lea & Febiger, 1991:323.)

Parasympathetic (Craniosacral) Division of the Autonomic Nervous System

Table 4-2. Parasympathetic (Craniosacral) Division of the Autonomic Nervous System

CRANIAL

Preganglionic fibers		Postganglionic fibers	
Cells of Origin	**Travel Via Cranial Nerve**	**Cells of Origin**	**Organ Innervated**
Endinger-Westphal nucleus (midbrain)	III	Ciliary ganglion	Ciliary muscle and iris of eye
Superior salivatory nucleus (pons)	VII	Pterygopalatine (sphenopalatine) ganglion	Lacrimal gland
		Submandibular ganglion	Submandibular and sublingual salivary glands
Inferior salivatory nucleus (medulla)	IX	Otic ganglion	Parotid salivary gland
Dorsal motor nucleus (vagus) (medulla)	X	Terminal ganglia in organs	Pharynx, larynx, trachea, bronchi, lungs, esophagus, heart, stomach, small intestine, liver, ascending and transverse colon, pancreas, kidneys (?)

SACRAL

Intermediolateral cell column in sacral cord S2-S4 (some references list only S3 and S4)	Pelvic splanchnic nerves	Terminal ganglia in organs innervated	Descending and pelvic colon, rectum, bladder, external genitalia

Color orange the preganglionic parasympathetic fibers (solid lines) and observe the brain stem location of the cranial nerves, which compose the cranial segment. This diagram shows only S3 and S4 as composing the sacral segment although S2 is often included as well; therefore, add a contribution from S2. Color the postganglionic fibers (broken lines) orange. These fibers are rather short because they originate near or in the terminal organ.

Parasympathetic (Craniosacral) Division of the Autonomic Nervous System

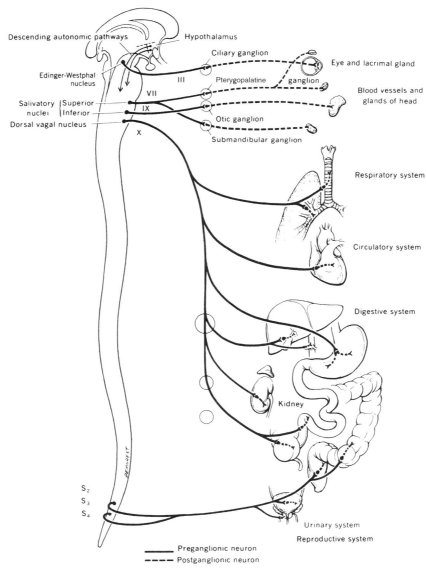

Descending autonomic pathways

Hypothalamus

Ciliary ganglion

Eye and lacrimal gland

Edinger-Westphal nucleus

III

Pterygopalatine ganglion

Blood vessels and glands of head

VII

Salivatory {Superior} nuclei {Inferior}

IX

Otic ganglion

Dorsal vagal nucleus

X

Submandibular ganglion

Respiratory system

Circulatory system

Digestive system

Kidney

S₂
S₃
S₄

Urinary system

Reproductive system

————— Preganglionic neuron
- - - - - Postganglionic neuron

(Reprinted with permission from Noback CR, Strominger NL, Demarest RJ. **The Human Nervous System.** Lea & Febiger, 1991:325.)

Dissection of the Left Hemisphere and Brain Stem From the Lateral Surface

This lateral view of the dissected left hemisphere and brain stem reveals a sweep of cortical efferent fibers en route to various subcortical targets. In their descent, they form the **corona radiata** (1), **internal capsule** (2), **base of the cerebral peduncle** (4), bundles of fibers in the **basal pons** (9), and the pyramids of the medulla. The **pyramidal decussation** (7) occurs at the junction of the medulla and spinal cord (foramen magnum).

Corticobulbar fibers terminate on nuclei in the tegmentum of the brain stem affecting cortical control, both crossed and uncrossed, over cranial nerve motor nuclei.

About 15% of the corticospinal fibers do not cross but continue caudally in the ventral funiculus of the spinal cord to motor neurons controlling trunk musculature. About 85% of the corticospinal fibers cross in the pyramidal decussation at the junction of the medulla and spinal cord and form the lateral corticospinal tract in the lateral funiculus. These terminate on interneurons or motor neurons controlling the limbs contralateral to the hemisphere of origin.

Additionally, the massive array of fibers shown include corticopontine fibers arising in frontal (frontopontine), parietal (parietopontine), occipital (occipitopontine), and temporal (temporo-pontine) lobes. These terminate in the pontine nuclei of the basal region of the pons. Ponto-cerebellar fibers arise from the pontine nuclei. Most of these fibers cross to enter the cerebellum through the contralateral **middle cerebellar peduncle** (5). This peduncle uniquely relates the cerebral cortex to the cerebellum; the **inferior cerebellar peduncle** (6) mainly interconnects nuclei in the spinal cord and medulla to the cerebellum.

The **olive** (8) is a structure lateral to the pyramid on the ventral surface of the medulla oblongata.

Prominently shown in this dissection are the **optic radiations** (3) from the lateral geniculate nucleus of the thalamus to the calcarine cortex, area 17, in the occipital lobe. Ventral to the frontal lobes, the cut **optic nerve** (14) can be seen continuing posteriorly to the **chiasm** (13). The **olfactory bulb** and **tract** (15) are also ventral in relation to the frontal lobe.

The **column** of the **fornix** (11) terminates mainly in the **mamillary body** of the hypothalamus (10). Note that it is immediately posterior to the **anterior commissure** (12), and recall that both the column of the fornix and the anterior commissure are anterior to the interventricular foramen.

One thing here is worth a great deal, to pass thy life in truth and justice,
with a benevolent disposition even to liars and unjust men. – Marcus Aurelius

Dissection of the Left Hemisphere and Brain Stem From the Lateral Surface

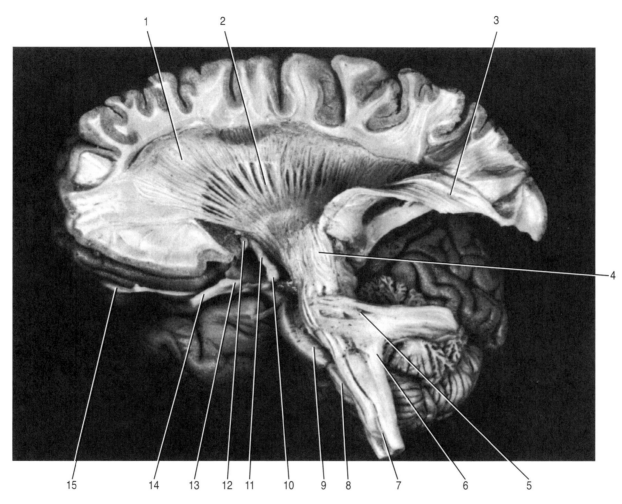

1. Corona radiata
2. Internal capsule
3. Optic radiations
4. Cerebral peduncle
5. Middle cerebellar peduncle
6. Inferior cerebellar peduncle
7. Pyramidal decussation
8. Olive
9. Basal pons, right
10. Mamillary body of hypothalamus
11. Fornix, column
12. Anterior commissure
13. Optic chiasm
14. Optic nerve
15. Olfactory bulb and tract

(Reprinted with permission from Ludwig E, Klingler J. **Atlas Cerebri Humani.** S. Karger, Basel, Switzerland, 1956, Table 23.)

Dissection of the Left Hemisphere From the Medial Surface With Brain Stem and Cerebellum Cut Midsagittally

The **ventricular system, brain stem** and **cerebellum** are focused on here because occipital lobe structures and centrally located pathways in the internal capsule have been defined and depicted in previous illustrations. This medial view shows the **thalamus** (6), **head** of the **caudate nucleus** (17), and the fibers of the **internal capsule** (15). Not visible in this dissection is the lenticular nucleus (globus pallidus and putamen), which is lateral to the fibers of the internal capsule.

Left and right lateral ventricles connect to the midline third ventricle through left and right interventricular foramina (of Monro). The **pineal gland** (5), a diencephalic structure, lies posterior to the third ventricle and is a useful landmark for defining the posterior commissure caudal to it and the habenular commissure rostral to it. Bordered by the thalami laterally and the hypothalamus laterally and ventrally, the third ventricle is connected to the fourth ventricle via the narrow cerebral aqueduct (of Sylvius). Midbrain structures dorsal to the cerebral aqueduct are collectively called the tectum. Ventral to the aqueduct is the tegmentum, which contains all ascending sensory pathways, some descending motor pathways, cranial nerve nuclei, and other important subcortical nuclei.

The **red nucleus** (19) and **substantia nigra** (20) are prominent nuclei in the tegmentum of the midbrain. Caudally the tegmental region extends into the pons and the medulla. The basal region of the pons is more extensive than are the basal regions of the midbrain rostrally and the medulla caudally. This region contains corticobulbar and corticospinal fibers as well as corticopontine fibers, pontine nuclei, and pontocerebellar fibers, and its uniqueness relates to its function as a way station or a bridge relating the cerebral cortex to the cerebellar cortex.

Dorsal to both the **pons** (23) and the **medulla oblongata** (24) and ventral to the cerebellum lies the **fourth ventricle** (25). Thus the posterior fossa of the cranium, which is roofed over by the tentorium cerebelli, houses the cerebellum, fourth ventricle, and the brain stem. The ventricular system contains the choroid plexuses, which continuously produce cerebrospinal fluid. Choroid plexuses are found in the floor of the lateral ventricles and in the roof of the third ventricle and are attached to the inferior medullary velum of the fourth ventricle. The only route of escape from the ventricular system is through the single midline foramen of Magendie or the lateral foramina of Luschka. These apertures permit passage of CSF into the subarachnoid space. Tumors in the cerebellum or in the brain stem may block these exit apertures and result in hydrocephalus.

Dissection of the Left Hemisphere From the Medial Surface With Brain Stem and Cerebellum Cut Midsagittally

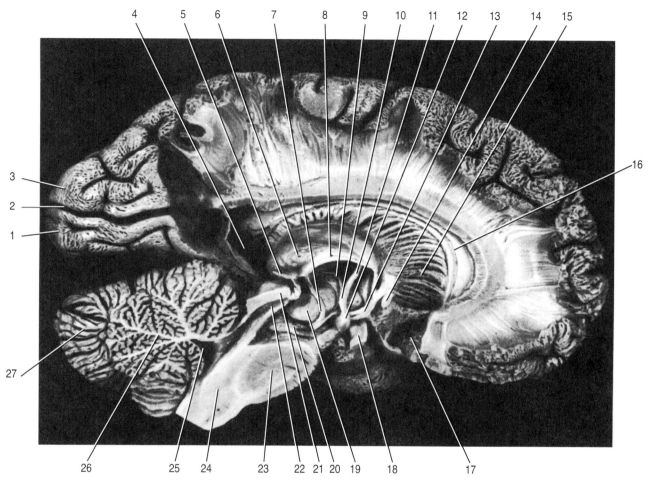

1. Lingual gyrus
2. Calcarine sulcus
3. Cuneus
4. Lateral ventricle
5. Pineal gland
6. Thalamus
7. Fasciculus retroflexus
8. Stria medullaris thalami
9. Mamillotegmental fasciculus
10. Principal mamillary fasciculus
11. Mamillothalamic fasciculus
12. Mamillary body of hypothalamus
13. Fornix, column
14. Anterior commissure
15. Internal capsule
16. Corpus callosum
17. Caudate, head
18. Optic tract
19. Red nucleus
20. Substantia nigra
21. Tectum
22. Cerebral aqueduct
23. Base of pons
24. Medulla oblongata
25. Fourth ventricle
26. Cerebellar vermis
27. Cerebellar hemisphere

(Reprinted with permission from Ludwig E, Klingler J. **Atlas Cerebri Humani.** S. Karger, Basel, Switzerland, 1956, Table 39.)

Chapter Four Study Questions

Directions: Each question below contains four or five suggested answers. Choose the **one best** response to each question.

1. **Which pathway transmits pain, temperature, and nondiscriminative touch impulses that ultimately reach the postcentral gyrus in the parietal lobe?**
    (a) Dorsal column
    (b) Medial lemniscus
    (c) Lateral lemniscus
    (d) Spinotectal
    (e) Spinothalamic

2. **Which statement is incorrect?**
    (a) The ventral spinocerebellar tract traverses the superior cerebellar peduncle.
    (b) The spinothalamic tract ascends in the brain stem tegmentum.
    (c) The corticopontine fibers descend through the base of the cerebral peduncle.
    (d) The medial lemniscus is an uncrossed pathway.
    (e) The corticospinal fibers descend in the base of the cerebral peduncle.

3. **Sensory information from the face ascends through the tegmentum of the brain stem to the ventral posteromedial nucleus of the thalamus via the**
    (a) Medial lemniscus
    (b) Dorsal longitudinal fasciculus
    (c) Dorsal and ventral trigeminothalamic tracts
    (d) Gracile fasciculus
    (e) Medial longitudinal fasciculus

4. **Second order neurons that transmit discriminative touch from the face are located in the**
    (a) Spinal nucleus of V
    (b) Chief sensory nucleus
    (c) Mesencephalic nucleus
    (d) Pterygopalatine ganglion
    (e) Superior salivatory nucleus

5. **The route through which pontocerebellar fibers reach the cerebellum is the**
    (a) Lateral lemniscus
    (b) Inferior cerebellar peduncle
    (c) Middle cerebellar peduncle
    (d) Superior cerebellar peduncle
    (e) Medial lemniscus

6. **Which cranial nerve motor nuclei are in the midbrain?**
    (a) The mesencephalic nucleus
    (b) Oculomotor
    (c) Trochlear
    (d) Oculomotor, trochlear and mesencephalic
    (e) Oculomotor and trochlear

7. **The column of the fornix terminates predominantly in the**
    (a) Habenula
    (b) Mamillary body
    (c) Pineal gland
    (d) Telencephalon
    (e) Subthalamus

8. **Which of these sequences correctly describes the descent of the corticospinal fibers?**
    (a) Corona radiata, posterior limb of the internal capsule, cerebral peduncle, basal pons, pyramid
    (b) Anterior limb of internal capsule, cerebral peduncle, basal pons, pyramid
    (c) Corona radiata, posterior limb of the internal capsule, tegmentum of the midbrain, basal pons, pyramid
    (d) Corona radiata, posterior limb of the internal capsule, cerebral peduncle, tegmentum of the pons, pyramid

9. **Which of the following parasympathetic preganglionic and postganglionic relations is a mismatch?**
    (a) Edinger-Westphal:ciliary ganglion
    (b) Dorsal motor nucleus (of X): terminal ganglia in organs
    (c) Superior salivatory nucleus:pterygopalatine ganglion
    (d) Inferior salivatory nucleus:otic ganglion
    (e) None of the above

10. **Pelvic splanchnic nerves transmit parasympathetic preganglionic impulses to terminal ganglia in the descending colon, and to the urinary and reproductive systems. The origin of these preganglionic fibers is from**
    (a) T1-L2
    (b) S2-S4
    (c) Dorsal motor nucleus (vagus)
    (d) Inferior salivatory nucleus
    (e) Inferior mesenteric ganglion

11. **The destination of corticobulbar fibers is**
    (a) Exclusively to motor neurons
    (b) Exclusively to sensory neurons
    (c) To contralateral and ipsilateral targets
    (d) Exclusively to ipsilateral targets
    (e) Exclusively to contralateral targets

Case History
A 45-year-old woman saw her family physician with the complaint of constant pain localized to the left upper face. The painful area was red and there were several vesicles over the left eyebrow.

12. **This history is most compatible with**
    (a) Trigeminal neuralgia
    (b) Tic douloureux
    (c) Ophthalmic herpes zoster
    (d) Maxillary herpes zoster
    (e) Mandibular herpes zoster

Answers and Explanations for Chapter Four Study Questions

1. **e** [pages 128 and 129] Fibers from dorsal root ganglion cells (1°) relay in the nucleus proprius (2°), cross in the ventral white commissure, and ascend to the ventral posterolateral nucleus (3°) of the thalamus. Axons from 3° neurons ascend through the posterior limb of the internal capsule to transmit pain, temperature, and nondiscriminative touch to the postcentral gyrus. The dorsal column–medial lemniscal system mediates proprioception, vibration, pressure, and discriminative touch. The lateral lemniscus is an auditory pathway. Spinotectal fibers terminate in the brain stem.

2. **d** [pages 126 and 132] Fibers from neurons in the gracile and cuneate nuclei in the caudal medulla swing ventrally, cross the midline, and ascend as the medial lemniscus through the tegmentum of the brain stem. Therefore, lesions of these fibers result in deficits contralateral and caudal to the site of the lesion. All other statements are true.

3. **c** [page 130] Second order fibers from the spinal nucleus, from the chief sensory nucleus, and from the mesencephalic nucleus transmit pain, temperature, and nondiscriminative touch and discriminative touch and proprioception from the face, respectively. Uncrossed fibers ascend in the dorsal, crossed fibers in the ventral trigeminothalamic tracts. They relay in the ventral posteromedial nucleus of the thalamus, which projects to the face area of the postcentral gyrus. The medial lemniscus transmits sensory input from the body, the dorsal longitudinal fasciculus contains ascending and descending fibers integrating autonomic activity, the gracile fasciculus is in the spinal cord, and the medial longitudinal fasciculus coordinates eye and head movements.

4. **b** [page 130] Central processes from large first order neurons in the trigeminal ganglion terminate on second order neurons in the chief sensory nucleus, which project via uncrossed dorsal and crossed ventral trigeminothalamic tracts to the ventral posteromedial nucleus of the thalamus. The spinal nucleus mediates pain, temperature, and nondiscriminative touch; and the mesencephalic nucleus mediates proprioception. The pterygopalatine ganglion and the superior salivatory nucleus are sources of parasympathetic postganglionic fibers and preganglionic fibers, respectively.

5. **c** [pages 126 and 148] The middle cerebellar peduncle is composed exclusively of fibers, which, through a relay in the basal pons, relate the cerebral cortex to the cerebellum. Some fibers from the arcuate nucleus (page 69) enter the MCP; however, arcuatocerebellar fibers are analogous to pontocerebellar fibers. The lateral lemniscus is an auditory pathway. The inferior cerebellar peduncle contains numerous pathways, most of which are afferent to the cerebellum from the spinal cord and medulla; however, efferent projections reach the brain stem through this peduncle also. The superior cerebellar peduncle is essentially an efferent route but it contains afferents to the cerebellum as well. The medial lemniscus traverses the brain stem, transmitting information from the body.

6. **e** [pages 126, 142] The oculomotor and trochlear nuclei are in the midbrain tegmentum at the level of the superior colliculi and inferior colliculi, respectively. The mesencephalic nucleus conducts sensory (proprioceptive) impulses and has no motor component.

7. **b** [page 148] Temporal lobe output via the fornix, mainly from pyramidal cells in the hippocampus, terminate predominantly in the mamillary body of the hypothalamus. The habenula receives the stria terminalis, the pineal is an endocrine gland, a minor complement of fibers reach basal and medial forebrain regions of the telencephalon via the fornix. The subthalamus is involved in motor circuits.

8. **a** [pages 127, 137, 143, and 149] Fibers form a radiating crown (corona radiata) as they descend from the cortex to the internal capsule (posterior limb). Together with the corticobulbar fibers the corticospinal fibers occupy the mid-region of the base of the cerebral peduncle. Corticospinal fibers spread out in the basal region of the pons and cluster again in the pyramid of the medulla. The lateral corticospinal tract crosses and descends in the lateral funiculus of the spinal cord. The ventral tract continues without crossing and descends in the ventral funiculus of the spinal cord.

9. **e** [page 147] All of the relations are correct. The two-neuron chain in **a** innervates the ciliary muscle and iris of the eye, in **b** visceral structures extending from the pharynx to the transverse colon are innervated via the vagus and terminal ganglia, **c** innervates the lacrimal gland, and **d** innervates blood vessels and glands of the head including the parotid.

10. **b** [page 147] Within the spinal cord, parasympathetic neurons are located only at S2-S4 levels. Preganglionic neurons are in the lateral horn at T1-L2 spinal levels; however, these are sympathetic. The dorsal motor nucleus is a preganglionic nucleus and projects axons to terminal ganglia of the viscera but only as caudal as the junction of the transverse and descending colon. The inferior mesenteric ganglion sends **postganglionic sympathetic** innervation to the lower colon and the urinary and reproductive systems.

11. **c** [page 140] The paramount destination of corticobulbar fibers is to contralateral motor nuclei in the brain stem. There are also ipsilateral projections (lower facial nucleus is an exception) to motor nuclei as well as corticobulbar fibers, which modulate sensory input, usually on the 2° neuron in the pathway.

Case History

12. **c** [pages 48 and 130] Both **a** and **b** answers are synonymous and refer to paroxysms of sharp intermittent pain that occur most frequently in CN V2 and CN V3 divisions of the trigeminal. Constant pain and vesicles localized to a dermatome or to the distribution of a cranial nerve unilaterally is suggestive of herpes zoster (shingles), which is caused by a viral inflammation of a dorsal root or cranial nerve ganglion. The topographic area affected is innervated by the ophthalmic division of CN V; corneal scars may result.

CHAPTER 5 Forebrain at the Level of the Striatum and Nucleus Accumbens

Definitions

The **forebrain** is derived from the prosencephalon (the most rostral subdivision of the embryonic brain) and includes the cerebrum and the diencephalon. The caudate and putamen are among the subcortical neuronal masses referred to as the **basal ganglia,** which are embedded in the lower parts of each cerebral hemisphere. (Ganglia is actually a misnomer; the term describes clusters of neurons outside the CNS.) The **caudate nucleus** and the **putamen** make up the **striatum** or **dorsal striatum**. The **nucleus accumbens** is ventromedial to the striatum and is referred to as ventral striatum because of its location, neural connections, and neurochemistry. The **ventral striatum** also contains the ventral divisions of both the caudate and putamen and the **substantia innominata**. The latter is an area in the anterior forebrain adjacent to the anterior perforated substance. It contains large, deeply staining cells that make up the basal nucleus of Meynert as well as several other nuclei. The nucleus accumbens receives projections from the cingulate and temporal gyri and from the piriform area, which is an olfactory relay center in the anterior temporal lobe medial to the rhinal sulcus. It includes the uncus and lateral olfactory stria and the anterior part of the parahippocampal gyrus including the entorhinal area. Projections from the nucleus accumbens reach the precommissural septum (see below) and other regions.

These large nuclear masses, the basal ganglia, are interconnected with the cerebral cortex, thalamus, and brain stem and play a significant role in motor control. Fibers ascending to and descending from the cerebral cortex pass through or between the basal ganglia and the thalamus. Bridges of neurons connecting the caudate and putamen across the internal capsule account for the striated appearance, hence the terms striatum and **corpus striatum**. The latter includes the **striatum** and the **globus pallidus** (pallidum; paleostriatum). In anatomic usage, the term basal ganglia most often refers to the corpus striatum. In early texts, less was known regarding function, and the **amygdala** and **claustrum** were included as well (see below for clinical terminology). The **anterior limb of the internal capsule** refers to the fibers **bounded medially** by the **head of the caudate nucleus** and **laterally** by the **lenticular nucleus** (**putamen** and **globus pallidus,** see below).

Structural and Functional Features

The phylogenetically related caudate and putamen are connected by cellular bridges across the anterior limb of the internal capsule. The head of the caudate nucleus forms the **lateral wall** of the **anterior (frontal) horn of the lateral ventricle**. The **corpus callosum** connects similar neocortical areas of the two hemispheres. The **cingulum** and the **superior occipitofrontal fasciculus** contain **associational fibers** confined to one hemisphere. The internal capsule largely contains **projection fibers,** which establish **reciprocal connections** between the **cerebral cortex** and **subcortical centers**. Specifically, the anterior limb of the internal capsule contains **corticopontine fibers** and reciprocal connections between the **mediodorsal thalamic nucleus** and the **prefrontal cortex** (**thalamocortical** and **corticothalamic fibers**). Projections from the anterior nucleus of the thalamus reach the cingulum through the **anterior limb**, and corticostriate fibers also pass through the an-

terior limb. As fibers fan out in the white matter of the **telencephalon,** they form a radiating crown, the **corona radiata**. This section is anterior to the **globus pallidus**. The **claustrum** is a neuronal strip between the cortex of the **insula** and the putamen. Fibers between the putamen and claustrum make up the **external capsule**. Fibers traversing lateral to the claustrum and **medial** to the **insula** compose the **extreme** capsule.

The **septum pellucidum** forms the **medial wall** of the **lateral ventricles**. The **septal nuclei** and the **gyrus rectus** lie **ventral** to the septum pellucidum. The septal nuclei are in front of the anterior commissure in the subcallosal area named the precommissural septum. This area is continuous with the internal portion of the globus pallidus, thus, these **precommissural septal nuclei** are referred to as the **ventral pallidum**. The **anterior cerebral arteries** lie within the interhemispheric fissure. The **cingulate gyrus** lies adjacent to the falx cerebri, which lies within the fissure.

Clinical Correlations . . . .

As used by many clinicians, the term basal ganglia encompasses the **corpus striatum,** the **subthalamic nucleus,** and the **substantia nigra**. This reflects involvement of circuitry of additional structures that, like the corpus striatum, are central to **motor control**. Lesions of these structures result in **unwanted involuntary movements** as opposed to paralysis. In patients with **Huntington's disease,** athetoid (slow, writhing) movements, choreiform (sudden, jerky) movements, and progressive mental deterioration are characteristically observed and are attended by marked neuronal degeneration in the striatum and cerebral cortex. The loss of neurons is often particularly evident in the **caudate nucleus** because it borders the ventricle.

A more common basal ganglia disorder is **Parkinson's disease**. It is characterized by tremor at rest, muscular rigidity, slowness of movements (bradykinesia), and postural instability. Degeneration of the pars compacta cells of the **substantia nigra** can be demonstrated at autopsy. Axons from these **dopaminergic** cells form the **nigrostriatal pathway** and innervate the ipsilateral caudate and putamen. **Resting tremor** that ceases with movement is distinguished from **intention tremor** that occurs only during movement. The latter is pathognomonic of cerebellar dysfunction.

On the right, color the CAU and PU (including bridges of neurons among ICap fibers) green. Color the NAcc yellow.

Forebrain at the Level of the Striatum and Nucleus Accumbens

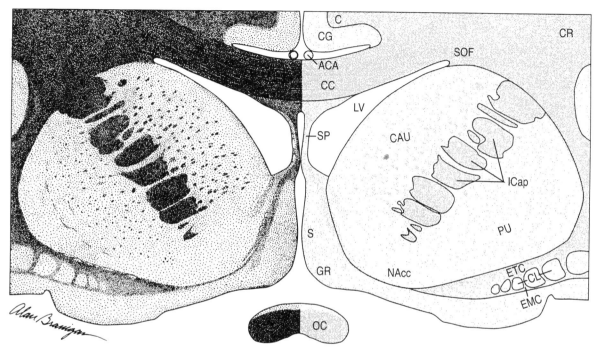

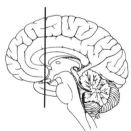

ACA	Anterior cerebral artery
C	Cingulum
CAU	Caudate nucleus (head)
CC	Corpus callosum
CG	Cingulate gyrus
CL	Claustrum
CR	Corona radiata
EMC	Extreme capsule
ETC	External capsule
GR	Gyrus rectus
ICap	Internal capsule (anterior limb), fibers
LV	Lateral ventricle (anterior horn)
NAcc	Nucleus accumbens
OC	Optic chiasm
PU	Putamen
S	Septal nuclei
SOF	Superior occipitofrontal fasciculus
SP	Septum pellucidum

Forebrain at the Level of the Anterior Nucleus of the Thalamus

Definitions

This section resembles that on page 155 only in the dorsal region, which contains the **cingulum, cingulate gyrus, anterior cerebral artery, corpus callosum, lateral ventricle, superior occipitofrontal fasciculus,** and **corona radiata.** The **thalamus** and **hypothalamus,** demarcated by the **hypothalamic sulcus,** form the **walls** of the **third ventricle. The posterior limb of the internal capsule** lies between the **thalamus medially** and the **lenticular nucleus laterally.** The **fornix** is a bundle of fibers that **connects** the **hippocampal formation** of the temporal lobe with the septal area, anterior thalamus, and hypothalamus. From caudal to rostral, the main parts of the fornix are the **crus,** the **body,** and the **column** (page 169). The crus is continuous with the fimbria in the temporal lobe. It arches upward and medially and is continuous with the body under the **splenium** of the **corpus callosum.** The body passes forward in the **free edge** of the **septum pellucidum** to a point above the **anterior commissure.** The column is that part which **turns backward** and **downward** behind the anterior commissure to terminate in the **hypothalamus** (mainly in the **mamillary body**). A small bundle of fornix fibers descends precommissurally en route to the septal nuclei. The column divides the hypothalamus into **medial** and **lateral** zones. The **tuber cinereum** is a slight elevation between the mamillary bodies posteriorly and the optic chiasm anteriorly. This **section** is posterior to the optic chiasm but **transects** the **optic tracts** as they **encircle** the **cerebral peduncles** en route to the **lateral geniculate nuclei** of the thalami.

Fibers in the **anterior commissure** traverse the midline in the lamina terminalis, a structure that forms the rostral wall of the third ventricle. There is a component of the anterior commissure that is functionally similar to the corpus callosum in that it connects the middle and inferior temporal gyri of the two hemispheres that are neocortical (six-layered). Other fibers in the commissure, not functionally analogous to the corpus callosum, connect **olfactory areas** of the temporal lobes, which are allocortical (three-layered).

Structural and Functional Features

Observe the tufts of **choroid plexus** in the **floor of the lateral ventricles** and in the **roof of the third ventricle.** The subfornical organ is one of several highly vascularized tissues located in midline ventricular positions (circumventricular) that lack a blood-brain barrier. It lies between the columns of the fornix in the anterior wall of the third ventricle. The **neurons of the subfornical organ** function as **primary afferent receptors.** These osmoregulatory neurons respond to small changes in the osmolality of the blood and, in turn, project to the vasopressin-producing cells in the hypothalamus, thus contributing to **body fluid regulation.** Additionally, the subfornical organ has connections with the limbic lobe through which it is involved in the behavioral thirst drive.

The **anterior nucleus of the thalamus** underlies the **anterior thalamic tubercle.** The **anterior nucleus** is bordered ventromedially by the **stria medullaris thalami,** dorsolaterally by the **stria terminalis,** and laterally by the **internal medullary lamina** (page 161). The anterior nucleus **receives mamillothalamic projections** and **projects** to the **cingulate gyrus**; thus, it is pivotal to limbic system connections. The **stria medullaris thalami** runs along the dorsal medial border of the thalamus from the **interventricular foramen** to the **habenula.** It reciprocally connects septal and hypothalamic areas with the habenular nucleus. The **internal cerebral vein** lies superior to the stria medullaris.

The **stria terminalis** is a nerve fiber bundle that extends along the **medial border** of the **body of the caudate nucleus.** It reciprocally connects the **amygdala** and the medial hypothalamus. The amygdala is a subcortical neuronal mass located in the **temporal lobe** anterior to the inferior horn of the lateral ventricle (pages 169 and 175). The **ventroanterior nucleus** lies between the **anterior nucleus** and the **posterior limb of the internal capsule.** The lenticular nucleus borders the posterior limb of the internal capsule laterally. It comprises the **internal** and **external** segments of the **globus pallidus** and the **putamen.** The internal capsule and lenticular nucleus are also discussed on pages 158 and 164.

Clinical Correlations . . . .

Obstruction of the interventricular foramen occurs rarely, but may occur due to a cyst of the choroid plexus, resulting in **unilateral dilation** of the **lateral ventricle.** Lesions of the **fornix** deprive the hypothalamus of hippocampal input from the temporal lobe and have been associated with **amnesia.**

On the right color the CAU and PU green, the GPI and GPE red, the AN and VA blue, the HYM orange, the HYL brown, and the BN(M) yellow. Color the AGD with vertical yellow stripes.

Forebrain at the Level of the Anterior Nucleus of the Thalamus

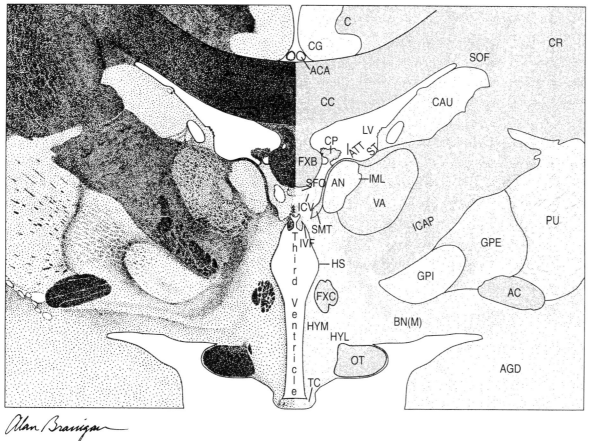

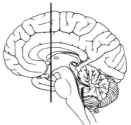

AC	Anterior commissure
ACA	Anterior cerebral artery
AGD	Amygdala
AN	Anterior nucleus of thalamus
ATT	Anterior tubercle of thalamus
BN(M)	Basal nucleus (of Meynert)
C	Cingulum
CAU	Caudate nucleus (body)
CC	Corpus callosum
CG	Cingulate gyrus
CP	Choroid plexus
CR	Corona radiata
FXB	Body of the fornix
FXC	Columns of the fornix
GPE	Globus pallidus (external)
GPI	Globus pallidus (internal)
HS	Hypothalamic sulcus
HYL	Hypothalamus (lateral)
HYM	Hypothalamus (medial)
ICap	Internal capsule (anterior limb)
ICV	Internal cerebral vein
IML	Internal medullary lamina
IVF	Interventricular foramen (of Monro)
LV	Lateral ventricle
OT	Optic tract
PU	Putamen
SFO	Subfornical organ
SMT	Stria medullaris thalami
SOF	Superior occipitofrontal fasciculus
ST	Stria terminalis
TC	Tuber cinereum
VA	Ventroanterior nucleus of thalamus

Forebrain at the Level of the Midthalamus

Definitions

Many of the structures in and around the **lateral ventricles** in the previous section are also present at this level. The **interthalamic adhesion (massa intermedia)**, evident in this brain, is an inconsistent structure of gray matter that joins the thalami across the **third ventricle**. Its absence in 20–30% of brains has no significance. Thalamic nuclei prominent at midthalamic level include the **laterodorsal**, **mediodorsal**, and **ventrolateral** nuclei. Input-output connections of these and other thalamic nuclei are depicted on page 161. A significant structure between the thalamus and the lenticular nucleus is the **posterior limb** of the **internal capsule. Thalamocortical fibers from the VPL and VPM nuclei traverse the posterior limb en route to the somatosensory cortex, and corticospinal fibers also pass via the posterior limb.** The lateral surface of the thalamus is covered by the **external medullary lamina** (a thin layer of nerve fibers) and the **thalamic reticular nucleus** (a thin sheet of nerve cells between the external medullary lamina and the **internal capsule**). The external medullary lamina of fibers is made up of thalamocortical and corticothalamic fibers passing in and out of the internal capsule. Most of the thalamic nuclei project to various cortical areas, but the thalamic reticular nucleus does not (page 161). It receives collaterals from thalamocortical and corticothalamic fibers and, in turn, projects to other thalamic nuclei. These connections are consistent with the suggested role of the thalamic reticular nucleus of modulating the output of individual thalamic nuclei.

Structural and Functional Features

Internal (medial) and **external (lateral)** segments of the **globus pallidus** are wedged between the **putamen** and the posterior limb of the internal capsule. Descending fibers in the posterior limb continue into the **basis pedunculi** of the midbrain. The elongated structure lying medially against the internal capsule, adjacent to the **substantia nigra** of the midbrain, is the **subthalamic nucleus.** It receives inhibitory projections from the external segment of the ipsilateral globus pallidus and sends excitatory projections to the internal segment of the globus pallidus. The subthalamic nucleus, therefore, modulates the output of the basal ganglia. The internal segment of the globus pallidus directly inhibits the thalamic nuclei involved in motor integration, i.e., the ventroanterior and ventrolateral nuclei.

The **mamillary bodies** define the posterior limit of the **hypothalamus.** Each body contains several nuclei. This part of the hypothalamus is integrated into the limbic system. It receives projections from the hippocampus and septal area through the fornix and sends projections to the cingulate gyrus via the anterior nucleus of the thalamus (Papez circuit, page 168). This circuitry plays a role in learning and in processing memory. The **mamillothalamic tract** contains fibers from the medial mamillary nucleus, which ascend through the **internal medullary lamina** to reach the anterior nucleus of the thalamus.

Two fiber bundles are prominent in the region rostral to the subthalamic nucleus. The **thalamic fasciculus** consists of fibers that originate in the globus pallidus, the dentate nucleus of the cerebellum, and the red nucleus and terminate mainly in the ventroanterior and ventrolateral nuclei of the thalamus. The **lenticular fasciculus** consists of fibers that originate in the lenticular nucleus and terminate in several motor-related nuclei including the ventroanterior and ventrolateral nuclei of the thalamus. At this level, the **optic tract** lies dorsomedial to the **hippocampus** of the temporal lobe.

Clinical Correlations . . . .

Cerebrovascular accidents occasionally damage the **subthalamic nucleus,** which sends excitatory projections to the internal segment of the globus pallidus. This results in a loss of excitation in this segment, which, if excited, inhibits the activity of the ventrolateral and ventroanterior nuclei of the thalamus. The net result is increased output from the motor cortex resulting in **violent flinging, uncontrollable, ballistic movements** of the **contralateral extremities**. Lateralized ballistic movements are described as **hemiballistic. Chronic alcohol abuse** results in degenerative changes in the **mamillary nuclei of the hypothalamus** and in the **mediodorsal nuclei of the thalamus.** Memory impairment in alcoholics (amnesic syndrome) is attributed to the chronic toxic effect of alcohol on these structures.

 On the right color the CAU and PU green, the GPI and GPE red, and the thalamus (LD, MD, VL) blue.

To be aware in youth of the advantages of age, to preserve in age the advantages of youth, each of these is one and the same good fortune. – Goethe

158

Forebrain at the Level of the Midthalamus

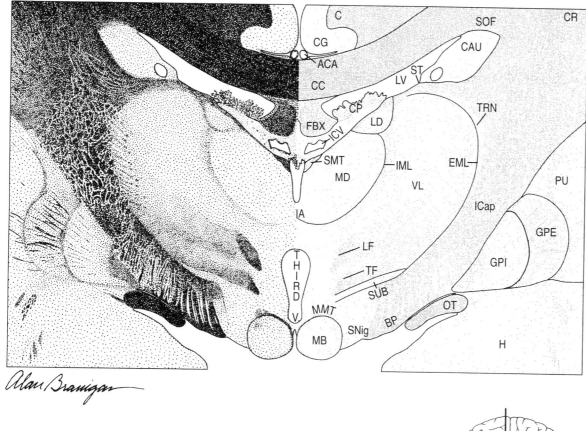

ACA	Anterior cerebral artery
BP	Basis pedunculi
C	Cingulum
CAU	Caudate nucleus (head)
CC	Corpus callosum
CG	Cingulate gyrus
CP	Choroid plexus
CR	Corona radiata
EML	External medullary lamina of thalamus
FXB	Body of the fornix
GPE	Globus pallidus (external)
GPI	Globus pallidus (internal)
H	Hippocampus
IA	Interthalamic adhesion
ICap	Internal capsule (posterior limb)
ICV	Internal cerebral vein
IML	Internal medullary lamina of thalamus
LD	Laterodorsal nucleus
LF	Lenticular fasciculus
LV	Lateral ventricle
MB	Mamillary body
MD	Mediodorsal nucleus
MMT	Mamillothalamic tract
OT	Optic tract
PU	Putamen
SMT	Stria medullaris thalami
SNig	Substantia nigra
SOF	Superior occipitofrontal fasciculus
SUB	Subthalamic nucleus
TF	Thalamic fasciculus
TRN	Thalamic reticular nucleus
VL	Ventrolateral nucleus

Thalamic Nuclei

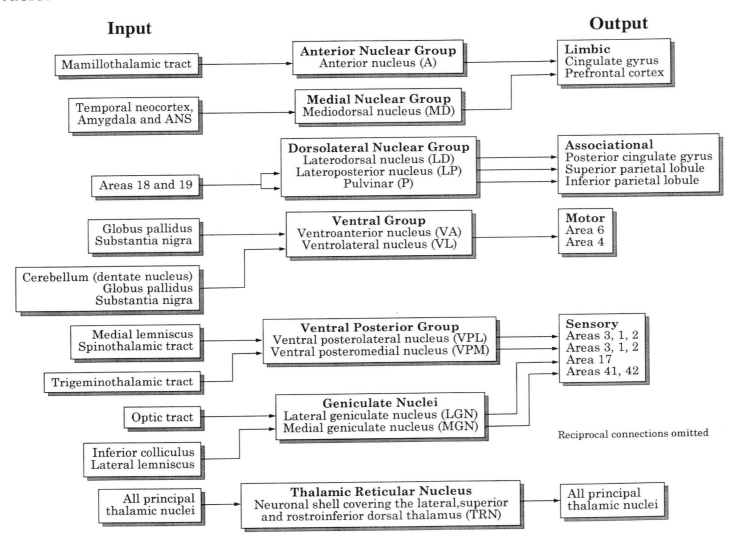

Input

Output

Mamillothalamic tract	**Anterior Nuclear Group** Anterior nucleus (A)	**Limbic** Cingulate gyrus Prefrontal cortex
Temporal neocortex, Amygdala and ANS	**Medial Nuclear Group** Mediodorsal nucleus (MD)	
Areas 18 and 19	**Dorsolateral Nuclear Group** Laterodorsal nucleus (LD) Lateroposterior nucleus (LP) Pulvinar (P)	**Associational** Posterior cingulate gyrus Superior parietal lobule Inferior parietal lobule
Globus pallidus Substantia nigra	**Ventral Group** Ventroanterior nucleus (VA) Ventrolateral nucleus (VL)	**Motor** Area 6 Area 4
Cerebellum (dentate nucleus) Globus pallidus Substantia nigra		
Medial lemniscus Spinothalamic tract	**Ventral Posterior Group** Ventral posterolateral nucleus (VPL) Ventral posteromedial nucleus (VPM)	**Sensory** Areas 3, 1, 2 Areas 3, 1, 2 Area 17 Areas 41, 42
Trigeminothalamic tract		
Optic tract	**Geniculate Nuclei** Lateral geniculate nucleus (LGN) Medial geniculate nucleus (MGN)	
Inferior colliculus Lateral lemniscus		
All principal thalamic nuclei	**Thalamic Reticular Nucleus** Neuronal shell covering the lateral,superior and rostroinferior dorsal thalamus (TRN)	All principal thalamic nuclei

Reciprocal connections omitted

On the right, color the IML orange; the MD purple; the A yellow; the LD, LP, and P green; the VA and VL red; the VPM, VPL, MGN, and LGN blue; and the TRN brown.

Thalamic Nuclei

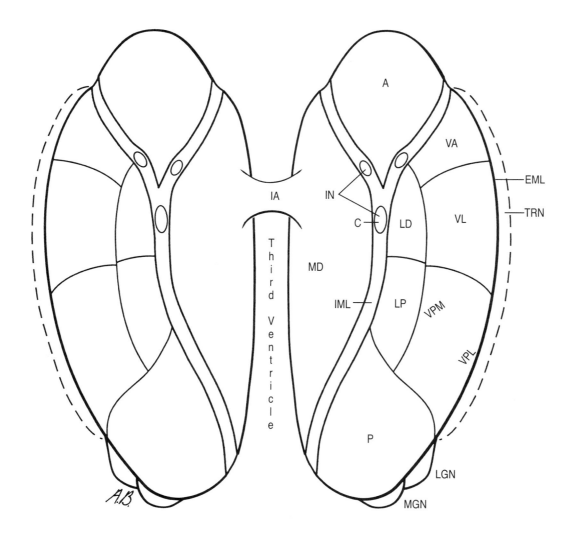

A	Anterior nucleus
C	Centromedian nucleus
EML	External medullary lamina
IA	Interthalamic adhesion
IML	Internal medullary lamina
IN	Intralaminar nuclei
LD	Lateral dorsal nucleus
LGN	Lateral geniculate nucleus
LP	Lateral posterior nucleus
MD	Mediodorsal nucleus
MGN	Medial geniculate nucleus
P	Pulvinar
TRN	Thalamic reticular nucleus
VA	Ventroanterior nucleus
VL	Ventrolateral nucleus
VPL	Ventral posterolateral nucleus
VPM	Ventral posteromedial nucleus

Hypothalamic Nuclei

Definitions

The diencephalon is divided into four regions: **dorsal thalamus** (syn: **thalamus**), **epithalamus, ventral thalamus**, and **hypothalamus**. As shown on page 160, the individual nuclei of the **thalamus** project to specific regions of the ipsilateral neocortex. The **epithalamus** consists of the habenular nuclei, the stria medullaris, the pineal gland, and part of the posterior commissure. The **ventral thalamus** (syn: subthalamus) is that part of the diencephalon located ventral to the dorsal thalamus and caudolateral to the hypothalamus. It consists of the subthalamic nucleus, the zona incerta, the nucleus of the field of Forel, the entopeduncular nucleus and the rostral extension of the red nucleus and substantia nigra. The ventral thalamus is not to be confused with the ventral nuclei of the dorsal thalamus. The **hypothalamus** is located on either side of the third ventricle, just ventral to the hypothalamic sulcus. The latter is a distinct groove in the wall of the ventricle (page 157).

Structural and Functional Features

The small size of the hypothalamus belies its functional importance. Its functions are related to regulation of temperature; food and water intake; sexual behavior and reproduction; circadian rhythms; and emotions including fear, rage, aversion, pleasure, and reward. As previously discussed, the **column of the fornix** divides the hypothalamus into **medial** and **lateral zones**. In a coronal plane, the hypothalamus has three zones: **periventricular, medial**, and **lateral**. It also has three areas in a midsagittal plane: **anterior** or **chiasmatic, middle** or **tuberal**, and **posterior** or **mamillary**. In the diagrams below, note that areas and nuclei are distinguished by a difference in the degree of shading. In the **anterior zone**, the preoptic area and the anterior area contain ill-defined small nuclear groups; both areas are involved in sexual and reproductive behavior. The anterior zone of the hypothalamus also contains the prominent **paraventricular** and **supraoptic nuclei** whose neurohormone secretions travel through axons that form the neurohypophysial tract. The terminals of these axons release **oxytocin** and **vasopressin (antidiuretic hormone, ADH)** adjacent to capillaries in the neurohypophysis. ADH contracts small blood vessels, raises blood pressure, and reduces the excretion of urine by the kidneys, hence its name. The ADH-producing cells are sensitive to circulating plasma osmolality as are cells of the organum vasculosum, subfornical organ (page 157), and periventricular nucleus.

Oxytocin stimulates contraction of the myoepithelial cells of the **mammary glands** (milk-ejection reflex) and of the myometrial cells of the uterus (contractions at parturition). The oxytocin-producing cells receive afferents from serotonergic neurons of the midbrain raphe and from neurons in the hypothalamic arcuate nuclei. The **suprachiasmatic** nucleus is also in the anterior region. It receives input from the **retina** and from the **lateral geniculate nucleus** and, as the pineal gland, is implicated in **circadian rhythms**.

The middle hypothalamus contains the **arcuate**, the **ventromedial**, and the **dorsomedial nuclei**. Both the **ventromedial** and **dorsomedial** nuclei play a role in **food intake.** Caloric intake is thought to be monitored by glucose-sensitive cells in the ventromedial nucleus. The ventromedial nucleus has afferent and efferent connections with the amygdala, the reticular formation, the periaqueductal gray, and other CNS regions. The function of the adenohypophysis (AH) is under the humoral control of the hypothalamus. Hypothalamic cells in the tuberal region (periventricular and arcuate nuclei) synthesize and release hypothalamic hypophysiotropic hormones (HHHs) into the hypophysial portal vessels in the median eminence. Within the AH, HHHs stimulate or inhibit the release of AH hormones, which have widespread endocrine functions.

In the **posterior** or **mamillary region,** a complex of nuclei form a breast-like elevation, the mamillary bodies, on the ventral surface of the hypothalamus. The mamillary nuclei receive the fornix and project to the anterior nuclei of the thalamus via the myelinated mamillothalamic tract. Most hypothalamic connections are reciprocal and are unmyelinated or lightly myelinated. The medial forebrain bundle, for example, is a diffuse array of small fibers that traverses the lateral hypothalamus in an anteroposterior direction, interconnecting the hypothalamus with the brain stem and basal forebrain. The dorsal longitudinal fasciculus provides another efferent route between the hypothalamus and the brain stem. Its fibers terminate on parasympathetic nuclei and other brain stem centers (page 168). Like most pathways, it is a reciprocal one.

In summary, the **hypothalamus** modifies the synthesis and release of hypophysial hormones through neuronal and vascular links. It regulates **autonomic functions** via efferent fibers to the brain stem and spinal cord. In general, the **anterior** and **medial regions** of the hypothalamus are associated with **parasympathetic** activity, whereas the **posterior** and lateral regions are concerned with **sympathetic** responses. Finally, through limbic system connections, the hypothalamus is integrated into **cortical circuits** that **mediate emotional behavioral responses**.

Clinical Correlations . . . .

(See Page 174)

On the medial view, color the anterior area yellow, the middle area orange, the posterior area purple, and the thalamus blue. On the coronal section, color the thalamus blue, PEVN and ARN dark green, the VMN and DMN orange, the LHA brown, the CAU and putamen green, and the GPI and GPE red.

There is a graciousness of the heart; it is related to love.
It is the source of the most natural graciousness of outward conduct. – Goethe

Medial View of the Hypothalamus

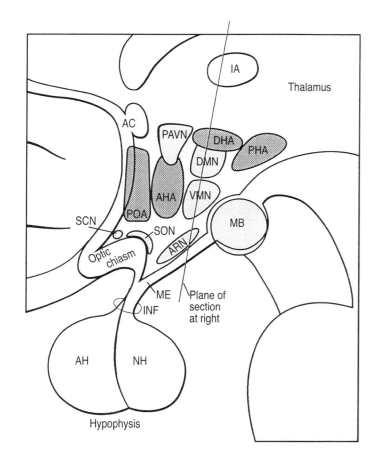

CORONAL SECTION

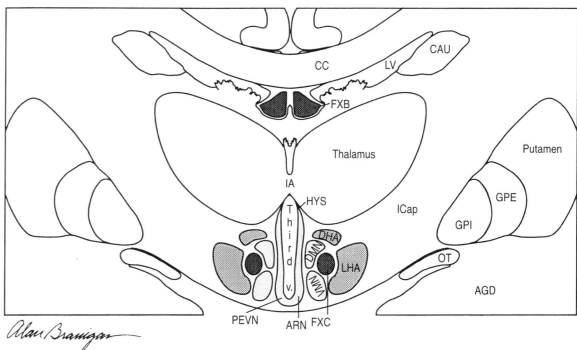

AC	Anterior commissure	DMN	Dorsomedial nucleus	INF	Infundibulum	PEVN	Periventricular nucleus
AGD	Amygdala	FXB	Fornix (body)	LHA	Lateral hypothalamic area	PHA	Posterior hypothalamic area
AH	Adenohypophysis	FXC	Fornix (column)	LV	Lateral ventricle	POA	Preoptic area
AHA	Anterior hypothalamic area	GPE	Globus pallidus (external)	MB	Mamillary body	SCN	Suprachiasmatic nucleus
ARN	Arcuate nucleus	GPI	Globus pallidus (internal)	ME	Median eminence	SON	Supraoptic nucleus
CAU	Caudate (body)	HYS	Hypothalamic sulcus	NH	Neurohypophysis	VMN	Ventromedial nucleus
CC	Corpus callosum	IA	Interthalamic adhesion	OT	Optic tract		
DHA	Dorsal hypothalamic area	ICap	Internal capsule (posterior limb)	PAVN	Paraventricular nucleus		

A Horizontal Section of the Brain Through the Basal Ganglia, Thalamus, and Internal Capsule

Note: Many of these structures have been discussed relative to their appearance in coronal views. Boundaries of the internal capsule are repeated in reference to this horizontal dissection with a schematic diagram of all components of the right internal capsule.

Definitions
The **glomus choroideum** is an expanded portion of the choroid plexus in the collateral trigone of the lateral ventricle. The **trigone** or **atrium** is the junction of the body and the inferior and posterior horns of the lateral ventricle. Recall that the putamen and globus pallidus make up the lenticular nucleus.

Structural and Functional Features
Note the oval dark head of the **caudate nucleus** (2) together with the equally dark **putamen** (6). The pallor of the globus pallidus is due to its being traversed by numerous myelinated fibers. The putamen (6) and **globus pallidus** (7) are topographically related, lying lateral to the internal capsule. Note the head of the caudate nucleus bulging into the **anterior horn of the lateral ventricle** (24).

Observe the **internal capsule** (3), bordered by the caudate nucleus and **thalamus** (10) medially and by the lenticular nucleus laterally. It mainly contains projection fibers, both ascending (corticopetal) and descending (corticofugal) fibers. The **anterior limb** of the capsule lies between the caudate nucleus medially and the lenticular laterally. It contains frontal corticopontine fibers and thalamic radiations both from the anterior nucleus and the mediodorsal nucleus. The **genu** (knee) is at the bend between the anterior and posterior limbs. It comprises the corticobulbar fibers from areas 3,1,2 and the thalamocortical projections to areas 4 and 6. The **posterior limb** lies between the thalamus medially and the lenticular nucleus laterally. Among its fibers are the corticospinal tract (motor) and the thalamocortical radiations (sensory). The posterior limb also contains corticothalamic fibers and other corticofugal fibers including many to the basal pons (corticopontine; parieto-occipito-temporopontine). The retrolenticular portion of the internal capsule contains **optic radiations** (14) (geniculocalcarine fibers) from the lateral geniculate nucleus (LGN) to the occipital lobe, whereas the sublenticular portion contains fibers that originate in the medial geniculate nucleus (MGN) of the thalamus and terminate in the temporal lobe.

Projection fibers in the internal capsule are distinguished from the corpus callosal fibers as follows: The former connect the cortex to subcortical centers whereas the latter connect like areas in the two hemispheres. The **genu of the corpus callosum** (1) contains numerous fibers connecting frontal cortices whereas the **genu of the internal capsule** (3) contains corticobulbar fibers.

Observe the **external capsule** (9) between the putamen (6) and **claustrum** (5) and the **extreme capsule** (8) between the claustrum and the **insula** (4). The insula lies in the depth of the lateral fissure.

In the posterior corners of the lateral wall on either side of the **third ventricle** (20) lie the **habenulae** (11), which are protuberances that contain the habenular nuclei. These nuclei are connected across the midline rostral to the pineal gland via the habenular commissure. Another subcortical commissure is the **posterior commissure** (19), located caudal to the pineal. It is partly composed of fibers interconnecting the two pretectal nuclei at the junction of the midbrain and diencephalon.

The **velum interpositum** (18) is pia mater and connective tissue located between the corpus callosum dorsally and the dorsal thalamus, roof of the third ventricle, and pineal gland ventrally. The internal cerebral veins pass through it en route to becoming a single great cerebral vein (of Galen), which is continuous with the straight sinus.

This asymmetric section reveals the **hippocampus** (13) on the right. This horizontal (axial) view clearly demonstrates the **anterior horns of the lateral ventricles** (24) in the frontal lobe and the **posterior horns** (15) extending into the occipital lobes. Note the **interventricular foramina** (22) connecting the lateral ventricles with the **third ventricle** (20), which, in this specimen as in the previous coronal ones, contains a connecting bridge between the thalami—the **interthalamic adhesion** (21). Both the column of the **fornix** (23) and the **crux** (17) are apparent as is the **glomus choroideum** (16).

Clinical Correlations . . . .

Vascular lesions are discussed in Chapter 6. The glomus choroideum may **calcify** and serve as a radiographic landmark in the **collateral trigone** of the **lateral ventricle** (12).

In the diagram of the right internal capsule, color green the caudate and putamen; color red the globus pallidus; and color blue the thalamus, medial geniculate nucleus (MGN), the lateral geniculate nucleus (LGN), and sublenticular and retrolenticular pathways.

A Horizontal Section of the Brain Through the Basal Ganglia, Thalamus, and Internal Capsule

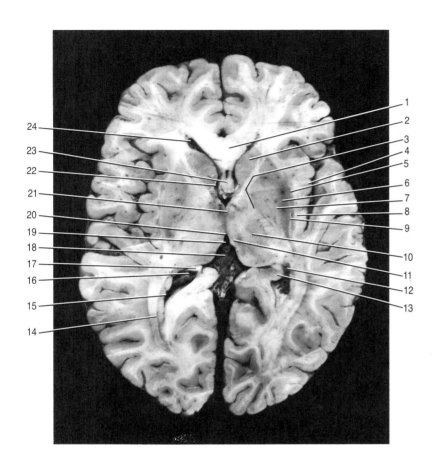

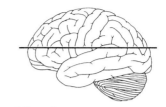

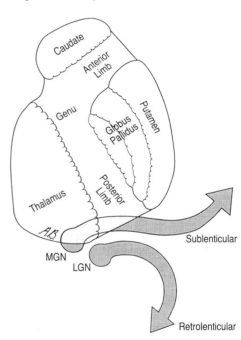

Right Internal Capsule

1. Corpus callosum (genu)
2. Caudate nucleus (head)
3. Internal capsule (anterior limb, genu, and posterior limb)
4. Insula
5. Claustrum
6. Putamen
7. Globus pallidus
8. Extreme capsule
9. External capsule
10. Thalamus
11. Habenula
12. Lateral ventricle (collateral trigone)
13. Hippocampus
14. Optic radiations
15. Lateral ventricle (posterior horn)
16. Glomus choroideum
17. Fornix (crux)
18. Velum interpositum
19. Posterior commissure (position of)
20. Third ventricle
21. Interthalamic adhesion
22. Interventricular foramen
23. Fornix (column)
24. Lateral ventricle (anterior horn)

Limbic System Structures: Dissection of the Right Hemisphere From the Medial Surface, Thalamic Radiations Exposed

Definitions

The terms **limbic lobe** and **limbic system** are derived from the Latin word *limbus,* meaning border. Limbic lobe refers to gyri that form a rim around the rostral part of the brain stem and adjoining forebrain. Limbic lobe is not a "lobe" in the anatomic sense. The limbic lobe of the cortex consists of the **cingulate** and **parahippocampal gyri**. Limbic system encompasses the "lobe" and functionally related **subcortical structures**. This dissection reveals many limbic nuclei and fiber tracts whose intricate connections mainly funnel sensory information to the hypothalamus. Through the hypothalamus, the limbic system modulates autonomic nervous system (ANS) and endocrine activity and indirectly influences the immune system.

Structural and Functional Features

Compare this dissection with those on pages 171 and 173 to appreciate the differences in medial versus lateral structures. As previously noted, the **thalamus** (4,5) forms the upper part of the lateral wall of the third ventricle. The caudate nucleus has been removed. The **mediodorsal nucleus** (5) of the thalamus has reciprocal connections with the **prefrontal cortex** (1) through the anterior limb of the internal capsule, as does the **anterior nucleus** (4) whose fibers, via the anterior thalamic radiation, project to the **cingulate gyrus** (2). The **cingulum** (3) is an association bundle of fibers located mainly within the cingulate gyrus. The mediodorsal nucleus also has connections to the amygdala and olfactory cortex. Anteriorly the corpus callosum (6) has been cut away to reveal the **thalamic radiations** (1,2). The **splenium** (7) (bulbous posterior extent) is robust with fibers, especially with occipital interconnections. Posterior to the splenium of the **corpus callosum** (7) is the continuation of the cut surface of the cingulate gyrus. The cingulate gyrus extends from the subcallosal region beneath the rostrum of the corpus callosum and passes behind the splenium of the corpus callosum where it continues as the isthmus (narrow passage) and merges into the parahippocampal gyrus. Thus, the cingulate gyrus encircles the corpus callosum and encompasses temporal as well as frontal and parietal cortices on the medial surface of the hemisphere.

On the medial surface, the **parieto-occipital sulcus** (8) defines parietal and occipital lobe boundaries, and the **calcarine sulcus** (10) marks area 17, which receives the terminal optic radiations. The occipital lobe is more extensive on the medial surface than on the lateral, and almost all of the primary visual cortex is located medially on the banks of, and in the depth of, the calcarine sulcus. The wedge-shaped gyrus above the calcarine sulcus is the **cuneus** (9), whereas the lin-

gual gyrus (11) of the occipital lobe lies below the sulcus and is continuous with the **parahippocampal gyrus** (12) of the temporal lobe. Fibers in the **fornix** (body) (13) bend ventrally, posterior to the **anterior commissure** (20) and anterior to the interventricular foramen. Fibers of the **fornix** (column) (19) pass through the **hypothalamus** (17) and terminate mainly in the **mamillary body** (18). The fornix therefore relays information from the **hippocampus** (16) to the hypothalamus. A further connection is made from the mamillary body of the hypothalamus via the **mamillothalamic fasciculus** (15) to the **anterior nucleus of the thalamus** (4) and to the cingulate gyrus. Note the relation of the **hippocampus** (15) to the **inferior horn of the lateral ventricle** (14).

The functions of the limbic lobe are very complex. The **cingulate cortical region** appears to **integrate sensory information** received from neocortical association areas and from subcortical structures. **Limbic system output** is from the hippocampal formation via the **fornix** to the **hypothalamus,** which elicits **endocrine** and **ANS participation** in the response. Although the limbic system is interconnected with the thalamus and hypothalamus for visceral and emotional behavior, its connection with the **cerebral cortex** implicates the system in **cognitive behavior**. In summary, limbic system activities include modulation of sympathetic and parasympathetic activity in relation to autonomic demands, addition of emotional coloring to behavioral output, mediation of sexual activity and overt aggression, and playing a role in learning and memory. In a sense, drive and motivation, i.e., the will, can be attributed to the limbic system.

Clinical Correlations . . . .

Destruction of the **mediodorsal nucleus of the thalamus** or of its **projections** to the ipsilateral prefrontal cortex can result in **neuropsychological dysfunctions** similar to those observed in prefrontal lobe damage. Symptoms of a unilateral lesion vary relative to whether the left or the right hemisphere is involved. A **more pronounced deficit** follows a lesion to the **dominant hemisphere. Characteristic behavioral changes include a lack of tact, a loss of social inhibition, and a loss of initiative (apathy).**

 On the diagram on the right, color the cingulate and parahippocampal gyri yellow.

Limbic System Structures: Dissection of the Right Hemisphere From the Medial Surface, Thalamic Radiations Exposed

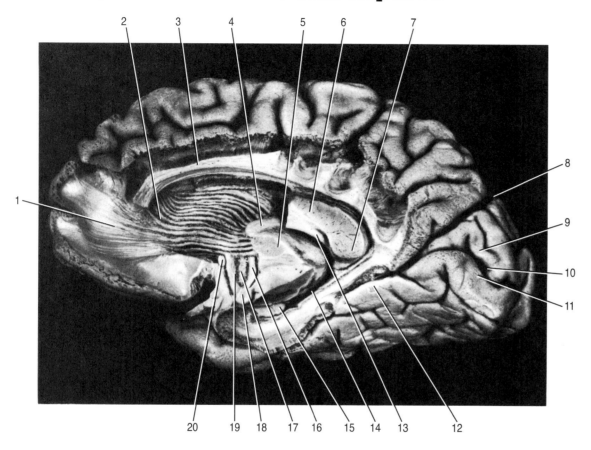

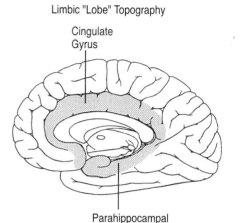

Limbic "Lobe" Topography

Cingulate Gyrus

Parahippocampal Gyrus

1. Thalamic radiations to prefrontal cortex via internal capsule
2. Thalamic radiations to cingulate gyrus
3. Cingulum
4. Anterior thalamic nucleus
5. Mediodorsal nucleus of thalamus
6. Corpus callosum (body)
7. Corpus callosum (splenium)
8. Parieto-occipital sulcus
9. Cuneus
10. Calcarine sulcus
11. Lingual gyrus
12. Parahippocampal gyrus
13. Fornix (body)
14. Lateral ventricle (inferior horn)
15. Hippocampus
16. Mamillothalamic fasciculus
17. Hypothalamus
18. Mamillary body of hypothalamus
19. Fornix (column)
20. Anterior commissure

(Reprinted with permission from Ludwig E, Klingler J. **Atlas Cerebri Humani.** Basel, Switzerland: S. Karger, 1956 Table 56.)

Limbic System Connections

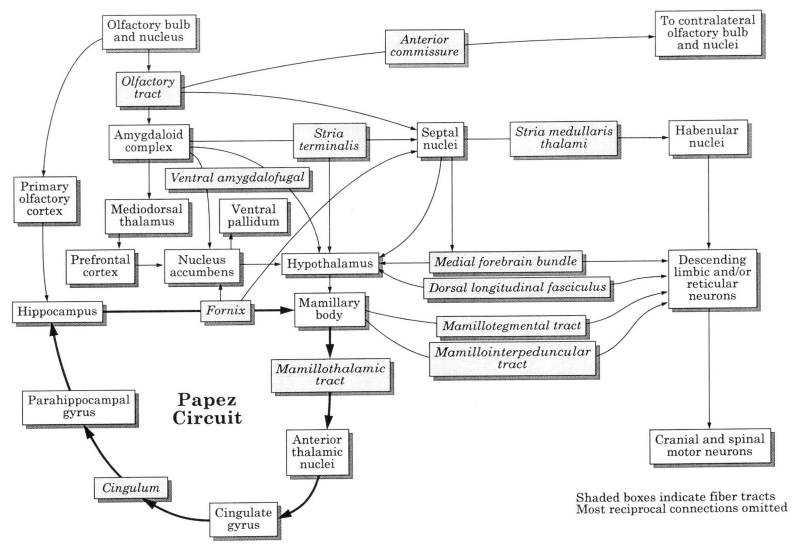

Papez Circuit

Shaded boxes indicate fiber tracts
Most reciprocal connections omitted

 Color OLB, OLT, LS, and POC brown; AC blue; AGD orange; H and MB purple; DG green; FXCR, FXB, FXC, and HC red; and AN yellow.

Limbic System Connections

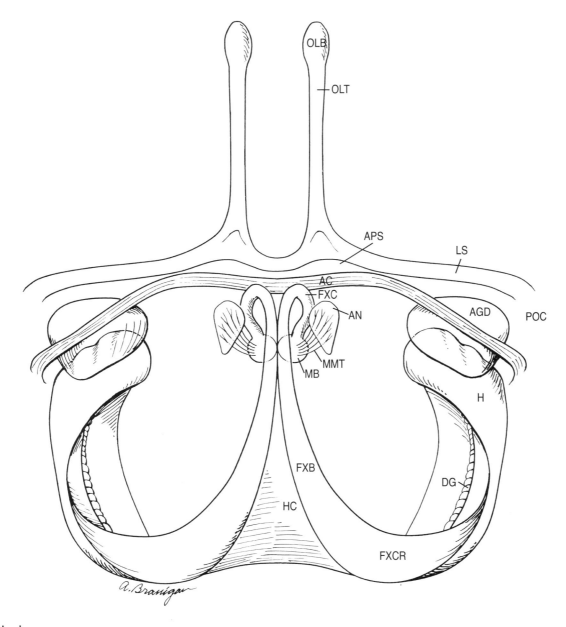

AC	Anterior commissure
AGD	Amygdala
AN	Anterior nucleus of thalamus
APS	Anterior perforated substance
DG	Dentate gyrus
FXB	Fornix (body)
FXC	Fornix (column)
FXCR	Fornix (crux)
H	Hippocampus
HC	Hippocampal commissure
LS	Lateral stria
MB	Mamillary body
MMT	Mamillothalamic tract
OLB	Olfactory bulb
OLT	Olfactory tract
POC	Primary olfactory cortex

Dissection of the Right Hemisphere From the Lateral Surface, Putamen and Hippocampus Exposed

Definitions

The **hippocampus** (8) (Latin for sea horse) is a **primitive,** three-layered cortical structure that projects into the **inferior horn** of the **lateral ventricle** (10). The **hippocampal formation** includes the hippocampus, dentate gyrus, and the subiculum. The **dentate gyrus** is a scalloped band of **cortex** composed of **three layers.** The middle layer consists of densely packed, small granule cells. The **subiculum** is **five-layered cortex** apposed to the dentate gyrus. The **amygdala** is described as an almond-shaped nucleus partly beneath the uncus. "Extended amygdala" encompasses the central and medial nuclei of the amygdala and cells traversing the sublenticular part of the substantia innominata, the bed nucleus of the stria terminalis, and part of the nucleus accumbens.

Structural and Functional Features

In this dissection, the **lenticular nucleus (putamen** [2] and **globus pallidus)** is intact, and one can visually appreciate the terms **sublenticular** (6) and **retrolenticular** (9). The globus pallidus is not apparent in this view because it lies wedged between the putamen laterally and the internal capsule medially. Appreciate that medial to the **anterior limb** (1) of the **internal capsule** lies the head of the caudate nucleus and medial to the **posterior limb** (7) lies the thalamus. Note this lateral view of the **atrium** (11).

In addition to the hippocampus, other structures related to the inferior horn of the lateral ventricle are the **amygdala** (4) and the **tail of the caudate nucleus** (5). The tail is superior and the amygdala is anterior to the inferior horn. The amygdala contains a corticomedial nuclear group with olfactory and subcortical connections and a basolateral nuclear group with cortical connections. The amygdala receives processed information from neocortical association areas and contributes to limbic circuitry via projections to the hippocampus, septal nuclei, and hypothalamus.

The uncinate **fasciculus** (3) is described on page 40. A medial view of the caudate nucleus is on page 175.

Anteriorly the hippocampus is marked by shallow grooves that give it the appearance of an animal's paw, thus the term "pes" hippocampus (page 170). The **hippocampus** receives **afferent** fibers from the **amygdala, claustrum, septal area, thalamus, hypothalamus,** and **entorhinal cortex;** it also receives projections from chemically defined brain stem nuclei. **Dopaminergic fibers** from the ventral tegmental midbrain nucleus, **serotonergic fibers** from the raphe nucleus, and **noradrenergic fibers** from the locus ceruleus innervate it. A recurrent circuit from the parahippocampal gyrus to the hippocampus, to the hypothalamus (via the fornix) and thalamus (via mamillothalamic tract) is completed by thalamocortical projections (anterior nucleus) back to the cingulate cortex (Papez circuit, page 168). The cingulate cortex receives extensive connections from prefrontal and parietal association areas.

In a coronal plane, the hippocampus resembles a ram's horn (Ammon's horn; cornu ammonis [CA]). Pyramidal cells whose axons make up the major efferent outflow are topographically designated as regions CA1, CA2, CA3, and CA4. Cells in the **CA1 region** (Sommer's sector) are particularly vulnerable to **anoxia** and **ischemia.**

Clinical Correlations . . . .

The hippocampal formation appears to be essential in memory mechanisms. The mamillary nuclei of the hypothalamus receive a major portion of fibers emanating from the hippocampus. **Lesions** have been demonstrated in the **mamillary nuclei** in patients experiencing **amnesia. Bilateral trauma** to the temporal poles in the middle cranial fossae can damage the underlying **hippocampi** and cause amnesia.

Pathologic changes appear early in the **hippocampal formation** in patients with **Alzheimer's disease;** loss of neurons in the CA1 region is implicated. Diminished cholinergic innervation is a feature of Alzheimer's disease involving the large cholinergic cells in the basal nucleus of Meynert in particular. The temporal lobe, especially the medial aspect, has a low threshold for hyperexcitability, either endogenously or due to scar formation. In **temporal lobe epilepsy,** the most pronounced site of cellular degeneration is the CA1 region. Anoxia due to cardiorespiratory arrest can result in **anterograde amnesia** as a result of ischemia and neuronal damage in the CA1 region.

Dissection of the Right Hemisphere From the Lateral Surface, Putamen and Hippocampus Exposed

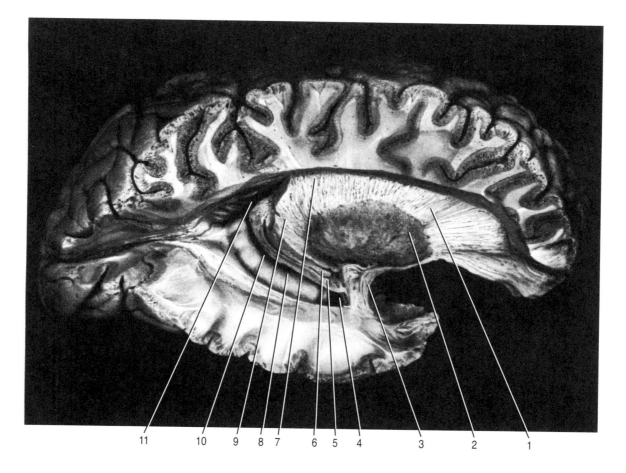

1. Internal capsule (anterior limb)
2. Putamen
3. Uncinate fasciculus
4. Amygdala (location of)
5. Caudate (tail)
6. Internal capsule (sublenticular)
7. Internal capsule (posterior limb)
8. Hippocampus
9. Internal capsule (retrolenticular)
10. Lateral ventricle (inferior horn)
11. Lateral ventricle (atrium)

(Reprinted with permission from Ludwig E and Klingler J. **Atlas of Cerebri Humani.** Basel, Switzerland: S. Karger, 1956 Table 16.)

Chapter 5   **The Forebrain**

Dissection of the Right Hemisphere From the Lateral Surface, Internal Capsule and Optic Radiations Exposed

Definitions

Only the rostral stem of the lateral **sulcus** (6) is apparent in this dissection. The lateral sulcus separates the temporal lobe inferiorly from the frontal and parietal lobes superiorly. Inferiorly from the **lateral sulcus** (6), the gyri of the **temporal lobe** (7), are the **parahippocampal**, the **medial occipitotemporal**, and the **lateral occipitotemporal**. Relate this dissection to the medial view on page 25 and to the inferior view on page 27.

Structural and Functional Features

Commissural fibers of the **corpus callosum** (4) are oriented in a transverse plane connecting left and right hemispheres. Mainly, however, this dissection reveals projection fibers in the **corona radiata** (1) and **internal capsule** (2,3). "Corona radiata" refers to projection fibers as they fan out from the **internal capsule** (2) to approach the cerebral cortex. "Internal capsule" describes the same mass of fibers as they pass between the caudate nucleus and thalamus medially and the lenticular nucleus laterally (pages 165 and 167). Removing the lenticular nucleus (**globus pallidus** [5], medially, and putamen, laterally) leaves the imprint of these structures on the course of the fibers.

Projection fibers make connections primarily in a rostral-to-caudal or caudal-to-rostral plane. The **optic radiations** (8) are thalamocortical fibers of the visual system that exemplify projection fibers running in an anterior-to-posterior plane. They arise from cells in the lateral geniculate nucleus in a sublenticular position, and pass in a retrolenticular direction en route to the calcarine cortex, area 17, in the occipital lobe.

Clinical Correlations . . . .

Tumors and **vascular accidents** of the temporal lobe may **disrupt** the **optic radiations.** Visual field organization is maintained in a point-to-point fashion in the lateral geniculate nucleus, in the lamination of the geniculocalcarine fibers and in their cortical termination along the calcarine sulcus. **Tumors** result in a gradual, **insidious onset** of visual field deficits whereas **vascular lesions** are often characterized by a sudden, frightening **loss of visual function** (page 190).

Gnosis is the Greek word for knowledge. Agnosia is the inability to understand the significance of sensory stimuli. The inability to recognize a familiar face, **prosopagnosia**, is a **rare visual memory disorder** involving **bilateral lesions** of the **parahippocampal** and **medial occipitotemporal gyri**. Although the visual receptive striate cortex may be intact, damage to regions involved in processing visual input can result in both **prosopagnosia** and **achromatopsia** (color blindness). The inferomedial temporal cortex is supplied by the posterior cerebral artery.

The dense concentration of fibers in the internal capsule—corticospinal, corticobulbar, corticopontine, corticonigral, thalamocortical, etc.—renders this region a **strategic passage where even a small lesion can result in extensive dysfunction.** The ischemic or hemorrhagic nature of vascular lesions of the internal capsule is best understood in relation to the vascular anatomy, which is discussed in Chapter 6. A relevant case history at the end of this chapter (questions and explanations) is included to whet student interest in that important subject.

The real in us is silent; the acquired is talkative. – Kahlil Gibran

Dissection of the Right Hemisphere From the Lateral Surface, Internal Capsule and Optic Radiations Exposed

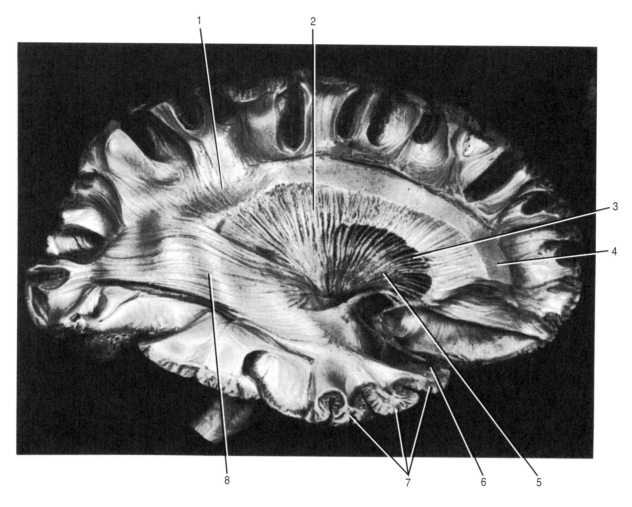

1. Corona radiata
2. Internal capsule (posterior limb)
3. Internal capsule (anterior limb)
4. Corpus callosum
5. Impressions made by the globus pallidus
6. Lateral sulcus
7. Gyri of temporal lobe
8. Optic radiations

(Reprinted with permission from Ludwig E and Klingler J. **Atlas of Cerebri Humani.** Basel, Switzerland: S. Karger, 1956 Table 21.)

Dissection of the Right Hemisphere From the Medial Surface, Caudate Nucleus and Limbic Structures Exposed

Definitions

The **fasciculus retroflexus** (9) (habenulointerpeduncular tract) is a major discharge bundle from the habenula. It passes through the edge of the red nucleus to terminate in the interpeduncular nucleus of the **midbrain**. The **cerebral peduncle** (10) is also a midbrain structure. Recall that it is the ventral part of each half of the midbrain, minus the tectum.

Structural and Functional Features

The caudate nucleus is C-shaped with a large "head" (2), which lies in the floor and lateral wall of the **lateral ventricle** (1). It has a tapering "body" that ends in a "tail" (7) in relation to the inferior horn of the lateral ventricle. Because the caudate nucleus and the thalamus are medial to the internal capsule, the fibers of the capsule cannot be seen. This plane of section shows the **corpus callosum** (3) forming the rostral and dorsal limits of the lateral ventricle.

Connections of the diencephalon are again visually defined here, including the column of the **fornix** (13), **mamillothalamic fasciculus** (11), and **fasciculus retroflexus** (9). The **mamillary body** (12), in the posterior hypothalamus, receives most of the fibers of the fornix and projects through the mamillothalamic fasciculus to the anterior nucleus of the thalamus. The **habenular nuclei** (6) connect across the midline rostral to the pineal gland in the habenular commissure. The **stria medullaris thalami** (5) extends along the dorsal medial border of the dorsal thalamus from the habenula to the interventricular foramen and is composed of fibers from the fornix (mainly), stria terminalis, and the medial forebrain bundle. The **posterior commissure** (8), caudal to the pineal gland, contains fibers connecting the pretectal nuclei and fibers from certain midbrain nuclei that project into the contralateral medial longitudinal fasciculus. The position of the pineal gland is midsagittal, however, it was removed in the dissection.

Output from the **amygdala** (14) is through the ventral amygdalofugal pathway and the stria terminalis. The amygdala projects to the hypothalamus, the septal area, the mediodorsal nucleus of the thalamus, the dorsal motor nucleus of the vagus, and other brain stem nuclei as well as to the prefrontal and premotor cortex.

Anterior to the column of the fornix at the interventricular foramen is the cut surface of the **anterior commissure** (15). This bundle of **fibers** crosses the median plane in the lamina terminalis and consists primarily of **interconnections between the olfactory bulbs, amygdaloid nuclei, anterior perforated substances, parahippocampal gyri, and neocortical areas of the temporal lobes** (pages 157 and 169).

The **cingulum** (4) is an association bundle of fibers located mainly within the cingulate gyrus. An important pathway of the limbic system, it receives projections from the anterior nucleus of the thalamus and it interconnects frontal, parietal, and temporal cortices. Positron emission tomography (PET) studies show that **nociceptive** (painful) **stimuli** consistently activate the **anterior portion of the cingulate gyrus.**

Clinical Correlations . . . .

Lesions of the mamillary nuclei have been discussed relative to chronic alcoholism and subsequent amnesia. **Neurons** surrounding the mamillary bodies in the **posterior hypothalamus** project to brain stem and spinal cord centers controlling **sympathetic activity of the ANS.** Lesions of the posterior hypothalamus may result in temperature control disruption and Horner's syndrome (page 122). Precise localization of function in the hypothalamus is difficult because of the density of nuclear groups and the plethora of afferent and efferent fibers. Hence, **reference to areas** rather than to specific nuclei is generally appropriate in discussing hypothalamic **clinical deficits. Loss of appetite** may accompany lesions of the **lateral hypothalamus.** A **satiety center** in the **medial hypothalamic area**, if lesioned, can result in **hyperphagia** and **obesity. Diabetes insipidus** (symptoms are polydipsia and polyuria) is related to **destructive lesions** of the **supraoptic** or **paraventricular nuclei** in the anterior zone or of the **infundibulum** or **neurohypophysis.** Lesions of the anterior hypothalamus can disrupt temperature and sleep-wake control centers.

Bilateral damage to the amygdalae produces the Klüver-Bucy syndrome. This condition involves the following abnormalities: psychic blindness or visual agnosia (normal visual fields but inability to recognize common objects), oral tendencies, emotional changes associated with anger or fear, indiscriminate sexual behavior, and, indiscriminate dietary habits.

Damage to the cingulate gyrus can result in **apathy** and **indifference to pain.** Cingulotomies have been preformed on patients experiencing intractable pain.

Transfer of learning from one hemisphere to the other occurs through commissural pathways. To confine epileptic discharge to one hemisphere, the corpus callosum is sometimes severed. Disconnecting the hemispheres changes behavior in subtle ways. Generally, however, "split-brain" patients function quite normally after an initial adjustment period.

Dissection of the Right Hemisphere From the Medial Surface, Caudate Nucleus and Limbic Structures Exposed

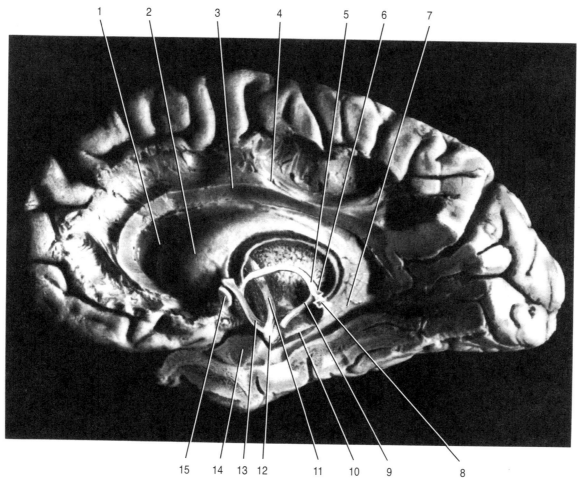

1. Lateral ventricle
2. Caudate (head)
3. Corpus callosum
4. Cingulum
5. Stria medullaris thalami
6. Habenula
7. Caudate (tail)
8. Posterior commissure
9. Fasciculus retroflexus
10. Cerebral peduncle (cut surface)
11. Mamillothalamic fasciculus
12. Mamillary body of hypothalamus
13. Fornix (column)
14. Amygdala
15. Anterior commissure

(Reprinted with permission from Ludwig E and Klingler J. **Atlas of Cerebri Humani.** Basel, Switzerland: S. Karger, 1956 Table 40.)

Chapter Five Study Questions

Questions 1–11
Directions: Each question below contains four or five suggested answers. Choose the **one best** response to each question.

1. Which of the following fiber connections is classified as an associational pathway?
    - (a) Dorsal longitudinal fasciculus
    - (b) Superior occipitofrontal fasciculus
    - (c) Hippocampal commissure
    - (d) Internal capsule
    - (e) Corona radiata

2. The anterior limb of the internal capsule contains all of the following fibers except
    - (a) Thalamocortical
    - (b) Corticothalamic
    - (c) Corticostriate
    - (d) Corticopontine
    - (e) Corticospinal

3. All of the following are associated with pathology of the basal ganglia except
    - (a) Tremor at rest
    - (b) Chorea
    - (c) Athetosis
    - (d) Intention tremor
    - (e) Postural instability

4. Huntington's disease is characterized by neuronal degeneration in which of the following structures?
    - (a) Striatum
    - (b) Globus pallidus, internal segment
    - (c) Globus pallidus, external segment
    - (d) Substantia nigra
    - (e) Thalamus

5. A pathway that extends along the medial border of the caudate nucleus and reciprocally connects the amygdala and the hypothalamus is the
    - (a) Ventral amygdalofugal
    - (b) Stria medullaris thalami
    - (c) Fornix
    - (d) Stria terminalis
    - (e) Medial forebrain bundle

6. The following are associated with degenerative changes in the CAI region of the hippocampus except
    - (a) Obesity
    - (b) Epilepsy
    - (c) Amnesia following cardiorespiratory arrest
    - (d) Alzheimer's disease
    - (e) b and c

7. A diencephalic structure that plays a key role in modulating ANS and endocrine activity is the
    - (a) Amygdala
    - (b) Septum (septal nuclei)
    - (c) Hypothalamus
    - (d) Nucleus accumbens
    - (e) Substantia innominata

8. Bilateral cortical damage to the inferomedial temporal cortex may result in
    - (a) Hemianesthesia
    - (b) Hemiplegia
    - (c) Broca's (expressive) aphasia
    - (d) Wernicke's (receptive) aphasia
    - (e) Prosopagnosia

9. Positron emission tomography (PET) studies show that nociceptive stimuli activate the anterior region of the
    - (a) Temporal lobe
    - (b) Dorsolateral frontal lobe
    - (c) Cingulate gyrus
    - (d) Inferior parietal lobule
    - (e) Insula

10. The structure that divides the hypothalamus into medial and lateral zones is the
    - (a) Anterior commissure
    - (b) Fornix (column)
    - (c) Fornix (body)
    - (d) Dorsal longitudinal fasciculus (DLF)
    - (e) Medial forebrain bundle (MFB)

11. Which of the following is the correct sequence for processing and relaying information?
    - (a) Mamillary body, cingulate gyrus, anterior nucleus of the thalamus, parahippocampal gyrus, hippocampus
    - (b) Cingulate gyrus, parahippocampal gyrus, hippocampus, anterior nucleus of the thalamus, mamillary body
    - (c) Cingulate gyrus, hippocampus, parahippocampal gyrus, mamillary body, anterior nucleus of the thalamus
    - (d) Cingulate gyrus, mamillary body, parahippocampal gyrus, hippocampus, anterior nucleus of the thalamus
    - (e) Anterior nucleus of the thalamus, cingulate gyrus, parahippocampal gyrus, hippocampus, mamillary body

Answers and Explanations for Chapter Five Study Questions

1. **b** [page 154] The superior occipitofrontal fasciculus is an association bundle located along the caudate nucleus medial to the interdigitating fibers of the internal capsule and corpus callosum. Its fibers interconnect the cortex of the occipital and temporal lobes and the frontal lobe and insula within the same hemisphere. The dorsal longitudinal fasciculus (DLF) is located in the brain stem and contains fibers mainly from the hypothalamus and dorsal tegmental nucleus and some from the habenula. These terminate on cranial parasympathetic nuclei and other brain stem motor nuclei. The DLF also contains ascending fibers. Most of the fibers in the fornix do not cross; however, those that do, reach the opposite hemisphere via the hippocampal commissure. The corona radiata and the internal capsule contain projection fibers between the cerebral cortex and subcortical structures.

2. **e** [page 154] Corticospinal fibers pass through the posterior limb of the internal capsule, which is more prone to vascular damage than is the anterior limb. Reciprocal connections between the cortex and both the anterior and the mediodorsal nuclei of the thalamus pass through the anterior limb. Corticopontine fibers traverse the anterior (frontopontine) and the posterior (parieto-occipital and temporopontine) limbs. Reciprocal connections also traverse the anterior limb between the cortex and striatum (corticostriate and striatocortical).

3. **d** [page 154] Intention tremor is characteristic of cerebellar damage. Degeneration of striatal neurons in Huntington's disease can result in athetoid or choreiform movements. Postural instability, resting tremor, slowness of movement (bradykinesia), and muscular rigidity characterize Parkinson's disease.

4. **a** [page 154] There is degeneration of neurons in the striatum and in the cerebral cortex in patients with Huntington's disease. Lesions of the globus pallidus result in hypokinesia without tremor at rest. Both the striatum and substantia nigra are implicated in Parkinson's disease. The thalamus is interposed between the cerebral cortex and the basal ganglia. Disruption of circuits through the ventroanterior and ventrolateral nuclei of the thalamus may also result in abnormal motor responses; however, this is different from the neuronal degeneration in Huntington's disease.

5. **d** [pages 156 and 168] Specifically, the stria terminalis connects the amygdala and the medial hypothalamus and also contains connections between the two amygdalae. The amygdala and hypothalamus are connected via a more direct, sublenticular route through the ventral amygdalofugal pathway. The stria medullaris thalami runs along the dorsal medial border of the thalamus from the interventricular foramen to the habenula and reciprocally connects septal and hypothalamic areas with the habenular nucleus. Finally, the medial forebrain bundle connects the hypothalamus with the brain stem and spinal cord.

6. **a** [pages 170 and 174] A lesion in the medial hypothalamic area can result in obesity. Anoxia and ischemia due to cardiac arrest damages the CAI cells of the hippocampus as do epilepsy and Alzheimer's disease. Diminished cholinergic innervation seems also to be involved in Alzheimer's disease.

7. **c** [page 162] The hypothalamus is important in regulating visceral function and in modulating endocrine activities through its neural and vascular connections to the hypophysis. The other structures may indirectly modulate these activities (to a lesser extent or through hypothalamic connections). The amygdala, septal nuclei, nucleus accumbens, and substantia innominata are telencephalic structures in the basal forebrain.

8. **e** [page 172] Prosopagnosia, a rare memory disorder, is the inability to recognize a familiar face. Multimodal processing areas of the parahippocampal and medial occipitotemporal gyri integrate present visual stimuli with stored memories. Hemianesthesia and hemiplegia may result from damage to various loci but not the medial inferotemporal area. Broca's aphasia is a frontal lobe phenomenon, and Wernicke's aphasia involves the posterior region of the superior temporal gyrus and the angular gyrus of the parietal lobe.

9. **c** [page 174] A lesion of the anterior region of the cingulate gyrus, located in the medial frontal lobe, can result in indifference to pain. The other regions listed are not involved in processing painful stimuli. The thalamus, however, receives sensory pathways and can, if lesioned, be a locus of intractable pain.

10. **b** [pages 162 and 168] The column of the fornix divides the hypothalamus into medial and lateral zones. The body of the fornix runs midline in the free edge of the septum pellucidum. The anterior commissure crosses the midline in the rostral wall of the third ventricle. The DLF interconnects the hypothalamus with autonomic brain stem nuclei and the MFB is composed of diffuse unmyelinated or lightly myelinated fibers that traverse the lateral hypothalamus in an anteroposterior direction. It interconnects the hypothalamus with the basal forebrain and brain stem. In myelin-stained sections the fornix is easily identified because it, in contrast to the DLF and MFB, contains large, heavily myelinated fibers.

11. **e** [page 168] Sensory stimuli that reach the anterior nucleus of the thalamus are projected to the cingulate gyrus via the anterior limb of the internal capsule and the cingulum. The cingulate gyrus receives input from association areas in the frontal, parietal, and temporal lobes. It projects to the parahippocampal gyrus via the cingulum. The circuit is completed with input from the parahippocampal gyrus to the hippocampus and then, via the fornix, to the mamillary body of the hypothalamus. Finally, the circuit is completed via the mamillothalamic tract to the anterior thalamic nucleus. This describes the Papez circuit of the limbic system.

Study Questions (continued)

Question 12

12. **Dysfunction of which of the following hypothalamic nuclei is likely to result in diabetes insipidus?**
    (a) Suprachiasmatic
    (b) Dorsomedial
    (c) Ventromedial
    (d) Mamillary nuclei
    (e) Supraoptic

Questions 13–17

Directions: Match each of the numbered statements with the appropriate lettered area in the figure.

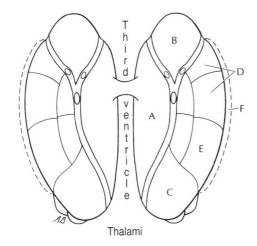

Thalami

13. **Has reciprocal connections with all principal thalamic nuclei**
14. **Projects to the somatosensory cortex**
15. **Projects to the prefrontal cortex**
16. **Receives the mamillothalamic tract**
17. **Projects to areas 4 and 6**

Questions 18–27

Directions: Match each of the numbered statements with the appropriate lettered area in the figures. A given structure has the same letter in both views. More than one lettered area may apply to the numbered statement.

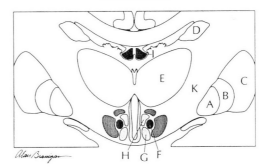 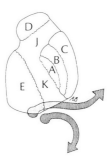

Middle Hypothalamus
Coronal Section

Right Internal Capsule

18. **Caudate nucleus**
19. **Thalamus**
20. **Fibers originate predominantly in the hippocampus**
21. **Lenticular nucleus**
22. **Ventromedial nucleus**
23. **Striatum**
24. **Corpus striatum**
25. **Receives input from the subthalamic nucleus**
26. **Projects to ventroanterior and ventrolateral thalamic nuclei**
27. **Posterior limb of the internal capsule**

Case History

While shoveling snow for two hours, a 57-year-old sedentary hypertensive man experienced a sudden onset of dizziness and malaise. With his wife's help he got undressed and went to bed, thinking that he was just exhausted. Subsequently, he developed what his neurologist described as a wild, flailing movement of his left arm.

28. **What one word describes this bizarre and rare disorder?**
29. **Damage of which brain structure causes this abnormality?**
30. **Is it likely that the lesion is in the left or right hemisphere?**
31. **What clue suggests the cause of this damage?**
32. **Is this a basal ganglia lesion?**

Answers and Explanations for Chapter Five Study Questions (continued)

12. **e** [pages 156 and 162] Terminals from axons whose cell bodies are in the supraoptic and paraventricular nuclei release oxytocin and vasopressin in the neurohypophysis. A deficiency of vasopressin, the antidiuretic hormone, causes diabetes insipidus. This disorder is marked by profuse secretion of urine (polyuria) and intense thirst (polydipsia). The suprachiasmatic nucleus synchronizes bodily rhythms with external light stimuli received from the retina. The dorsomedial and ventromedial nuclei of the hypothalamus play a role in food intake and the mamillary nuclei receive various afferents including the majority of the fornix fibers. Lesions of the fornix or of the mamillary nuclei may result in amnesia.

13. **f** [page 160] A significant feature of the thalamic reticular nucleus is that it receives collaterals from thalamocortical fibers from all principal thalamic nuclei and projects back to these nuclei. Its role is therefore modulatory.

14. **e** [page 160] The ventral posterior nucleus receives the somatosensory information from the face (VPM) and body (VPL) and projects to areas 3,1,2.

15. **a** [page 160] The mediodorsal nucleus reciprocally connects with the prefrontal cortex. Lesions of these fibers result in dysfunction comparable to that seen in patients with prefrontal lesions.

16. **b** [page 168] The mamillothalamic tract ascends with other fibers in the intramedullary lamina and terminates in the anterior nucleus of the thalamus.

17. **d** [page 168] The ventroanterior and ventrolateral thalamic nuclei receive projections from the internal segment of the globus pallidus and from the cerebellum. These nuclei project to areas 4 and 6.

18. **d** [pages 158 and 164] The caudate nucleus forms the floor and lateral wall of the lateral ventricle and is medial to the anterior limb of the internal capsule.

19. **e** [pages 158 and 164] The thalamus forms the upper lateral wall of the third ventricle and is medial to the posterior limb of the internal capsule.

20. **f** and **i** [pages 162 and 168] The myelinated fibers of the fornix take origin from the hippocampal formation, particularly, the hippocampus. **F** identifies the column and **I** the body of the fornix.

21. **a, b,** and **c** [pages 158 and 164] The lens-shaped structure that lies lateral to the internal capsule is composed of the putamen (C) and both the external (B) and internal (A) segments of the globus pallidus.

22. **g** [page 162] The ventromedial nucleus is medial to the column of the fornix and plays a role in food intake.

23. **c** and **d** [page 154] The striatum includes the putamen (C) and caudate nucleus (D).

24. **a, b, c,** and **d** [pages 156 and 164] The corpus striatum includes the striatum (C, D) plus the globus pallidus (A, B).

25. **a** [page 158] The internal segment of the globus pallidus receives projections from the subthalamic nucleus.

26. **a** [page 158] The internal segment of the globus pallidus projects to the VA/VL thalamic nuclei.

27. **k** [pages 158 and 164] The posterior limb of the internal capsule is easily identified in horizontal sections because of its posterior location. Its definition as that part of the internal capsule that is bordered medially by the thalamus is helpful relative to identifying it in coronal sections.

Case History

28. **Hemiballism describes this movement.**

29. **Damage to the subthalamic nucleus located in the ventral thalamus of the diencephalon causes contralateral hemiballism.**

30. **The lesion would be in the right hemisphere because motor circuits control movement of the contralateral limbs.**

31. **The clue of sudden onset of symptoms during exertion in a sedentary, hypertensive individual suggests a hemorrhagic vascular lesion. Subthalamic lesions usually are hemorrhagic.**

32. **Semantics is a problem in answering this question. Basal ganglia circuitry is definitely involved. An anatomist may view only the subcortical, telencephalic neuronal masses involved in motor control as basal ganglia. The subthalamic nucleus and the substantia nigra are involved in the outflow circuitry from the basal ganglia; however, neither is a telencephalic structure. Clinically, they are considered basal ganglia because of their connections and because pathology involving either can result in motor dysfunction. Although the amygdala and claustrum are subcortical telencephalic structures, they do not participate in the circuits linking the ipsilateral basal ganglia, thalamus, and motor cortex. Current texts seem not to include them as basal ganglia.**

CHAPTER 6 Circle of Willis

Table 6.1 Artery Location   Incidence of Congenital Aneurysms

Anterior Circulation 80%
Internal carotid artery (ICA).. 30%
    Ophthalmic
    Posterior communicating artery (PCoA)
    Anterior choroidal artery (AChA)
• Anterior cerebral artery (ACA) 25%
    Anterior communicating artery (ACoA)
• Middle cerebral artery (MCA) 25%
Posterior Circulation 20%
• Vertebral artery (VA)
• Posterior spinal artery (PSA)
    May originate from the vertebral as shown or from PICA
• Posterior inferior cerebellar artery (PICA)
• Anterior spinal artery (ASA)
• Basilar artery (BA)
• Anterior inferior cerebellar artery (AICA)
• Internal auditory artery (labyrinthine artery)
• Superior cerebellar artery (SCA)
• Posterior cerebral artery (PCA)

Definitions
The **internal carotid system** makes up the **anterior circulation** because its branches nourish the rostral areas of the cerebral hemispheres. The **vertebral-basilar** system supplies the brainstem, cerebellum, and the inferior and posterior surfaces of the cerebrum. This is referred to as the **posterior circulation.**

Structural and Functional Features
The **arterial circle (of Willis)** at the base of the brain surrounds the optic chiasm, the infundibulum, and the mamillary bodies. It lies mainly in the interpeduncular cistern. The **anterior communicating artery** (ACoA) connects the left and right anterior cerebral artery (ACA); thus, an overlapping blood supply exists between the paired internal carotids. The larger terminal branch of the internal carotid artery (ICA) is the **middle cerebral artery** (MCA), which is a direct continuation of the **ICA**. The anterior circulation is joined to the posterior circulation by the paired

posterior communicating arteries (PCoAs), which connect to the **posterior cerebral arteries** (PCAs). The **vertebral arteries** (often unequal in size) ascend through the foramen magnum and unite at the lower border of the pons to form the single, large **basilar artery** in the midline groove on the ventral surface of the pons. At the upper border of the pons, the basilar bifurcates into left and right **PCAs,** which ascend over the tentorium cerebelli, circle around the cerebral peduncle, and reach the inferomedial temporal and the medial occipital cortices. The final branch caudal to the bifurcation is the **superior cerebellar artery** (SCA).

Learning the anterior and posterior circulation as separate entities and then connecting the two facilitates understanding the alternate paths of the overlapping blood supply made possible by the circle of Willis. If the initial segment of the **PCA** is developmentally hypoplastic, the PCA may be supplied by blood flowing through the **PCoA** from the anterior circulation. The genetic predisposition to aneurysms varies between the posterior and anterior circulation (chart at left). An aneurysm of the internal carotid can be seen in an angiogram on page 197, as can the **ACA** and **MCA** on a coronal view.

Clinical Correlations . . . .

The **oculomotor nerve** passes between the **SCA** and the **PCA** and is vulnerable to aneurysms of either. A supratentorial mass herniating through the tentorial notch is likely to compress the oculomotor nerve. Small-caliber vessels arising from the circle of Willis are termed "end" arteries. They lack anastomoses and tend to rupture due to hypertension.

Color to Learn

Throughout this chapter use red for coloring the arterial blood supply. For proprioceptive learning, color the internal carotids on each side. Note the diameter of the lumen and how short the intracranial segment is. Color the ophthalmic artery. Color each **ACA** from its origin and each **MCA** while comparing their size. Color the recurrent artery of Heubner. Color the anterior choroidal and lateral striate arteries. Join left and right components of the anterior circulation by coloring the anterior communicating artery. Color the entire vertebral-basilar system, giving close attention to the size of each vessel, especially the pontine branches. Connect the anterior and posterior circulations by coloring the **PCoA.** Finally, color all the striate arteries of the circle of Willis.

Circle of Willis

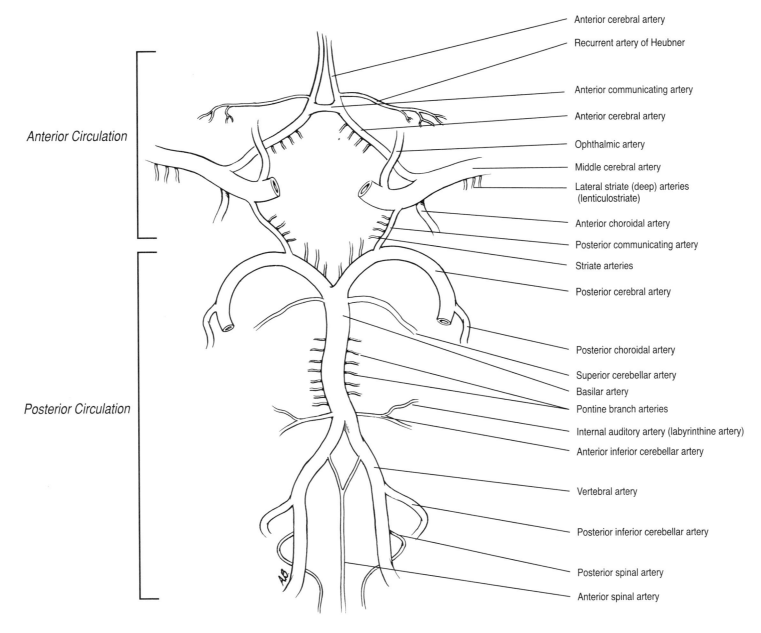

Anterior Circulation

Posterior Circulation

Anterior cerebral artery

Recurrent artery of Heubner

Anterior communicating artery

Anterior cerebral artery

Ophthalmic artery

Middle cerebral artery

Lateral striate (deep) arteries (lenticulostriate)

Anterior choroidal artery

Posterior communicating artery

Striate arteries

Posterior cerebral artery

Posterior choroidal artery

Superior cerebellar artery

Basilar artery

Pontine branch arteries

Internal auditory artery (labyrinthine artery)

Anterior inferior cerebellar artery

Vertebral artery

Posterior inferior cerebellar artery

Posterior spinal artery

Anterior spinal artery

General Blood Supply of the Brain

Definitions

The **left common carotid artery** arises from the **arch of the aorta** whereas the right one arises from the **brachiocephalic artery.** The **internal carotid artery** (ICA), a terminal branch of the common carotid artery, enters the middle cranial fossa of the skull through the carotid canal. It undergoes a series of bends termed "carotid siphon" running forward in the cavernous venous sinus. The internal carotid system, with assistance from the vertebral-basilar system, supplies the cerebral hemispheres.

Structural and Functional Features

The **ICA** pierces the dura mater, courses backward under the optic nerve, and turns upward lateral to the optic chiasm. Under the anterior perforated space, it divides into the **ACA** and **MCA.** Before its terminal bifurcation, it gives rise to the **hypophysial,** the **ophthalmic,** and the **PCoAs.** The **anterior choroidal** almost always branches from the ICA; however, it may arise from the MCA. The **vertebral arteries** arise from the subclavian, ascend in the foramina of the transverse processes of C1-C6 vertebrae, and enter the skull through the foramen magnum. They run forward beneath the medulla and join to form the **basilar artery** at the caudal border of the pons. Fine branches directly off the vertebrals supply the medulla. A single **anterior spinal artery** is formed from a contribution from each vertebral artery. A **posterior spinal artery** on each side arises from either the **vertebral** or the **posterior inferior cerebellar artery** (PICA). The latter is the largest branch of the vertebral and has a tortuous course to reach the inferior vermis, intracerebellar (central, deep) nuclei of the cerebellum, and the choroid plexus of the fourth ventricle. Important **medullary branches** arise from **PICA** to irrigate the dorsolateral region the medulla.

The **basilar artery** gives off three named branches and numerous pontine arteries before its terminal bifurcation into the PCAs at the rostral border of the pons. The **anterior inferior cerebellar artery** (AICA) arises from the caudal basilar to supply portions of the pontine tegmentum and middle surface of the cerebellum. It assists in the supply of the intracerebellar nuclei as well as the upper medulla and lower pons.

The **labyrinthine artery** usually arises from AICA. In less than 20% of brains it arises from the basilar. It courses through the internal auditory meatus to supply cranial nerves VII (facial) and

VIII (vestibulocochlear). Pontine branches are "end" arteries with small lumen branching off an artery with a large lumen (basilar) that penetrate the pons to supply its ventral portion containing the corticospinal, corticobulbar, corticopontine tracts and the pontine tegmentum. A branch close to the terminal bifurcation of the basilar is the **superior cerebellar artery** (SCA), which supplies rostral portions of the pons, the inferior colliculi of the mesencephalon, and the superior cerebellar peduncle in addition to the superior surface of the cerebellar hemisphere.

Clinical Correlations . . . .

Carotid endarterectomy is a surgical procedure to remove blockages from the internal carotid arteries that furnish the major blood supply to the cerebrum. This can reduce the risk of stroke in patients who have emboli or plaque that causes temporary (transient) weakness or numbness on one side of the face, arm, or leg. **Transient monocular blindness** is a sign that should not be ignored. It involves the central artery of the retina and may reflect ipsilateral internal carotid involvement that is amenable to treatment. Lesions of the vertebral-basilar system in the infratentorial compartment were discussed in Chapter 3.

Color the left vertebral-basilar system first on the frontal view, then on the lateral view. Give attention to the terminal bifurcation of the basilar into the PCAs. Color the left common carotid on the frontal view, observing how its origin off the aorta differs from the right. Continue coloring and note the extracranial bifurcation of the common carotid and the course of the "carotid siphon." On the lateral view, follow the course of the PICA, the AICA, and the SCA to their terminal inferior, middle, and superior surfaces of the cerebellum, respectfully. Color the branches of the MCA in the lateral sulcus. Color the ACA of the right hemisphere. Connect the posterior and anterior circulation by coloring the anterior and posterior communicating arteries. Color the left PCA along the cerebral peduncle to its cut surface. Finally, color the terminal branches of the right PCA.

General Blood Supply of the Brain

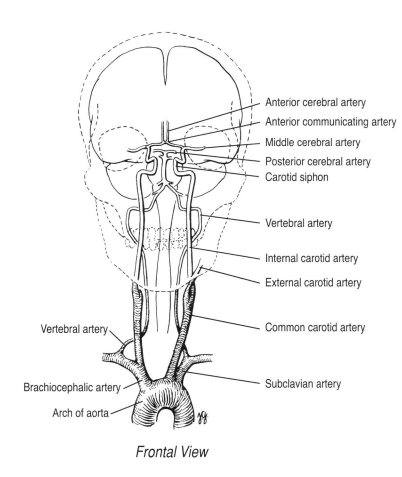

Anterior cerebral artery

Anterior communicating artery

Middle cerebral artery

Posterior cerebral artery

Carotid siphon

Vertebral artery

Internal carotid artery

External carotid artery

Common carotid artery

Subclavian artery

Vertebral artery

Brachiocephalic artery

Arch of aorta

Frontal View

Arch of the Aorta

Source and course of the large arteries that supply the brain.

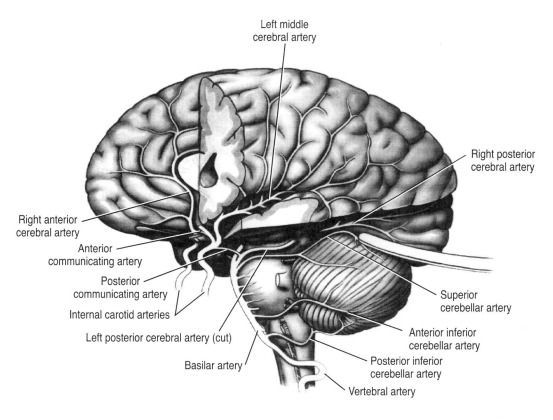

Left middle cerebral artery

Right posterior cerebral artery

Right anterior cerebral artery

Anterior communicating artery

Posterior communicating artery

Internal carotid arteries

Left posterior cerebral artery (cut)

Basilar artery

Superior cerebellar artery

Anterior inferior cerebellar artery

Posterior inferior cerebellar artery

Vertebral artery

Lateral View

Arterial Supply of the Brain

Semidiagrammatic figure showing the two major arteries, the internal carotid artery and the vertebral artery, carrying blood to the brain. Part of the left hemisphere has been removed in order to show the distribution of the anterior and posterior cerebral arteries on the medial side of the hemisphere. The three main cerebellar arteries are also illustrated. (Reprinted with permission from Heimer, Lennart. **The Human Brain and Spinal Cord.** Springer-Verlag, New York, 1995:464. Art by Medical and Scientific Illustration, Crozet, Virginia.)

Blood Supply of Basal Ganglia, Thalamus, and Internal Capsule

Definitions

The diencephalic-telencephalic junction receives striate (syn: penetrating, perforating, deep, and central) branches from all three cerebral arteries—**anterior** (ACA), **middle** (MCA), and **posterior** (PCA). **Striate arteries** from the ACA reach ventral regions of the caudate nucleus and the anterior limb of the internal capsule whereas striate branches from the PCA supply the thalamus and contribute to the supply of the posterior limb of the internal capsule. The striate vessels are so named because of the striated appearance of this region created by gray strands across the internal capsule between the caudate nucleus and the putamen. The term **stroke** refers to the onset of neurologic signs and symptoms caused by a cessation of blood flow due to blockage of a cerebral artery by an **embolus** (ischemic infarction) or from a **hemorrhagic infarction** of cerebral tissue. **Transient ischemic attacks** (TIAs) precede a stroke and suggest serious cerebrovascular disease. **Aphasia** is a language disorder involving a loss of ability to comprehend or express the signs and symbols used in human communication. **Global aphasia** indicates that all aspects of speech and language are severely disturbed. **Dysarthria** is a faulty articulation of consonant and vowel sounds.

Structural and Functional Features

The **recurrent artery of Heubner** (medial striate artery) is the largest striate off the **ACA**. It and other **medial striate arteries** supply the striatum and ventral region of the **anterior limb** of the internal capsule. The **lateral striate (lenticulostriate) branches** from the **MCA** provide the main blood supply to the **basal ganglia** and to the **internal capsule**. **Thalamogeniculate arteries** from the **PCA** are the main source of supply to the thalamus and the posterior choroidal branch of the PCA supplies the ventral surface of the **posterior limb** of the internal capsule. The fact that striate vessels take origin from the circle of Willis and from the proximal segments of the ACA, MCA, and PCA and are **dead-end vessels** ("end" arteries) most distal in the vascular tree is a significant anatomic point. Small caliber striate arteries arise at right angles from parent vessels that have a larger lumen; therefore, end arteries lack the gradual diminution of lumen that is characteristic of arteries in general.

Clinical Correlations . . . .

For reasons cited above, the deep penetrating branches that supply the basal ganglia, thalamus, and internal capsule are especially prone to rupture in patients with degenerative changes due to cerebrovascular disease. Hypertension often contributes to **stroke.** Hemorrhagic lesions of the striate branches may result in **contralateral hemiplegia** due to destruction of the descending motor fibers in the posterior limb of the internal capsule. **Contralateral hemianesthesia** may result if the ascending thalamocortical fibers are also destroyed. Both **embolic** and **hemorrhagic strokes** are characterized by an **abrupt onset**. Massive bleeding into the **posterior limb** of the internal capsule or an occlusion of the stem of the **MCA** cause **contralateral hemiplegia** and **hemianesthesia** and **homonymous hemianopsia**. When the stem of the MCA is blocked in the dominant hemisphere, **global aphasia** occurs as well. Lesions in the internal capsule do not cause aphasia although **dysarthria** due to supranuclear lesions of corticobulbar fibers to cranial nerve nuclei may hinder speech.

Transient ischemic attacks (TIAs) present with a plethora of symptoms that vary relative to the artery that is temporarily occluded. A TIA can be a "wake-up call" of an existing plaque or thrombus. **Surgical or medical care needed may, if sought, avert a recurrence and potential irreversible damage.**

Color the caudate head, body, and tail purple and the putamen and the thalamus blue. Color the corona radiata, anterior, posterior, and retrolenticular parts of the internal capsule yellow. Color both parts of the globus pallidus brown, the amygdala green, and the claustrum orange. Finally color all of the arteries, always giving attention to the caliber of the vessel and the direction of flow. Use the same color scheme throughout because a given structure has the same number in all views.

Blood Supply of Basal Ganglia, Thalamus, and Internal Capsule

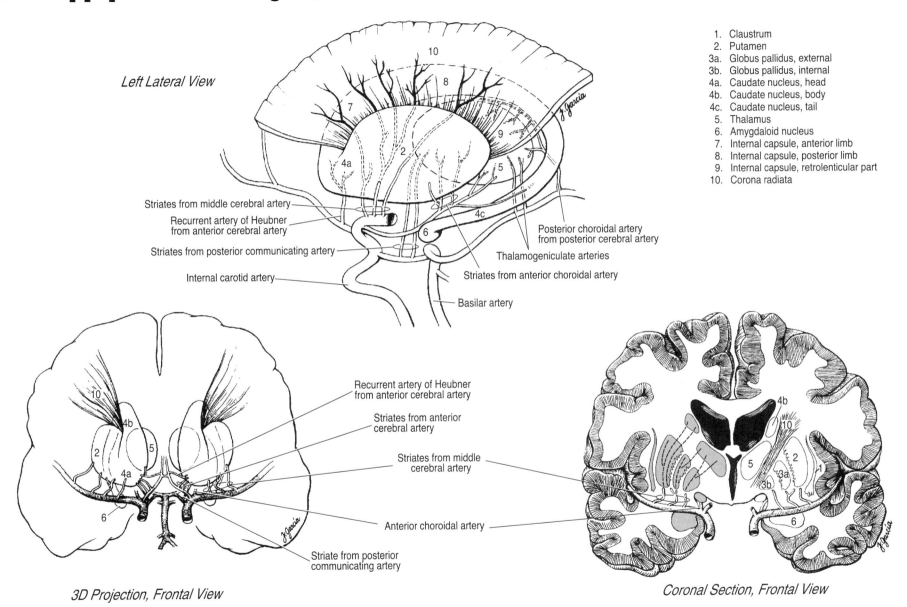

Left Lateral View

1. Claustrum
2. Putamen
3a. Globus pallidus, external
3b. Globus pallidus, internal
4a. Caudate nucleus, head
4b. Caudate nucleus, body
4c. Caudate nucleus, tail
5. Thalamus
6. Amygdaloid nucleus
7. Internal capsule, anterior limb
8. Internal capsule, posterior limb
9. Internal capsule, retrolenticular part
10. Corona radiata

Striates from middle cerebral artery

Recurrent artery of Heubner from anterior cerebral artery

Striates from posterior communicating artery

Internal carotid artery

Posterior choroidal artery from posterior cerebral artery

Thalamogeniculate arteries

Striates from anterior choroidal artery

Basilar artery

Recurrent artery of Heubner from anterior cerebral artery

Striates from anterior cerebral artery

Striates from middle cerebral artery

Anterior choroidal artery

Striate from posterior communicating artery

3D Projection, Frontal View

Coronal Section, Frontal View

Blood Supply of the Brain, Lateral View

Definitions

The direct continuation of the internal carotid artery lateral to the origin of the **anterior cerebral artery** (ACA) becomes the **stem** of the **middle cerebral artery** (MCA). Functional areas in the **MCA** territory and their Brodmann's classification are labeled on page 187. "Watershed" areas are **border zones** of anastomoses between the terminal branches of the MCA with the terminal branches of the **ACA** and **PCA,** which continue over from the medial surface of the hemisphere.

Structural and Functional Features

The MCA runs in the lateral sulcus where numerous branches ramify over the insula before they pass out to supply most of the dorsolateral surface of the **frontal, parietal,** and **temporal cortices.** In addition to furnishing the main supply to the **corpus striatum** and **internal capsule** via penetrating striate branches (pages 184 and 185). Meyer's loop fibers (page 191) are supplied by the MCA. As the striate arteries arise from the proximal segment, they enter the anterior perforated space. Because the striate arteries come off at right angles, they are not likely sites of embolic strokes; however, they are prone to hemorrhagic stroke or atherosclerotic occlusion.

Clinical Correlations . . . .

The functions supplied by the branches of the MCA are depicted on page 187. An **embolus** from the heart or from the internal carotid artery may **occlude** the stem of the MCA. Embolic strokes present with an abrupt onset. In a worst case scenario (as previously discussed on page 184), an embolic occlusion of the stem could result in **contralateral hemiplegia** and **hemianesthesia, homonymous hemianopsia,** and **global aphasia** if the lesion is in the dominant hemisphere. However, the extent of an ischemic infarction due to an embolic stroke or a hemorrhagic infarction involving the striate arteries is extremely **variable** and depends on the location of the insult and on the effectiveness of the collateral circulation. Initially one cannot know whether the pathology involving a vascular territory will be temporary or irreversible. Regions supplied by the terminal branches of the vascular tree in the **watershed zones** of anastomoses between the three major cerebral arteries are particularly

vulnerable to hypoxia under conditions of low blood pressure and cardiac arrest. An infarction occurring in this region may be called a border zone or a watershed zone infarct.

The middle meningeal artery arises from the maxillary artery off the external carotid artery. **Fractures** in the **frontotemporal region (pterion)** may **rupture the middle meningeal artery** and result in an **epidural hematoma.** Pressure of such a mass on the anterior speech area and on the motor and sensory cortices may cause **contralateral paresis** and **anesthesia** of the **face** and **arm** as well as **expressive aphasia** if the dominant hemisphere is involved. Note that the phenomenon of an epidural hematoma that presses on cerebral tissue in the MCA territory resembles a vascular lesion of the MCA per se. In the case of a hematoma external to the dura, however, the prognosis of recovery is good if the diagnosis of a mass-occupying lesion is made quickly and the hematoma is surgically evacuated.

In summary, three factors contribute to the high incidence of focal damage to the territories irrigated by branches of the MCA: **Emboli** from the **heart** and from the **carotid arteries** lodge in the MCA; the **vulnerability** of the **striates,** of which the MCA is the dominant source (page 184); and **trauma** to the dorsolateral hemispheric surface and the location of the middle meningeal artery make an epidural hematoma over the MCA territory more prevalent than on the superior, medial, and basal surfaces of the cerebrum.

First, color the stem of the MCA and the branch that runs inferiorly from the lateral sulcus to supply the temporal lobe. Color the other branches as they emanate from the surface of the insula to supply the frontal and parietal cortices, and observe the diminishing caliber of the vessels as they ramify over the dorsolateral surface of the hemisphere. Be aware of the probability of the course of an embolus. Note the extent to which terminal branches from the ACA and PCA meet the terminal branches of the MCA in the watershed zones. Finally, color the middle meningeal artery observing the frontal and parietal branches to supply the dura mater.

Nature does not give a man virtue: the process of becoming a good man is an art. – Seneca
186

Blood Supply of the Brain, Lateral View

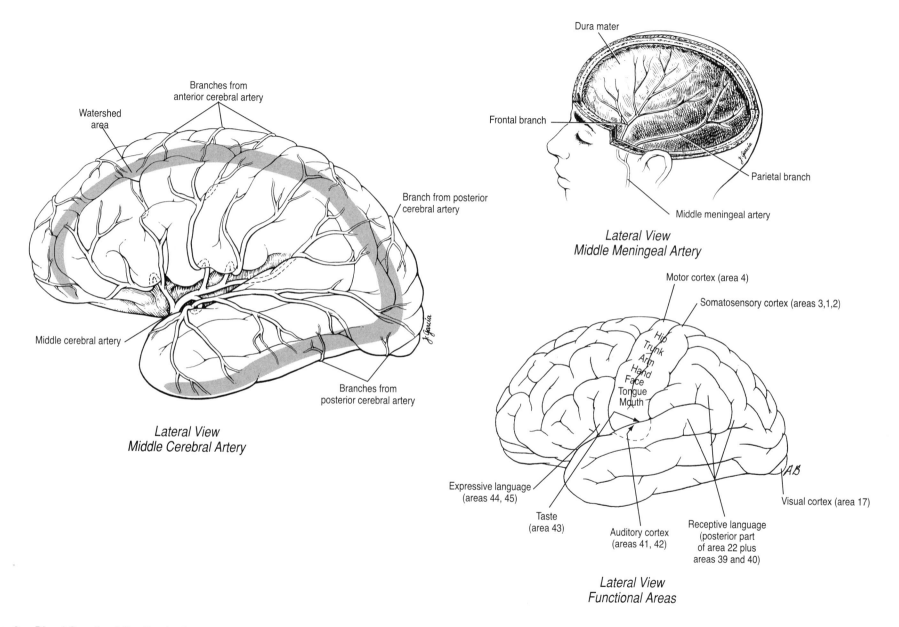

Watershed area

Branches from anterior cerebral artery

Branch from posterior cerebral artery

Middle cerebral artery

Branches from posterior cerebral artery

Lateral View
Middle Cerebral Artery

Dura mater

Frontal branch

Parietal branch

Middle meningeal artery

Lateral View
Middle Meningeal Artery

Motor cortex (area 4)

Somatosensory cortex (areas 3,1,2)

Hip
Trunk
Arm
Hand
Face
Tongue
Mouth

Visual cortex (area 17)

Expressive language (areas 44, 45)

Taste (area 43)

Auditory cortex (areas 41, 42)

Receptive language (posterior part of area 22 plus areas 39 and 40)

Lateral View
Functional Areas

Blood Supply of the Brain, Medial View

Definitions
The anterior cerebral artery (ACA) is the smaller terminal branch of the internal carotid artery. The **pericallosal artery** is the continuation of the main trunk of the ACA after it gives off the **callosomarginal** branch near the genu of the corpus callosum. The **posterior cerebral artery** (PCA) is a terminal branch of the basilar artery.

Structural and Functional Features
The **ACA** passes across the anterior perforating space where it gives off penetrating branches that contribute to the blood supply of the **striatum** and **internal capsule**. The main trunk curves upward over the genu of the corpus callosum, which it supplies as far posteriorly as the splenium. The unpaired **anterior communicating artery** connects the two anterior cerebral arteries, which then arch upward and run posteriorly in the interhemispheric fissure. **Cortical branches** of the ACA supply the **medial aspects of the frontal and parietal lobes** as well as the **orbital gyri** of the frontal lobe. **Thalamoperforating branches** from the **PCA** enter the posterior perforated space to supply the **thalamus** as it runs laterally along the rostral border of the pons. After receiving the posterior communicating artery, the PCA curves around the cerebral peduncles of the mesencephalon and gives off **thalamogeniculate** branches to supply the thalamus and **tectum**. The **posterior choroidal artery** arises from the PCA near the splenium to assist in the supply of the **choroid plexus** in the body of the **lateral ventricle** and the choroid plexus in the **third ventricle**.

Clinical Correlations ·

Because the motor and sensory functions of the lower limb are represented in the paracentral lobule (medial aspects of the precentral and postcentral gyri, respectively), **occlusion or hemorrhage** of the **ACA** may result in **contralateral lower limb dysfunction. Occlusion** of the blood supply to the **occipital lobe** results in **blindness** in the **contralateral field of vision** (homonymous hemianopsia). **Disruption** of blood supply to the **thalamus** may result in **altered sensation including spontaneous and agonizing pain (thalamic syndrome). The syndrome usually occurs during recovery from a thalamic infarct.**

Begin by coloring the internal carotid artery and observe the size of the ACA compared to the MCA as you color. Color the pericallosal artery to its junction with the PCA. Color the callosomarginal artery and its branches to the convexity of the hemisphere and observe their continuation onto the lateral surface. Note as you color the PCA that it ramifies over the inferomedial temporal and the medial occipital cortices and that it supplies the splenium of the corpus callosum and sends small "twigs" into the posterior parietal lobe. Finally, beginning at the internal carotid, color the posterior communicating artery to connect it with the PCA.

How far that little candle throws his beams! So shines a good deed in a naughty world. – Shakespeare

188

Blood Supply of the Brain, Medial View

Medial View

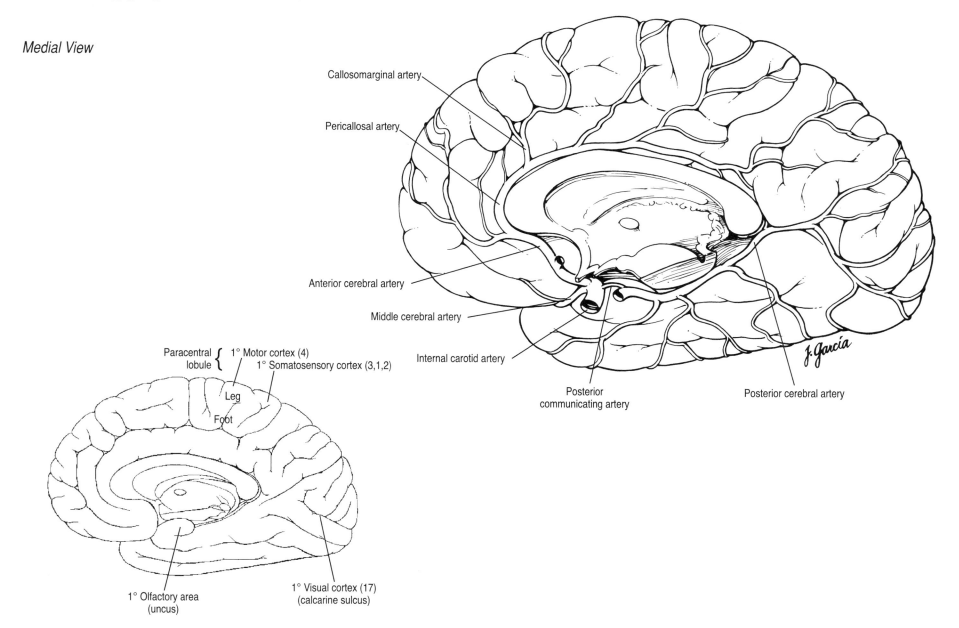

Callosomarginal artery

Pericallosal artery

Anterior cerebral artery

Middle cerebral artery

Internal carotid artery

Posterior communicating artery

Posterior cerebral artery

J. Garcia

Paracentral lobule { 1° Motor cortex (4)
1° Somatosensory cortex (3,1,2)

Leg

Foot

1° Olfactory area (uncus)

1° Visual cortex (17) (calcarine sulcus)

Blood Supply of the Visual System

Definitions
Terms related to the visual pathways and visual deficits were discussed and depicted on pages 90 and 91.

Structural and Functional Features
The visual system receives its blood supply from the **internal carotid** and from the **vertebral-basilar systems.** The **ophthalmic artery**, a branch of the internal carotid, gives rise to the **central artery of the retina,** which runs in the optic nerve. It is therefore surrounded by cerebrospinal fluid in the subarachnoid space because the optic nerve is ensheathed by the meninges. **Anterior and posterior choroidal arteries** branch off the **internal carotid (or MCA)** and the **posterior cerebral arteries (PCAs),** respectively. In addition to supplying the **choroid plexus,** they supply the **optic tract** and the **lateral geniculate nucleus,** a thalamic relay that gives rise to the geniculocalcarine tract (optic radiations). The PCA continues posteriorly to supply the **cuneus** and **lingual gyri** on the medial surface of the occipital lobe.

Clinical Correlations . . . .

An **occlusion** of the **PCA**, if complete, results in **homonymous hemianopsia** (page 91). **Cortical blindness** is a potential possibility if both PCAs are pushed against the tentorium cerebelli in the event of a mass herniating through the tentorial notch. Theoretically, cortical blindness could likewise result from **embolization** to the basilar bifurcation. An **acute onset** as is characteristic of an **embolus** could preclude effective **collateralization** from the internal carotid system via the posterior communicating arteries. **Lesions posterior** to the **lateral geniculate nucleus** spare the retinal input to the superior colliculus and pretectal area; thus, **reflex response** to light via the tectospinal tract and the pupillary response to light are preserved.

Color the internal carotid artery, noting the origins of the ophthalmic, posterior communicating, and anterior choroidal. Realize that the central artery of the retina is a branch of the ophthalmic. Connect "anterior" and "posterior" circulations by coloring the posterior communicating artery. Color the anterior choroidal and its branches to the optic tract and lateral geniculate body. As you color the PCA , note its anastomosis with the anterior choroidal and its twigs to the lateral geniculate body. Continue coloring the PCA and its cortical branches as it continues posteriorly to supply the medial occipital cortex and underlying white matter. Finally, color the MCA and its cortical branches to the geniculocalcarine tract.

Blood Supply of the Visual System

View of Inferior Surface

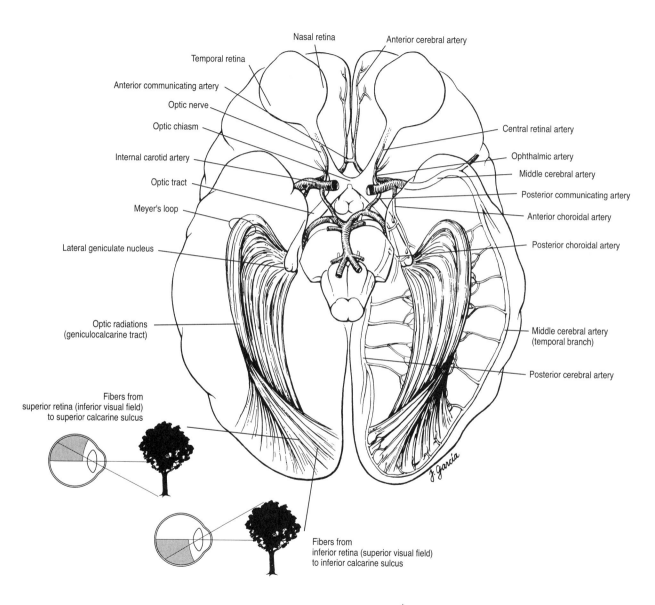

Nasal retina

Anterior cerebral artery

Temporal retina

Anterior communicating artery

Optic nerve

Optic chiasm

Central retinal artery

Internal carotid artery

Ophthalmic artery

Optic tract

Middle cerebral artery

Meyer's loop

Posterior communicating artery

Lateral geniculate nucleus

Anterior choroidal artery

Posterior choroidal artery

Optic radiations
(geniculocalcarine tract)

Middle cerebral artery
(temporal branch)

Posterior cerebral artery

Fibers from
superior retina (inferior visual field)
to superior calcarine sulcus

Fibers from
inferior retina (superior visual field)
to inferior calcarine sulcus

J. Garcia

Regional Blood Supply of the Main Cerebral Arteries

Table 6.2 Regional Blood Supply of the Main Cerebral Arteries

Artery	Area Supplied	Brodmann's Number if Applicable	Function
ACA	Medial and orbital prefrontal cortex Paracentral lobule Precuneus Cingulate gyrus Corpus callosum, genu, and body Striatum, ventral surface Anterior limb, internal capsule (assists MCA)	4;3,1,2 5,7	Initiative and emotional restraint Motor and sensory representation, contralateral leg Somesthetic association cortex Motivation and emotions Reciprocal connections: frontal, parietal, and temporal lobes Involved in motor circuity Anterior thalamic and corticopontine fibers

MCA	Precentral gyrus
	Premotor area
	Postcentral gyrus
	Frontal eye field
	Inferior frontal gyrus
	Opercular part, precentral gyrus
	Transverse temporal gyri
	Superior temporal gyrus
	   Posterior part
	Inferior parietal lobule
	   Supramarginal gyrus
	   Angular gyrus
	Prefrontal cortex
	Corpus striatum
	Internal capsule (main source is MCA)
	Anteromedial temporal lobe, including uncus
		4
		6
		3,1,2
		8
		44,45
		43
		41,42
		22
		
		40
		39
			Motor output, face, contralateral arm, trunk
			Motor planning and output
			Primary somatosensory cortex
			Contralateral conjugate deviation of the eyes
			Motor (expressive) speech (dominant hemisphere)
			Primary area of taste
			Primary auditory cortex
			Left hemisphere: understanding language
			Right hemisphere: understanding prosody
			
			Concentration, judgment and executive command
			Involved in motor circuitry
			Ascending and descending pathways
			Primary olfactory area

PCA	Thalamus Parahippocampal and medial occipitotemporal gyri Medial occipital lobe Corpus callosum, splenium Posterior limb, internal capsule (assists MCA)	17,18,19	Motor and sensory gateway to the cortex Facial recognition Primary visual cortex, visual association cortex Reciprocal connections: occipital lobes Ascending and descending pathways

 Color the arterial territories of all views as follows: middle cerebral, yellow; deep branches of MCA, yellow stripes; anterior cerebral, blue; and posterior cerebral, green.

Regional Blood Supply of the Main Cerebral Arteries

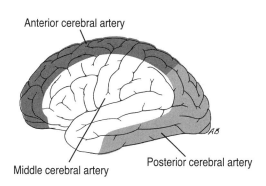

Anterior cerebral artery

Middle cerebral artery

Posterior cerebral artery

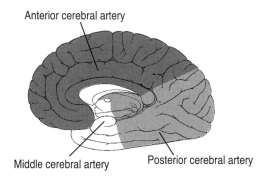

Anterior cerebral artery

Middle cerebral artery

Posterior cerebral artery

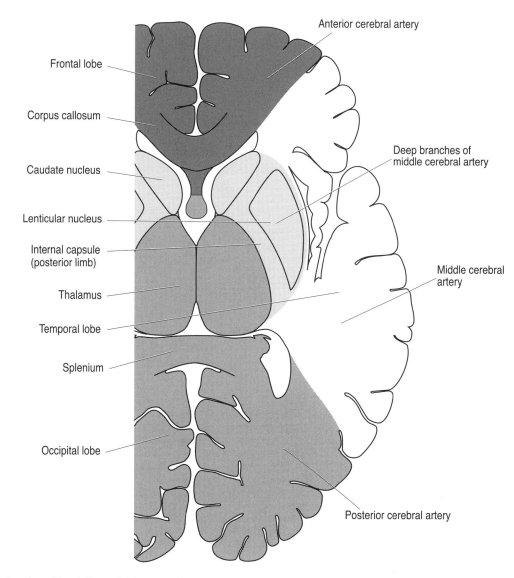

Anterior cerebral artery

Frontal lobe

Corpus callosum

Caudate nucleus

Lenticular nucleus

Internal capsule
(posterior limb)

Thalamus

Temporal lobe

Splenium

Occipital lobe

Deep branches of
middle cerebral artery

Middle cerebral
artery

Posterior cerebral artery

Diagram of the cerebral hemispheres showing the territories of the main cerebral vessels in dorsolateral (top left), medial (bottom left), and horizontal (right) views.

Computed Tomography Demonstration of Intracranial Hemorrhage

Definitions

Computerized axial tomography (CAT) is a procedure that utilizes x-ray absorption based on electron density. For images of the skull and its contents, the standard plane of the slices is parallel to the supraorbital line (25° to Reid's anthropologic baseline). All slices are parallel to each other (the angle slants inferiorly from anterior to posterior). This **favored axial (horizontal)** plane accounts for the initial use of the term CAT. **The baseline of Reid's angle prevents the exposure of the contents of the orbit to radiation**. The term "computed tomography" (CT) has replaced the CAT term because radiologists may select slices at other angles to the base of the skull, e.g., slices in the frontal (coronal) plane are indicated for visualization of the facial bones, orbits, and the pituitary gland.

Structural and Functional Features

Lesions vary in their ability to absorb or attenuate x-ray photons. They are **hypodense, isodense**, or **hyperdense** relative to the intrinsic density of the adjacent parenchyma.

Clinical Correlations

The most frequent cause of **intracranial hemorrhage** (ICH) is trauma. By virtue of the protein moiety (globin), intracranial blood has a high density on **CT**; therefore, CT is the **imaging modality of choice for evaluating acute ICH**. **Acute** is defined as less than 1 week, **subacute** as 1 week to 1 month, and **chronic** as more than 1 month. Whereas CT is superior to **MRI for early detection of ICH**, MRI sensitivity to the breakdown products of hemoglobin make it the ideal modality for evaluating the age and etiology of the lesion in later stages. The common use of the acronym ICH is in the context of a parenchymal hemorrhage, i.e., intracerebral. This, however, is a general term. Other types are specifically designated as subarachnoid, subdural, or epidural, all of which are intracranial hemorrhages. The incidence of spontaneous parenchymal ICH is higher in certain geographic regions, e.g., eastern North Carolina, probably because of the high incidence of undiagnosed (and thus untreated) hypertension.

Take it to heart and pass the word along: fair dealing brings more profit in the end. – Homer

Computed Tomography Demonstration of Intracranial Hemorrhage

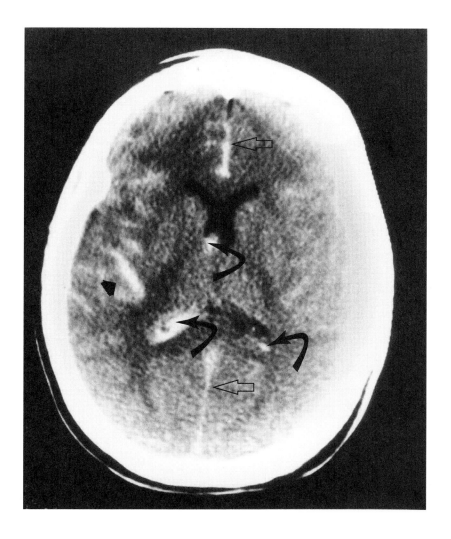

Hyperdense acute bleeding into subarachnoid space in the right lateral fissure (black arrow) and interhemispheric fissure (open arrows) and within the lateral ventricles (curved black arrows).

Unenhanced CT of trauma (37-year-old woman). (Courtesy of Dr. Michael D. Weaver, East Carolina University School of Medicine.)

Angiography, Aneurysms, and an Angiogram of an Internal Carotid Aneurysm

Definitions

Conventional angiography is a procedure based on the injection of a contrast medium into a vessel to render it visible by radiography. Recent and rapid advances have been made in **magnetic resonance angiography** (MRA), which requires no contrast medium and is therefore noninvasive. Nonetheless, at present, conventional angiography continues to be the definitive procedure of choice for evaluating the cerebral circulation.

Following the injection of a water-soluble organic radiolabeled iodine compound into the aortic arch, subclavian, carotid, or vertebral arteries, the radiopaque solution flows through the arteries, capillaries, and veins of the brain and head. Multiple timed exposures reveal the location of the radiopaque solution and produce a "road map" of the blood vessels.

The brain is isolated from the systemic circulation by an organ-specific protective mechanism, the blood-brain barrier (BBB). **The tight junctions (zonulae occludens) of brain endothelium preclude passage of high molecular weight substances.** The contrast medium does not gain access to cerebral parenchyma where the **BBB** is intact. **The choroid plexus and certain midline structures termed "circumventricular organs" (CVOs) lack this barrier that otherwise is found throughout the CNS.** Fenestrations in the capillaries of these highly vascularized organs permit interaction between circulating hormones and receptor sites in the **CVOs**. In addition to the choroid plexus, other structures that lack the BBB include the median eminence and neurohypophysis, vascular organ of the lamina terminalis, subfornical organ, subcommissural organ, pineal gland, and area postrema. The area postrema is an emetic center; other CVO chemoreceptors are also important for homeostasis. **Structures that lack a BBB show enhancement with contrast.**

Structural and Functional Features

Certain conditions—infarction, infection, abscess, and trauma—may disrupt the BBB. Neoplasms (tumors) develop neovascularity that lacks a BBB. It follows that the presence of a contrast medium in cerebral parenchyma, other than those areas lacking the BBB, indicates BBB disruption.

Aneurysms (focal dilatations of the arterial walls) are of multifactorial origin: congenital, atherosclerotic, traumatic, and mycotic. Congenital or "berry" aneurysms account for 80% of intracranial aneurysms and typically occur at arterial branches. (Page 180 contains details.) Subarachnoid hemorrhage (SAH), with resultant headache and photophobia, is the most common clinical manifestation of a ruptured aneurysm and may occur during exertion. The goal of the angiographer in evaluating a suspected aneurysm is not only to locate and define the neck of the aneurysm but also to evaluate for focal spasm and to examine the remainder of the anterior and posterior circulation for multiple aneurysms, which occur in 15–20% of cases.

Clinical Correlations . . . .

Arteriovenous malformation (AVM) is the most common type of vascular malformation. There are no intervening capillaries between the arteries and veins in these congenital anomalies, hence the blood flow is rapid. Aneurysms may coexist in this tangled, aberrant mass of vessels. **Risks** associated with **AVM** include **hemorrhage, ischemia**, and **epilepsy** (the latter being greater with a temporal lobe location because epilepsy often originates from temporal lobe foci).

Angiogram of an Internal Carotid Aneurysm

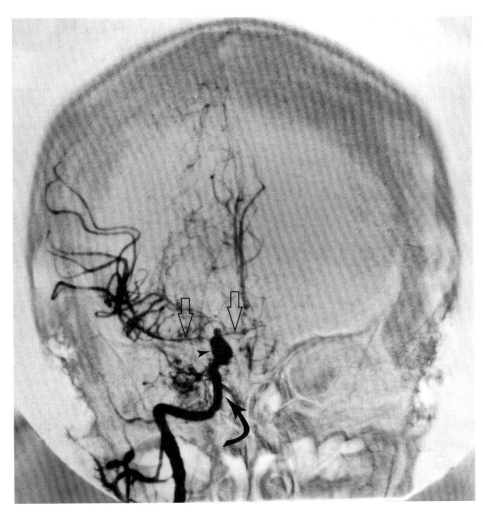

In addition to the aneurysm of the internal carotid artery (arrowhead), note the narrowing of the anterior and middle cerebral arteries (open arrows) which is evidence of focal spasm. Other points of interest are the carotid siphon (curved arrow) and the symmetry of the anterior cerebral arteries in the interhemispheric fissure on either side of the midline falx cerebri. There are numerous branches of the middle cerebral artery in the lateral (Sylvian) sulcus.

Congenital "berry" aneurysm (adult) of the internal carotid artery. (Courtesy of Dr. Michael D. Weaver, East Carolina University School of Medicine.)

Chapter Six Study Questions

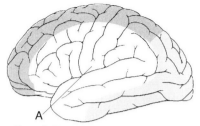
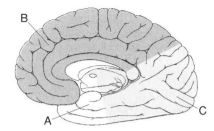

Questions 1–5

Directions: The letters above represent the vascular territories of the three major cerebral arteries. For each patient with neurologic abnormalities due to stroke, select the artery that is most likely to be involved. Each letter may be used more than once or not at all.

1. A 55-year-old right-handed woman is unable to understand spoken language in spite of the fact that her hearing is normal.

2. A 68-year-old right-handed man has weakness and hyperreflexia of the right arm. His sensation is normal. Despite weakness of the right lower facial muscles, his speech is fluent and appropriate.

3. A 72-year-old right-handed woman listens attentively to her examiner's questions and nods yes and no appropriately. She has no neurologic findings other than a slow, laborious, halting manner of speaking.

4. A 78-year-old right-handed man has paresis and anesthesia of the left leg. He has normal facial movements and normal strength in all other limbs.

5. A 58-year-old man has no vision in the hemifield contralateral to his lesion, i.e., has left homonymous hemianopsia.

Questions 6–10

Directions: Match the lettered artery in the coronal view of the blood supply with the numbered statement below.

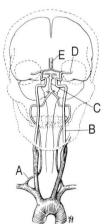

6. Traverses the cavernous venous sinus before piercing the dura and turning upward lateral to the optic chiasm

7. Its two terminal branches ascend over the tentorium cerebelli to supply the inferior temporal and medial occipital lobes bilaterally

8. Enters the cranium through the foramen magnum

9. Supplies the genu and body of the corpus callosum

10. Emboli from the heart tend to lodge in this artery or one of its branches

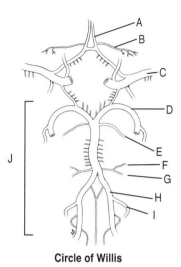

Circle of Willis

Questions 11–15

Directions: Match the lettered artery or arterial system in the diagram above with the numbered statement below.

11. Circles around the cerebral peduncle to provide the main source of blood supply to the thalamus

12. Supplies the superior surface of the cerebellum

13. In the majority of brains, this artery supplies the dorsolateral medulla.

14. This branch of the anterior cerebral artery, the only named medial striate artery, provides blood supply to the ventral striatum and ventral anterior limb of the internal capsule.

15. Furnishes the main blood supply to the internal capsule

Case History

16. A 78-year-old right-handed man has right hemiparesis including right lower face involvement. He also has hemianesthesia of the right side. He has normal comprehension of written and verbal commands and his speech is appropriate although somewhat hindered by the lower facial weakness. Which vessels are most likely to be involved?
    (a) Right lateral striate (lenticulostriate) arteries
    (b) Left lateral striate (lenticulostriate) arteries
    (c) Right middle cerebral artery
    (d) Left anterior cerebral artery
    (e) Right anterior cerebral artery

Answers and Explanations for Chapter Six Study Questions

1. **a** [page 187] The **receptive speech area** (Wernicke's) is in the superior temporal gyrus. Lesions here are devastating relative to social intercourse because fluent speech emanating from an intact Broca's area is nonsensical when one does not understand what is being said by oneself or by others. **Wernicke's area** is in the territory of the **middle cerebral artery** (MCA).

2. **a** [page 187] The precentral gyrus or motor cortex gives rise to about half of the corticospinal and corticobulbar fibers. The face, arm, and trunk are somatotopically organized with face fibers near the lateral sulcus and the hip at the convexity of the hemisphere. This territory is supplied by the **MCA.**

3. **a** [page 187] Only **Broca's area** in the posterior region of the inferior frontal gyrus (Brodmann's areas 44 and 45) is involved, which is the expressive speech area. One can compensate to an extent with gestures when there is understanding of what is being said because of the intactness of **Wernicke's area. Broca's area,** like most of the dorsolateral surface of the hemisphere, is **supplied** by the **MCA.**

4. **b** [pages 188 and 189] The motor and somesthetic areas of the leg are represented in the **paracentral lobule** on the **medial surface** of the **hemisphere,** which is supplied by the **anterior cerebral artery.**

5. **c** [page 191] Images from the **contralateral field** of vision are initially processed in the **medial occipital lobe,** which is supplied by the **posterior cerebral artery** (PCA). This man's lesion involves the right PCA.

6. **b, internal carotid artery** [page 182] Ipsilateral temporal retinal fibers are affected first by an aneurysm pressing on the lateral optic chiasm. Thirty percent of intracranial aneurysms involve the internal carotid artery.

7. **c, basilar artery** [page 180] The vulnerability of the posterior cerebral arteries, the terminal branches of the basilar, is a significant clinical point relative to herniation of a mass from the supratentorial compartment through the tentorial incisure.

8. **a, vertebral artery** [page 180] The vertebral arteries ascend through transverse processes of vertebrae C1-C6. After entering the skull through the foramen magnum, these vessels run medially (inferior to the medulla) and join at the medullopontine junction to form the basilar artery.

9. **e, anterior cerebral artery** [page 188] The main stem of the anterior cerebral artery, after giving rise to the callosomarginal branch, continues posteriorly as the pericallosal artery. In this position above the corpus callosum, it supplies all of it except the splenium, which is irrigated by the posterior cerebral artery. Fibers in the genu connect left and right frontal lobes. Frontal, parietal, and temporal lobes are reciprocally connected via fibers in the body.

10. **d, middle cerebral artery** [page 186] Emboli from the heart and from the common carotid artery travel into the middle cerebral, which is a direct continuation of the internal carotid artery.

11. **d, posterior cerebral artery** [pages 184, 191, and 193] Thalamoperforating branches of the PCA enter the posterior perforated space between the cerebral peduncles to supply the thalamus. Thalamogeniculate branches from the posterior choroidal (off PCA) contribute to the supply of the lateral geniculate nuclei which are thalamic nuclei. The anterior choroidal (from the MCA or internal carotid) also supplies the latter.

12. **e, superior cerebellar artery** (SCA) [page 182] The SCA is the last branch of the basilar before it bifurcates to form the posterior cerebral arteries. The SCA also supplies the rostral pons and the inferior colliculi of the mesencephalon.

13. **i, posterior inferior cerebellar artery** [page 182] Because of its long, looped course, this vessel is subject to thrombotic plaques. Its occlusion results in a lateral medullary syndrome. Additionally, it supplies the inferior cerebellum including the inferior vermis and central nuclei as well as the choroid plexus of the fourth ventricle.

14. **b, recurrent artery of Heubner** [page 184] This vessel enters the anterior perforated substance to reach the striatum and internal capsule.

15. **c, middle cerebral artery** (MCA) [pages 184, 192, and 193] Via lateral striate (lenticulostriate) arteries and the anterior choroidal artery, the MCA provides the **main source** of supply to the internal capsule, especially the genu and posterior limb where the clinically significant fibers to and from the face and body traverse. This includes ascending sensory tracts and descending motor tracts. Anteriorly and posteriorly the internal capsule receives branches from the anterior and posterior cerebral arteries, respectively.

Case History

16. **b** [page 184] Hemorrhage of the left lenticulostriate arteries into the internal capsule lesion corticobulbar and corticospinal fibers and ascending thalamocortical projections resulting in contralateral hemiparesis and hemianesthesia. The part of the facial motor nucleus controlling the muscles of the lower face receives only contralateral corticobulbar projections, which would also be damaged in the internal capsule, resulting in paralysis of facial musculature on the same side as the limb paresis. Control of the upper face remains intact due to intact ipsilateral corticobulbar innervation.

CHAPTER 7 Midline Sagittal T1 MRI Through the Cerebral Aqueduct

Definition

MRI is defined as a procedure that uses strong magnets to detect minute radio signals given off by the nuclei of brain molecules, typically protons, thus determining their location and providing precise images of the internal structure of the brain. Magnetic resonance produces superb sagittal, coronal, and axial images. The patient remains supine throughout the procedure. The image plane can be varied simply by changing gradients. The choice of image plane may be determined by the desire to highlight a particular anatomic structure. Slice thickness and intervals between slices also can be varied.

A pulse sequence is defined as one or more pulses of radio waves. Varying the pulse sequence produces different appearances of the same structure. Spin echo (SE) pulse is a series of alternating 90° and 180° pulses. It is the most commonly used pulse sequence. **Anatomic detail is clearer on T1-weighted images, whereas T2-weighted images are more sensitive in revealing pathology.** For example, **unenhanced T1- and T2-weighted images are often sufficient for confirming diagnoses.** Gray and white matter can be differentiated in T1-weighted images, and edematous and hemorrhagic lesions can be detected in T2-weighted sequences. In T1 MR images, compact bone has a dark signal, marrow-filled bone has a bright signal.

Structural and Functional Features

It has been stated that neurology depends on clinical–anatomic correlation more than any other specialty. Correlating the in situ brain with its representation by neuroimaging technology affords one a test of "applied neuroanatomy." After testing your knowledge by naming the labeled structures in this MRI, compare the in situ images to those of an anatomic specimen. This midline sagittal MRI is comparable to the actual brain dissection on page 37. All MR images presented in this chapter (pages 201 through 221) are T1-weighted images. They are of the same brain—that of a normal 20-year-old woman. The **hypointensity** of **CSF** is **black** on **T1-weighted images** in contrast to the **hyperintensity** of the **optic chiasm,** which is **white** due to its phospholipid content. The hypointense and hyperintense appearance of these structures is reversed on T2-weighted images, e.g., CSF appears white rather than black.

Visualization of structures in the **posterior cranial fossa** is difficult with CT because of interference of **bone artifacts.** Parts of the sphenoid and occipital bones make up the clivus, which extends from the dorsum sellae to the foramen magnum and forms the central floor of the posterior fossa. The posterior boundary of the posterior fossa is the occipital bone, the anterolateral boundary is the petrous pyramid of the temporal bone on each side. The **MRI technique** is especially useful in identifying pathology in the middle or posterior cranial fossae because it allows pictures that are **free** of **bone artifacts**.

MRI is useful in visualizing intracerebral pathology including demyelinating diseases such as multiple sclerosis, infarctions, and neoplasms.

Clinical Correlations . . . .

The posterior cranial fossa contains the cerebellum, medulla, pons, most of the midbrain, and the fourth ventricle. Cranial nerves III–XII emerge from the brain stem in the posterior fossa. The foramen magnum makes up its caudal opening and the tentorium cerebelli defines its upper limit. MRI is of particular significance in evaluating clinical impressions of any of the above structures, especially the **cerebellopontine angle** where **tumors** may develop on the posterior portion of the **vestibulocochlear** nerve.

Pituitary gland tumors that impinge on the optic chiasm can be visualized in a midline sagittal image.

In T2-weighted images, most **focal pathologies** and **congenital abnormalities,** including regions of cortical dysplasia, are well visualized.

Color dark blue the corpus callosum. Color purple the fornix and mamillary body. Color light blue the parietal lobe and thalamus. Color red the frontal lobe and the cerebellum vermis. Color yellow the occipital lobe and brain stem (medulla, pons, and midbrain, including tectum).

Midline Sagittal T1 MRI Through the Cerebral Aqueduct

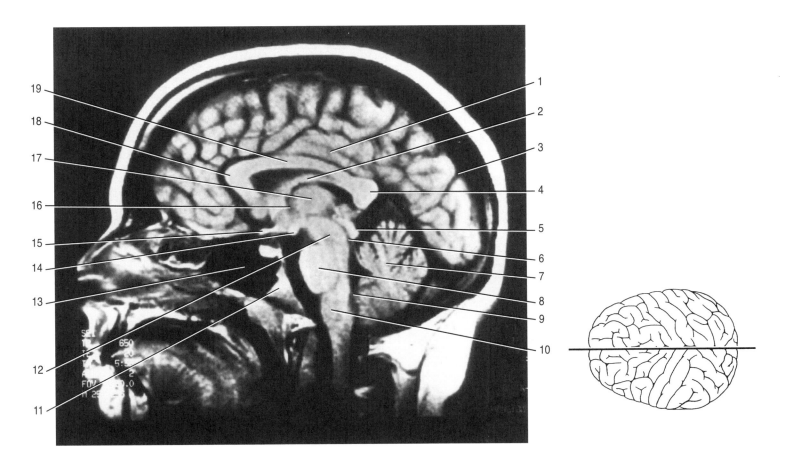

1. Cingulate gyrus
2. Fornix, body
3. Parieto-occipital sulcus
4. Corpus callosum, splenium
5. Tectum
6. Cerebral aqueduct
7. Cerebellum, vermis
8. Pons
9. Fourth ventricle
10. Medulla
11. Clivus
12. Tegmentum of midbrain
13. Sphenoid sinus
14. Mamillary body of hypothalamus
15. Optic chiasm
16. Interventricular foramen (of Monro)
17. Thalamus
18. Corpus callosum, genu
19. Corpus callosum, body

Normal brain (20-year-old woman).(Courtesy of Dr. Michael D. Weaver, East Carolina University, School of Medicine.)

Sagittal T1 MRI Through the Cerebral Peduncle

Definition

"Mass effect" is the change in position of brain structures as a result of an intracranial mass such as a neoplasm, abscess, or hematoma. The groove formed by the head of the caudate nucleus in relation to the thalamus is the **caudothalamic groove**. The **cisterna magna** (cerebellomedullary cistern) occupies the space between the cerebellum and medulla and receives CSF through the foramen of Magendie. It provides a source of CSF for diagnostic analysis when lumbar puncture is contraindicated, e.g., when intracranial pressure is elevated.

Structural and Functional Features

This off-center, i.e., parasagittal, section goes through the cerebral peduncle and the cerebellar tonsils. In this plane, the **caudothalamic groove** is of interest because **germinal matrix hemorrhages** occur here. The shape and extent of the body of the lateral ventricle can be appreciated in this particular plane of section.

Clinical Correlations . . . .

Space-occupying lesions in the posterior cranial fossa initially lead to a narrowing of the CSF spaces. If the obstruction in the CSF pathway is anywhere between the lateral ventricle and the cisterna magna, it is referred to as **obstructive** or **noncommunicating hydrocephalus**. **Communicating hydrocephalus** refers to a block in the CSF pathway between the cisterna magna and sites of absorption in blood vessels, i.e., in the subarachnoid space.

Space-occupying lesions cause displacement of cerebral structures through the tentorial incisure and through the foramen magnum. Note in this MRI the position of the cerebellar tonsil in relation to the foramen magnum. **Tonsillar displacement** through the foramen magnum into the spinal canal results in compression of the medulla and possibly to circulatory disturbances and respiratory arrest.

Cerebral parenchyma often atrophies with age. The decrease in the volume of the gyri and the increase, or widening, of the sulci can be visualized in T1 MR images as can the ventricular enlargement, which compensates for loss of brain mass.

Color dark blue the corpus callosum. Color light blue the parietal lobe and the thalamus. Color red the frontal lobe and draw red vertical lines through the cerebellum. Color yellow the occipital lobes, cerebral peduncle (of the midbrain), and pons. Color green the head of the caudate nucleus.

Behold, the fool saith, 'Put not all thine eggs in one basket'—which is but a manner of saying, 'Scatter your money and your attention;' but, the wise man saith,
'Put all your eggs in one basket and—WATCH THAT BASKET.' – Mark Twain

202

Sagittal T1 MRI Through the Cerebral Peduncle

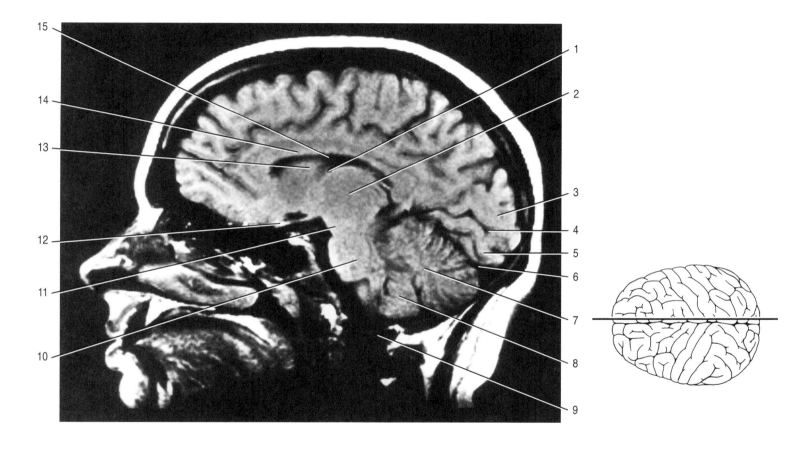

1. Caudothalamic groove
2. Thalamus
3. Occipital lobe, cuneus
4. Calcarine sulcus
5. Occipital lobe, lingual gyrus
6. Tentorium cerebelli
7. Cerebellum
8. Cerebellar tonsil
9. Foramen magnum
10. Pons
11. Cerebral peduncle
12. Optic tract
13. Caudate nucleus, head
14. Corpus callosum, body
15. Lateral ventricle, body

Normal brain (20-year-old woman). (Courtesy of Dr. Michael D. Weaver, East Carolina University, School of Medicine).

Sagittal T1 MRI Through the Lateral Ventricle, Inferior Horn

Definitions

Epilepsy is a chronic disorder of the CNS characterized by partial or complete loss of consciousness and sometimes convulsions; it is caused by a disturbance in the normal electrical rhythm of brain cells. About 30–40% of cases involve the **temporal lobe** (TLE), especially the hippocampus. **Schizophrenia** is a form of psychosis in which the patient is dissociated from the environment and deteriorates in character and personality. Although a diffuse reduction of cortical gray matter is characteristic, the atrophy appears to be greatest in the **temporal lobes**. **Contusions**, i.e., bruising of the brain, are characteristic of nonpenetrating head injury.

Structural and Functional Features

Anteroposterior orientation is provided by the orbit (globe) and cerebellum. Without benefit of surface markings, one can identify the five lobes—parietal, occipital, temporal, insula, and frontal—in this sagittal plane, deep to the lateral sulcus. This plane of section reveals the inferior and posterior horns of the lateral ventricle. **Note the low-intensity (black) signal from the eyeball in contrast to the high-intensity (white) signal from the intraorbital fat.** On T1 MR images, air in the sinuses has a low signal (dark) intensity.

Clinical Correlations . . . .

In the majority of patients with **TLE, T2-weighted scan sequences** reveal evidence of high-intensity lesions in the **medial temporal lobe.**

Morphometric studies frequently show volume loss in the hippocampus, a gyrus of the limbic system that projects into the inferior horn of the lateral ventricle (page 211, coronal view).

Imaging landmarks of reference for the temporal lobe are the lateral sulcus and the inferior horn of the lateral ventricle. Regarding **schizophrenia, ventricular enlargement,** especially of the **inferior horn,** accompanies the loss of temporal lobe gray matter.

Contusion of the temporal lobe occurs in deceleration injuries due to the position of the temporal lobe against bone in the middle cranial fossa. Contusions are not often found in the cerebellum or in the parietal and occipital lobes. Typically contusions are located in the **gyral crests** of parenchyma adjacent to bone including the frontal and temporal poles, the orbital surfaces of the frontal lobes, and the lateral and inferior surfaces of the temporal lobes.

 Color orange the insula. Color blue the parietal lobe. Color red the frontal lobe, and draw red vertical marks through the cerebellum. Color yellow the occipital lobe. Color green the temporal lobe.

In a free and just commonwealth, property rushes from the idle and imbecile to the industrious, brave, and persevering. – Ralph Waldo Emerson

204

Sagittal T1 MRI Through the Lateral Ventricle, Inferior Horn

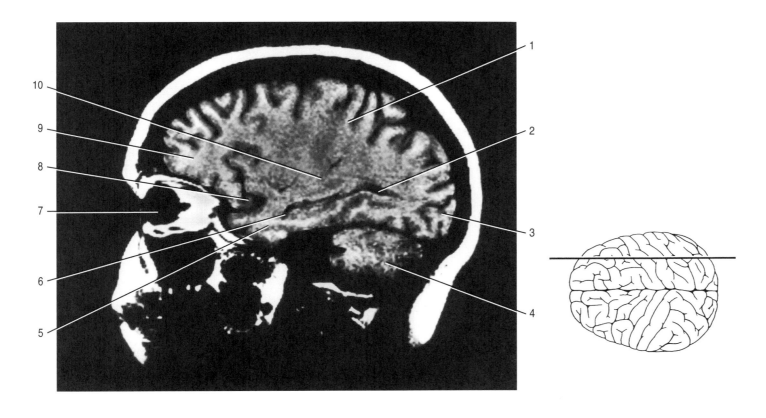

1. Parietal lobe
2. Lateral ventricle, posterior horn
3. Occipital lobe
4. Cerebellum
5. Temporal lobe

6. Lateral ventricle, inferior horn
7. Globe
8. Lateral sulcus
9. Frontal lobe
10. Insula

Normal brain (20-year-old woman). (Courtesy of Dr. Michael D. Weaver, East Carolina University, School of Medicine.)

Coronal T1 MRI Through the Lateral Ventricle, Anterior Horn

Definition

In typical cases of **Pick's disease,** marked atrophy affects the anterior portions of the frontal and temporal lobes. The cortical atrophy is accompanied by considerable enlargement of the anterior horns of the lateral ventricles.

Structural and Functional Features

Appreciating the **shape** of the **ventricular system** is essential to recognizing the plane of section. Coronal views reveal the bilateralism of the body and of the anterior, inferior, and posterior horns of the lateral ventricles. Interpreting **neural pathology** often involves assessing the size and position of the **ventricles**. For example, the shape of and identification of the anterior horns provide the clue that this section is through the frontal lobes, therefore, the corpus callosal component at this level is the genu. Note the cingulate gyrus above the corpus callosum and adjacent to the interhemispheric fissure. The falx cerebri occupies the fissure.

Clinical Correlations . . . .

In the form of **dementia** seen in **Pick's disease, changes in character and social behavior**, rather than impairment of memory and intellect, are the distinctive clinical features. The cause of the neurodegeneration is unknown. **Marked changes in mood are common.** MRI can be so characteristic as to confirm a tentative clinical impression (see above). The lateral sulcus is well visualized and separates frontal and temporal lobes.

Color dark blue the corpus callosum. Color red the frontal lobe. Color green the temporal lobe.

Coronal T1 MRI Through the Lateral Ventricle, Anterior Horn

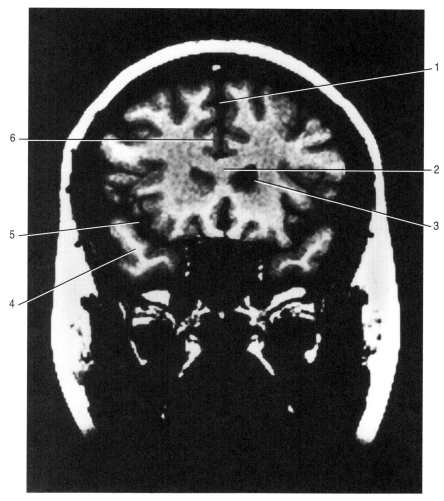

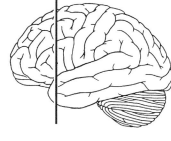

1. Interhemispheric fissure
2. Corpus callosum, genu
3. Lateral ventricle, anterior horn
4. Temporal lobe
5. Lateral sulcus
6. Cingulate gyrus of frontal lobe

(Normal brain (20-year-old woman). Courtesy of Dr. Michael D. Weaver, East Carolina University, School of Medicine.)

Coronal T1 MRI Through the Caudate Nucleus, Head

Definition

Dementia is a partial or complete deterioration of mind and it involves loss of intellectual faculties, memory, and reasoning power due to organic brain disease. Dementia is a component of several CNS diseases: Alzheimer's, Huntington's, Parkinson's, Pick's, AIDS, and prion disease. The latter includes the rare neurodegenerative disorders of Creutzfeldt-Jakob disease, Gerstmann-Sträussler-Sheinber syndrome, and kuru. Tumors and vascular lesions may also cause dementia.

Structural and Functional Features

Identification of the caudate nucleus is easy because it forms the wall and floor of the body of the lateral ventricle. Of particular interest in this view is the hyperintensity of the optic chiasm and the hypophysis (pituitary gland).

Clinical Correlations

Among the several causes of dementia, MRI reveals **pathology** most strikingly in Pick's disease (page 206) and in **Huntington's disease**. In addition to cortical atrophy, degeneration of neurons in the neostriatum (caudate and putamen) is seen in Huntington's disease and is particularly evident as a **loss of volume** in the **caudate nucleus** (probably because of its visibility adjacent to the ventricle). The neostriatal pathology accounts, in large part, for the abnormal choreiform movements characteristic of this disease.

Relative to dementia, MRI is primarily useful in **excluding space-occupying lesions, infarcts, lobar atrophy, infections**, etc., as the cause. Scans of older patients with Alzheimer's disease often do not show any more atrophy and ventricular enlargement than those of healthy persons of the same sex and age.

Color dark blue the corpus callosum. Color red the frontal lobe. Color green the caudate nucleus and the temporal lobe.

Coronal T1 MRI Through the Caudate Nucleus, Head

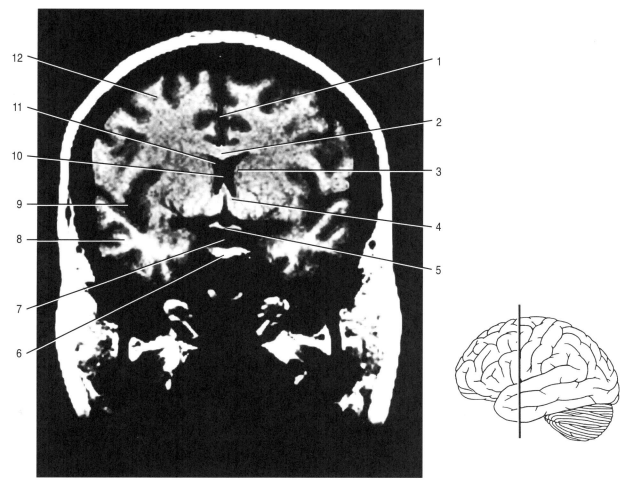

1. Interhemispheric fissure	5. Optic chiasm	9. Lateral sulcus
2. Corpus callosum, body	6. Hypophysis in sella turcica	10. Septum pellucidum
3. Caudate nucleus, head	7. Hypophysial stalk	11. Lateral ventricle, body
4. Septal area	8. Temporal lobe	12. Frontal lobe

Normal brain (20-year-old woman). (Courtesy of Dr. Michael D. Weaver, East Carolina University, School of Medicine.)

Coronal T1 MRI Through the Internal Capsule, Posterior Limb

Definitions

At this level, the body of the corpus callosum comprises **commissural** fibers connecting **similar** areas on the two sides of the frontal and parietal lobes. On the other hand, many of the descending fibers in the posterior limb of the internal capsule **decussate** and terminate on **dissimilar** structures in the brain stem or spinal cord, contralateral to their origin. **Lacunae** refers to multiple empty spaces or gaps due to multi-infarctions of small vessels.

Structural and Functional Features

The head of the caudate nucleus is no longer prominent but the thalamus appears in this MR plane. Note that the hippocampus lies within the temporal lobe, specifically adjacent to the inferior horn of the lateral ventricle. The thalamus lies medial to the posterior limb of the internal capsule, whereas the lenticular nucleus (page 165) forms its lateral border. (Lateral views of fibers of the internal capsule can be seen on pages 171 and 173.) This plane shows the continuation of the fibers in the pons of the brain stem, whereas the descent of fibers that originate in the cortex can be seen in the corona radiata, internal capsule, cerebral peduncle, and pyramidal decussation on page 149.

Clinical Correlations . . . .

Cerebrovascular accidents (CVAs) involving the lenticulostriate branches of the middle cerebral artery frequently interrupt fibers in the **posterior limb** of the **internal capsule.** On T2 images, multi-infarction disease (MID) is seen as signal hyperintensity of variable size and distribution. Hemorrhage and lacunar infarctions have a predilection for the basal ganglia and the posterior limb of the internal capsule. As was pointed out on page 194, CT is sensitive for **evaluating acute hemorrhage** whereas **MRI** is the modality of choice for demonstrating hemorrhagic lesions in later stages.

Color dark blue the corpus callosum. Color light blue the thalamus. Color purple the hippocampus and the fornix. Color yellow the midbrain and the pons. Color green the temporal lobe (inferior to the lateral sulcus) and observe in the reference diagram that this section is at the junction of the frontal and parietal lobes (to avoid ambiguity, do not color). Color the tail of the caudate nucleus green.

The latest Gospel in this world is, Know thy work and do it. – Carlyle

Coronal T1 MRI Through the Internal Capsule, Posterior Limb

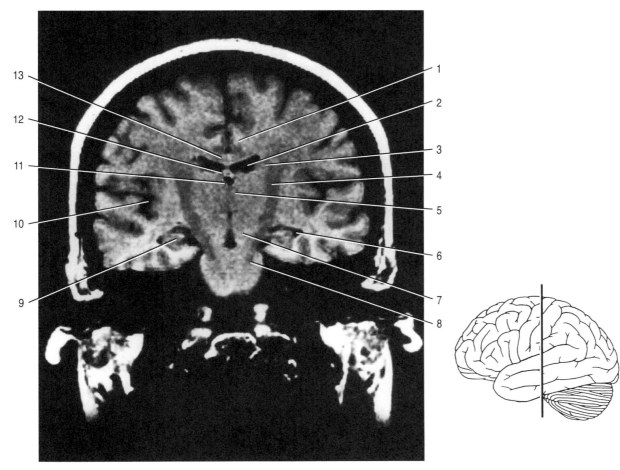

1. Cingulate gyrus
2. Lateral ventricle, body
3. Caudate, tail
4. Internal capsule, posterior limb
5. Thalamus
6. Lateral ventricle, inferior horn
7. Midbrain
8. Corticospinal fibers in the pons
9. Hippocampus
10. Lateral sulcus
11. Third ventricle
12. Fornix, body
13. Corpus callosum, body

Normal brain (20-year-old woman). (Courtesy of Dr. Michael D. Weaver, East Carolina University, School of Medicine.)

Coronal T1 MRI Through the Lateral Ventricle, Posterior Horn

Definition
The junction of the body, posterior and inferior horn of the lateral ventricle is the **atrium**, which defines lobar anatomy. The occipital lobe is posterior, the parietal lobe superior, and the temporal lobe inferolateral to the atrium.

Structural and Functional Features
Note the shape and distance of the posterior horns from the midline in contrast to the anterior horns on page 207. That single comparison enables one to determine the plane of section; the callosal component, therefore, in this section is the **splenium,** which contains **visual commissural fiber systems**.

Compare this exposure of the optic radiations to the lateral view (page 173). Although symmetry of the lateral ventricles has been stressed elsewhere, **asymmetry** of the posterior horns is normal; however, the reason for this is unclear. Recall that the fourth and third ventricles are single, midline structures.

Clinical Correlations . . . .

For reasons that are unclear, the **cerebellar vermis atrophies with chronic Dilantin use and with alcohol abuse**. Recall that lesions of the vermis produce an unsteady, ataxic gait whereas lesions of the cerebellar hemisphere are characterized by dysmetria, past pointing, adiadokokinesia, asynergy, and intention tremor involving the limbs ipsilateral to the lesion (page 114). A complete lesion of either the optic radiation or the medial surface of the occipital lobe results in contralateral homonymous hemianopsia (page 90).

Color dark blue the corpus callosum. Color red the vermis of the cerebellum and draw red vertical lines through the cerebellar hemisphere. Color the optic radiations and the occipital lobe (medial to posterior horn of lateral ventricle) yellow. Color the parietal lobe light blue and the temporal lobe green.

Coronal T1 MRI Through the Lateral Ventricle, Posterior Horn

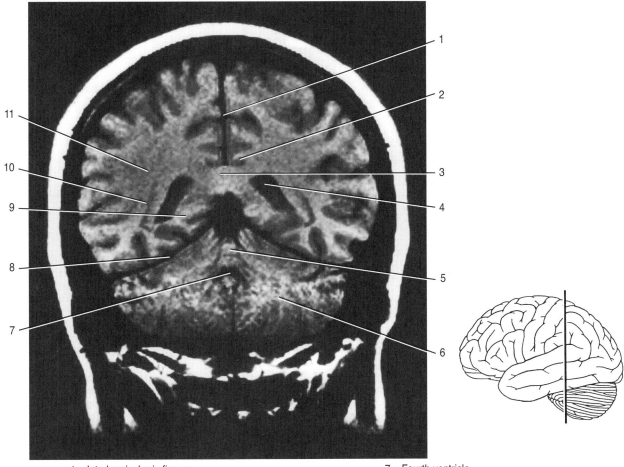

1. Interhemispheric fissure
2. Cingulate gyrus
3. Corpus callosum, splenium
4. Lateral ventricle, posterior horn
5. Cerebellum, vermis
6. Cerebellum, hemispheres
7. Fourth ventricle
8. Tentorium cerebelli in transverse fissure
9. Occipital lobe
10. Optic radiations
11. Parietal lobe

Normal brain (20-year-old woman). (Courtesy of Dr. Michael D. Weaver, East Carolina University, School of Medicine.)

Axial T1 MRI Through the Diencephalon

Definitions

Recall that the **anterior limb** of the **internal capsule** lies between the head of the caudate nucleus and the lenticular nucleus. The **genu** is between the anterior and posterior limbs of the internal capsule. The **posterior limb** lies between the thalamus and the lenticular nucleus.

Structural and Functional Features

The plane of this MRI should be compared to the dissection on page 165. Again, the lateral ventricles deserve attention. Note that the interventricular foramina join them with the third ventricle. Compare the configuration of the genu and the splenium of the corpus callosum.

Fibers passing between the frontal cortex and thalamus (**corticothalamic** and **thalamocortical**) and to pontine nuclei (**frontopontine**) compose the main constituents of the **anterior limb** of the internal capsule. The most important fibers in the **genu** are the corticobulbar fibers from the motor cortex to motor nuclei of the cranial nerves.

The **posterior limb** contains fibers to pontine nuclei (**parietopontine, occipitopontine, temporopontine**), sensory pathway fibers (thalamocortical), and fibers from the motor cortex to anterior motor horn cells of the spinal cord (corticospinal). There are other fiber systems that traverse the posterior limb; however, the thalamocortical and corticospinal are the most important clinically. The **sublenticular** part of the internal capsule contains auditory radiations from the medial geniculate nucleus to the **primary auditory cortex**. Fibers passing from the lateral geniculate nucleus begin in a **sublenticular** position and take a **retrolenticular** route to reach the visual area of the cortex. These constitute the **optic radiations** (geniculocalcarine tract).

Clinical Correlations ....

Hemorrhage gives a bright signal on T1 MR images. Intracranial hemorrhages are classified according to where they occur:

- epidural (extradural), subdural or subarachnoid spaces
- brain (intracerebral)
- ventricles (intraventricular)

The increased "mass effect" of epidural, subdural, and intracerebral hematomas usually **compresses** the **brain** and **raises** the **intracranial pressure**. **Subarachnoid hemorrhage** is often associated with contusions and intraventricular hemorrhage.

Most **epidural hematomas** are associated with **skull fractures**. Frequently the ruptured vessel is the **middle meningeal artery** following temporal bone fracture. If the focal pressure results in transtentorial herniation, death may result.

Subdural hematomas occur when **veins** crossing the subdural space rupture; blood spreads freely in the subdural space and may envelop the entire hemisphere. **The distinction to be made between subdural and epidural hematomas is an even increase in pressure versus focal pressure, respectively.**

Intracerebral hematomas occur within the brain, deep within the hemispheres. These hemorrhages are often multiple and their appearance on MR images is often delayed.

Color dark blue the corpus callosum. To emphasize the internal capsule, color orange the anterior limb, genu, and posterior limb of this important structure. Color the caudate nucleus green and the thalamus blue, and observe that these structures form the medial boundaries of the anterior and posterior limbs, respectively. The lenticular nucleus (putamen and globus pallidus) forms the lateral boundary of both limbs though it is not very visually distinct in this MRI. Compare with dissected specimen on page 165. Color red the frontal lobe, green the temporal lobe, yellow the occipital lobe, and orange the insula.

Axial T1 MRI Through the Diencephalon

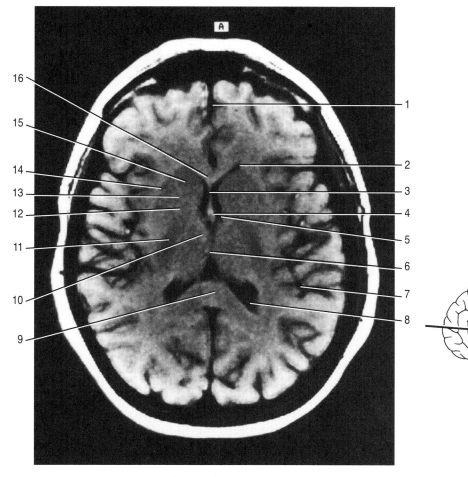

1. Interhemispheric fissure
2. Lateral ventricle, anterior horn
3. Septum pellucidum
4. Fornix, column
5. Interventricular foramen (of Monro)
6. Third ventricle
7. Lateral sulcus
8. Lateral ventricle, posterior horn
9. Corpus callosum, splenium
10. Thalamus
11. Internal capsule posterior limb
12. Internal capsule, genu
13. Internal capsule, anterior limb
14. Putamen
15. Caudate, head
16. Corpus callosum, genu

Normal brain (20-year-old woman). (Courtesy of Dr. Michael D. Weaver, East Carolina University, School of Medicine.)

Axial T1 MRI Through the Midbrain

Definitions

Some otherwise confusing terms can be made clear on brain stem cross sections. The **cerebral peduncle** refers to the midbrain minus the **tectum.** The tectum (roof) refers to the structures dorsal to the cerebral aqueduct (superior and inferior colliculi on each side number four, therefore, quadrigeminal plate). The **basis pedunculi** is the substantia nigra plus the most ventral region of the cerebral peduncle. The **tegmentum** is the area between the cerebral aqueduct and the basis pedunculi.

Structural and Functional Features

Recall that **cisterns** are expanded areas of the **subarachnoid space** (SAS) where the arachnoid spans irregularities on the surface of the brain. The **cisterna ambiens** is that part of the SAS that surrounds the midbrain. The cistern of the great cerebral vein is sometimes considered its dorsal part because it makes up the SAS dorsal to the superior colliculus. It is located between the splenium of the corpus callosum and the cerebellum and contains, not surprisingly, the great cerebral vein and the pineal gland. (synonyms: superior cistern; quadrigeminal cistern).

Clinical Correlations . . . .

The **cisterns** are continuous with one another and are filled with CSF. They show the same **hypointensity** as do the ventricles. Recall that stenosis of the cerebral aqueduct is a common cause of hydrocephalus. When it is obstructed, the lateral ventricles and the third ventricle become enlarged. (Discussion of uncal herniation involving the midbrain is on page 16.) Trauma to the temporal lobes against the sphenoid bones of the middle cranial fossae occurs in motor vehicle accidents. Bilateral damage to the hippocampi may cause memory impairment (page 116). The mesencephalic syndrome of Weber is described and depicted on pages 122 and 123.

Color the tectum, tegmentum, and cerebral peduncle of the midbrain yellow. Observe that cross sections of the brain stem in MRIs are upside down relative to the conventional way these sections are presented. Color purple the mamillary bodies. Color the occipital lobe yellow and the temporal lobe green.

I have my own stern claims and perfect circle.
It denies the name of duty to many offices that are called duties. – Ralph Waldo Emerson

216

Axial T1 MRI Through the Midbrain

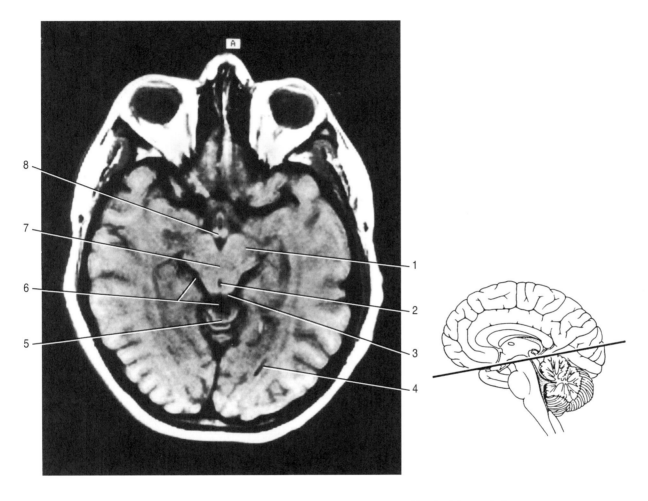

1. Cerebral peduncle
2. Cerebral aqueduct
3. Tectum
4. Lateral ventricle, posterior horn
5. Vermis of the cerebellum
6. Cisterna ambiens
7. Tegmentum of midbrain
8. Mamillary body of hypothalamus

Normal brain (20-year-old woman). (Courtesy of Dr. Michael D. Weaver, East Carolina University, School of Medicine.)

Axial T1 MRI Through the Pons

Definition

In the pons, the **tegmentum** is the region between the fourth ventricle and the basal pons, a region visually distinct because of the transversely coursing pontocerebellar fibers.

Structural and Functional Features

The pontine cistern cushions the pons and basilar artery from the bony clivus. The temporal lobe occupies the middle cranial fossa.

Clinical Correlations . . . .

Pontine and cerebellar **neoplasms** may **impair** or **block CSF** flow through the fourth ventricle. Increased intracranial pressure pushes the pons against the clivus and traps the abducens nerves between (page 98). The basal pontine syndrome is described and depicted on pages 122 and 123.

Color yellow the pons (basal region and tegmentum) and occipital lobe. Color green the temporal lobe. Color red the cerebellar vermis, and draw red vertical marks through the cerebellar hemispheres.

Fools and intelligent people are equally harmless.
It is half-fools and the half-intelligent who are the most dangerous. – Goethe

218

Axial T1 MRI Through the Pons

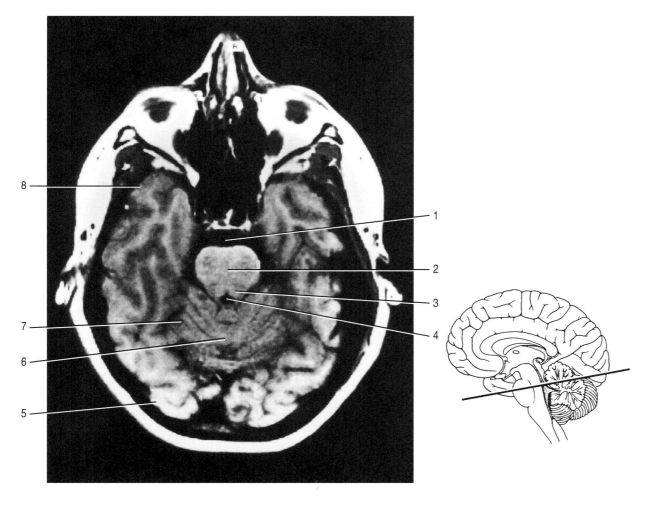

1. Pontine cistern
2. Pons, basal region
3. Tegmentum of pons
4. Fourth ventricle
5. Occipital lobe
6. Cerebellar vermis
7. Cerebellar hemispheres
8. Temporal lobe

Normal brain (20-year-old woman). (Courtesy of Dr. Michael D. Weaver, East Carolina University, School of Medicine.)

Axial T1 MRI Through the "Open" Medulla

Definition

That part of the medulla bordered posteriorly by the fourth ventricle is the "open" **medulla**. The caudal medulla contains a central canal continuous with the central canal of the spinal cord.

Structural and Functional Features

The median portion of the cerebellum between the two cerebellar hemispheres is the vermis. Fibers of CN IX–XII enter or exit from the medulla, and the two vertebral arteries lie on the ventral surface of the medulla. Cranial nerves VI, VII, and VIII exit at the junction of the medulla and pons.

Clinical Correlations . . . .

Herniation of the **cerebellar tonsils** through the foramen magnum is discussed on page 202. Medial and lateral medullary syndromes are presented on pages 122 and 123.

Color yellow the medulla. Color red the cerebellar vermis, and draw red vertical marks through the hemispheres. Recall that the contents of the posterior cranial fossa (brain stem and cerebellum) are in the infratentorial cranial compartment.

Against criticism we can neither protect nor defend ourselves;
we must act in despite of it, and gradually it resigns itself to this. – Goethe

220

Axial T1 MRI Through the "Open" Medulla

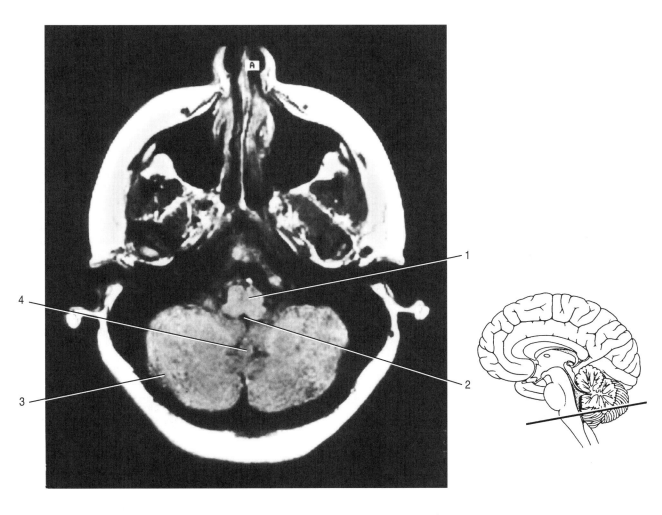

1. Medulla
2. Fourth ventricle
3. Cerebellar hemisphere
4. Cerebellar vermis

Normal brain (20-year-old woman). (Courtesy of Dr. Michael D. Weaver, East Carolina University, School of Medicine.)

Chapter 7 **T1 Magnetic Resonance Images (MRI)**

Chapter Seven Study Questions

Directions: Each question below contains four or five suggested answers. Choose the **one best** response to each question.

1. **On T1 MR images, the structure that has a bright signal is the**
    - (a) Sphenoid sinus
    - (b) Fourth ventricle
    - (c) Pontine cistern
    - (d) Clivus
    - (e) Parieto-occipital sulcus

2. **Which of the following T1 MR images is most suitable for visualizing a pituitary tumor?**
    - (a) Sagittal through the lateral ventricle, inferior horn
    - (b) Midline sagittal through the cerebral aqueduct
    - (c) Coronal through the lateral ventricle, posterior horn
    - (d) Axial through the diencephalon at midthalamic level
    - (e) Coronal through the internal capsule, posterior limb

3. **Which structure is not in the posterior cranial fossa?**
    - (a) Cranial nerve IX
    - (b) Medulla
    - (c) Pons
    - (d) Cerebellum
    - (e) Mamillary body

4. **Epilepsy originates predominantly from foci in the**
    - (a) Frontal lobe
    - (b) Insula
    - (c) Temporal lobe
    - (d) Occipital lobe
    - (e) Parietal lobe

5. **The brain of a patient with which of the following is most likely to show enlargement specifically of the inferior horn of the lateral ventricle?**
    - (a) Schizophrenia
    - (b) Pick's disease
    - (c) AIDS
    - (d) Parkinson's disease
    - (e) Huntington's disease

6. **Blood from ruptured veins usually accumulates in the**
    - (a) Epidural space
    - (b) Cisterna ambiens
    - (c) Subdural space
    - (d) Intracerebral parenchyma
    - (e) Ventricles

7. **The least likely site of a contusion is the**
    - (a) Frontal pole
    - (b) Orbital surface of the frontal lobe
    - (c) Temporal pole
    - (d) Medial surface of the parietal lobe

8. **Focal pathology of the pons is best visualized with**
    - (a) T1 MR images
    - (b) CT
    - (c) Radiographs
    - (d) Pneumoencephalograms
    - (e) T2 MR images

9. **Of the following, the most direct probable cause of respiratory arrest is**
    - (a) Herniation of the cerebellar tonsils
    - (b) Herniation of the uncus
    - (c) Increased intracranial pressure
    - (d) Epidural hematoma
    - (e) Blockage of the foramen of Magendie

10. **The value of MR imaging relative to dementia is primarily that of**
    - (a) Demonstrating gyral atrophy
    - (b) Excluding more definitive organic conditions
    - (c) Demonstrating ventricular enlargement
    - (d) Demonstrating sulci widening

Answers and Explanations for Chapter Seven Study Questions

1. **d** [page 200] Marrow-filled bone has a bright signal in contrast to compact bone, which has a dark signal. CSF that fills the ventricles and subarachnoid space is hypointense; therefore, the fourth ventricle, pontine cistern, and parieto-occipital sulcus give a dark signal as does the air within the sphenoid sinus.

2. **b** [page 200] The pituitary gland lies midline within the cranium; it enlarges upward because it is surrounded by bone in the sella turcica. It is covered over by the diaphragma sellae, which, though taut, offers less resistance than bone. The tumor impinges on the optic chiasm and tends to cause temporal field deficits. All other planes are unsuitable for pituitary visualization. The parasagittal image through the inferior horn of the lateral ventricle is too lateral; both coronal images are posterior to the pituitary and the axial image described is superior or above the pituitary gland.

3. **e** [page 200] The mamillary body is in the diencephalon and is located in the supratentorial compartment versus the medulla, pons, cerebellum, and glossopharyngeal nerve (IX), which are all in the infratentorial compartment in the posterior cranial fossa.

4. **c** [page 204] From 30–40% of cases of epilepsy originate in the temporal lobe; however, it may occur from foci in any lobe, especially when it is secondary to trauma.

5. **a** [page 204] Cortical atrophy and enlargement of the ventricle in the temporal lobe (inferior horn) is well documented in many patients who have schizophrenia. In Pick's disease and Huntington's disease, the enlargement usually is of the anterior horns of the lateral ventricle. In Parkinson's disease, the basal ganglia are also affected and the anterior horns of the lateral ventricles are likewise enlarged. The cortical atrophy is diffuse in the brains of patients who have AIDS; therefore, the ventricular enlargement would be general rather than localized.

6. **c** [page 214] Subdural hematoma usually occurs when the veins crossing the subdural space rupture. The accumulation of venous blood is diffuse rather than focal. Bleeding into the epidural space is typically arterial blood due to a fracture. Intracerebral and intraventricular bleeding is usually arterial as is that seen in the cisterna ambiens because it too is in the subarachnoid compartment.

7. **d** [page 204] The medial surface of the parietal lobe abuts the falx cerebri whereas the frontal and temporal poles and the orbital surface of the frontal lobe are adjacent to bone. In deceleration injuries, those areas adjacent to bone are vulnerable to contusions.

8. **e** [page 200] T1 MR images show normal anatomy; however, T2 MR images are more sensitive in revealing pathology. Because the pons rests on the bony clivus, MR images are more sensitive than CT images of structures in the posterior cranial fossa due to bone artifacts in the latter. Neither radiographs nor pneumoencephalograms are of value relative to intrinsic anatomy of the pons.

9. **a** [page 202] Tonsillar displacement through the foramen magnum compresses the medulla and may result in respiratory arrest. An epidural hematoma may result in increased intracranial pressure with resultant herniation of the uncus through the tentorial notch. These events may eventually result in crowding the posterior fossa to the extent that the tonsils are pushed downward. These events, however, are indirect in contrast to the more direct effect of the tonsillar herniation. Impairment of CSF flow due to blockage of the foramen of Magendie is also an indirect phenomenon.

10. **b** [page 208] Ruling out space-occupying lesions, infarcts, lobar atrophy, infections, etc. is the value of MR imaging in assessing a patient with dementia. Cortical atrophy (decrease in gyri and increase in sulci width) and ventricular enlargement are nonspecific findings in elderly individuals.

Index

Page numbers in *italics* indicate figures; page numbers with *t* indicate tables

A

Abducens nerves, 14, 98, *99*
Accessory (lateral) cuneate nucleus, 52, 62
Accessory nerves, 14, 108, *109*
Acetylcholine, 144
Achromatopsia, 172
Acupuncture, 62
Afferent fibers, 170
Afferent neurons, 48
Alar plate, 48
Alzheimer's disease, 170
Amygdala, 2, 154, 170, 174
Amygdaloid body, 88
Anencephaly, 4
Anesthesia, 186
Angiography of the internal carotid aneurysm, 196, *197*
Ansa, 50
Anterior cerebral arteries, 154, 156
Anterior commissure, *32, 33,* 36, *37,* 156, 166, 174
Anterior communicating artery, 180
Anterior frontal, *7*
Anterior limb, 170, 214
Anterior nucleus of thalamus, 166
Anterior olfactory nucleus, 88
Anterior perforated substance, 88
Anterior spinal artery, *51, 53, 55, 57*
Anterograde amnesia, 170
Anterolateral, 2
Aperture, 8
Aphasia, 40, 184
Arachnoid, 46
Arch of aorta, 182
Arcuate fasciculus, 40
Arcuate fibers, *32, 33*
Arcuate nucleus, 62, 162
Arnold-Chiari malformation, 10
Artery of Adamkiewicz, 58
Ascending rami, 20
Ascending reticular activating system (ARAS), 128, 134

Associational, 34
Association neurons, 48
Atrium, 164, 170, 212
Autonomic nervous system (ANS), 48
    parasympathetic division of, 146, *147*
    participation of, 166
    sympathetic division of, 144, *145*

B

Basal ganglia, 2, 154
    blood supply of, 184, *185*
    horizontal section of brain through, 164, *165*
Basal plate, 48
Basal vein (of Rosenthal), 12, *13*
Basilar artery, 180, 182
Basilar plexus, 12, *13, 15*
Basis pedunculi, 158, 216
Bilateral, 2
Bilateral damage, 52
Bilateral lesions, 172
Bilateral trauma, 170
Blindness, 188
Blink reflex, 96
Blood-brain barrier (BBB), 196
Blood supply
    of basal ganglia, 184, *185*
    of the brain, 182, *183*
        lateral view, 186, *187*
        medial view, 188, *189*
    of internal capsule, 184, *185*
    of main cerebral arteries, 192, *193*
    of spinal cord, 58, *59*
    of thalamus, 184, *185*
    of visual system, 190, *191*
Bone artifacts, 200
Brachiocephalic artery, 182
Brachium, 50
Brain
    blood supply of, 182, *183*
        lateral view, 186, *187*
        medial view, 188, *189*

development of mature, from the brain subdivisions, 4, *5*
    horizontal section of, through the basal ganglia, thalamus, and internal capsule, 164, *165*
    medial surface of, 36, *37*
Brain stem, 54
    basal view of, 114, *115*
    dissection of, from lateral surface, 148, *149*
    general organization of roof, 64
    lateral view of major pathways in the, 126, *127*
    lesions and syndromes, 122, *123*
    medial view of nuclei, 62, *63*
Bregma, 6, *7*
Broca's aphasia, 40
Broca's area, *32,* 38
Brodmann's areas, 28, 28*t, 29*
    lateral surface, 28, 28*t, 29,* 29
    medial surface, 30, 30*t, 31,* 31
Brown-Séquard syndrome, 56

C

Calcarine sulcus, 20, 36, *37,* 166
Callosal sulcus, 20, 36, *37*
Capsule, 50
Carotid arteries, 14, 186
Carotid endarterectomy, 182
Caudal, 2
Caudal medulla, 4
    at level of pyramidal (motor) decussation, 66, *67*
Caudal neuropores, 4
Caudal pons medullopontine junction, oblique section through, 74, *75*
Caudate nucleus, 2, *2, 3,* 154, 164
    coronal TI MRI through, 208, *209*
    exposure of, in dissection of right hemisphere, 174, *175*
Caudothalamic groove, 202
Cavernous sinus, 12, 14, *15*
Central artery of retina, 190

Central canal, 50, *51, 53, 55, 57*
Central lobe, 18
Central sulcus, 18, 20, 24, *35,* 38, *39*
Central tegmental tract, 62
Cerebellar artery, 182
Cerebellar peduncle, 148
Cerebellar tonsils, 220
Cerebellar vermis atrophies, 212
Cerebellopontine angle tumors, 74
Cerebellum, *5*
    basal view of, 114, *115*
Cerebral aqueduct, 4
    midline sagittal T1 MRI through, 200, *201*
    and periaqueductal gray, 27
Cerebral arteries, 16, 186
    regional blood supply of, 192, *193*
Cerebral cortex, 2, 34, 154, 166
    nonspecific input to diffuse areas of, 134
    specific input to primary somatosensory area of, 134
Cerebral hemispheres, 2, *5*
    dissection of left
        from lateral surface, 40, *41,* 148, *149*
        from medial surface, 150, *151*
    dissection of right
        from lateral surface, 170, *171*
            internal capsule and optic radiations exposed, 172, *173*
        from medial surface, 166, *167*
            caudate nucleus and limbic structures exposed, 174, *175*
    fibers of, 32, *32, 33,* 33
    lateral surface of left, showing sulci and gyri, 38, *39*
    lobes of, 18, *19*
    sulci of, 20, *21*
Cerebral peduncles, *5,* 156, 174, 216
    of midbrain, 27
    midline sagittal T1 MRI through, 202, *203*
Cerebral vein, *17*

Cerebrospinal fluid (CSF), 4
    production of, 8
    rhinorrhea, 88
    volume of, 8
Cerebrovascular accidents (CVAs), 210
Cerebrum, superior view of, 34, *35*
Cervical enlargement, spinal cord at, 56,
    57
Chemical stimulus, 88
Chief sensory (main) nucleus, 130
Choroidal artery, 188
Choroid plexus, 8, 188, 190
Ciliary muscle, 92
Cingulate, 166
Cingulate cortical region, 166
Cingulate gyrus, 24, 36, *37,* 154, 156, 166
Cingulate sulcus, 20, 36, *37*
Cingulum, *32, 33,* 154, 156, 166, 174
Circadian rhythms, 162
Circle of Willis, 180, *181*
Circumventricular organs (CVOs), 196
Cisterna ambiens, 216
Cisterna magna, 202
Cisterns, 8, 216
Claustrum, 154
Clinoid processes, 16, *17*
Clivus, *12,* 13, 114
Cognitive behavior, 166
Collateral sulcus, 20
Colliculus of midbrain, *27*
Color discrimination, 90
Commissural, 34
    fibers, *32*
Commissure, 50
    posterior, 92
Common carotid artery, 182
Communicating artery, 188
Communicating hydrocephalus, 10, 202
Computerized axial tomography (CAT),
    194
Conduction aphasia, *32*
Cones, 90
Confluence of sinuses, 12, *13, 15, 17*
Consensual reflex, 92

Contralateral, 2
Contralateral hemianesthesia, 184
Contralateral hemifield, 90
Contralateral hemiplegia, 184, 186
Contralateral leg, 36
Contralateral paresis, 186
Contralateral superior quadrantanopsia,
    90
Conus medullaris, 46
Conventional angiography, 196
Coronal suture, *7*
Corona radiata, 142, 154, 156, 172
Corporal planes, 2, *3*
Corpus callosum, *32, 33,* 36, 154, 156,
    166, 172, 174
Corpus striatum, 154, 186
Cortex, 170
Cortical blindness, 190
Cortical branches, 188
Cortical motor neurons, 138
Corticobulbar fibers, 126
Corticobulbar tract, 140, *141,* 142, *143*
Corticopontine fibers, 126, 154
Corticospinal, 52
Corticospinal fibers, *32,* 36, 126
    in base of pons, *37*
Corticospinal tract, 142, *143*
Cranial fossae, 14, *15*
Cranial nerves, 86*t*
    abducens, 98, *99*
    accessory, 108, *109*
    facial, 100, *101*
    glossopharyngeal, 104, *105*
    hypoglossal, 110, *111*
    intramedullary course of, 112, *113*
    nuclei and components, *87*
    oculomotor, 92, *93*
    olfactory, 88, *89*
    optic, 90, *91*
    trigeminal, 96, *97*
    trochlear, 94, *95*
    vagus, 106, *107*
    vestibulocochlear, 102, *103*
Cribriform plate, 14, *15,* 88

Crista galli, 14
Cross-sectional levels, 64, *65*
Cuneate fasciculus, 50, 54, *55, 57,* 58,
    126, 132
Cuneate nucleus, 62, 126, 132
Cuneocerebellar tract (CCT), 120, *121*
Cuneus, 24, 36, *37,* 166, 190

D
Dead-end vessels, 184
Decussation, *32,* 50
Degenerative diseases, 52
Dementia, 206
Demyelinating diseases, 52
Dentate gyrus, 170
Dermatome, 48
Descending herniation, 16, *17*
Descending pathways, convergence on
    motor neurons, 138, *139*
Descriptive terms, 2, *3*
Diabetes insipidus, 174
Diaphragma sellae, 14
Diencephalon, *2, 3,* 3, *4,* 5
    axial T1 MRI through, 214, *215*
    basal view of, 114, *115*
    third ventricle of, 8, 9, 11
Diencephalon bellum, 4
Direct pupillary light reflex, 92
Discriminative touch, 132, *133*
    sensation, 96
Distal, 2
Dopaminergic fibers, 170
Dopaminergic neurons, 82
Dorsal cochlear nucleus, rostral medulla
    at level of, 72, *73*
Dorsal column, 54
Dorsal column-medial lemniscal system,
    54, 132, *133*
Dorsal column-medial pathways, 130
Dorsal funiculus, *55, 57*
Dorsal funiculus fasciculus, *51*
Dorsal intermediate septum, *55, 57*
Dorsal longitudinal fasciculus, 62, 144
Dorsal median septum, *51, 53, 55, 57*

Dorsal nucleus of Clarke, 50, 52, *53, 55*
Dorsal roots, 46, 50, *51,* 52
    entry zone, *53, 55, 57*
Dorsal spinocerebellar tract (DSCT), 52,
    58, 126
Dorsal striatum, 154
Dorsal tegmental nucleus, 62
Dorsal thalamus, 162
Dorsal trigeminothalamic tract, 130
Dorsomedial nuclei, 162
Dural venous sinuses, *15*
Dura mater, 46
    venous sinuses of, 12, *13*
Dysarthria, 68, 184
Dysphagia, 68
Dysphonia, 68

E
Edinger-Westphal nucleus, 92
Efferent neurons, 48
Embolic stroke, 184
Embolus, 186
Emotional indifference, 26
Endocrine, 166
Ependymoma, 74
Epidural hematomas, 6, 26, 186, 214
Epidural space, 16
Epilepsy, 204
Epineurium, 46
Epithalamus, 2, *5,* 162
Expressive aphasia, 186
External hydrocephalus, 10
Extrapyramidal system, 142

F
Face, volitional control of, 140, *141*
Facial colliculus, pons at level of, 76, *77*
Facial nerves, 100, *101*
Falx cerebri, *13,* 14, *15,* 16
Fasciculus, 50, 170
Fasciculus interfascicularis, 54
Fasciculus retroflexus, 174
Fasciculus septomarginalis, 54
Fibers of cerebral hemispheres, 32, *32, 33*

Focal changes, 34
Fontanels in skull of neonate, 6, 7
Foramen magnum, 14, 15
Foramina, 88
Forebrain, 4, 5
　at the level of the anterior nucleus of
　　the thalamus, 156, 157
　at the level of the midthalamus, 158,
　　159
　at the level of the striatum and nucleus
　　accumbens, 154, 155
Fornix, 36, 37, 156, 166, 174
Fourth ventricle, 4, 8, 9, 11, 36, 37
Frontal bone, 7, 14
Frontal cortice, 186
Frontal gyrus, 24, 36
Frontal lobe, 18, 34
Frontal sulcus, 38
Functional segmentation, 46

G
Gaze center, 98
General somatic afferent (GSA) fibers,
　48, 130
General somatic efferent (GSE) fibers,
　48
General visceral afferent (GVA) fibers,
　48
General visceral efferent (GVE) fibers, 48
Geniculate nucleus, 190
Genu, 36, 164, 214
　of corpus callosum, 37, 164
　of internal capsule, 164
Germinal matrix hemorrhages, 202
Global aphasia, 40, 184, 186
Globus pallidus, 2, 154, 158, 164, 170,
　172
Glomeruli, 88
Glomus choroideum, 164
Glossopharyngeal nerves, 104, 105
Gracile, 54
Gracile fasciculus, 50, 55, 57, 58, 126,
　132
Gracile nucleus, 62, 126, 132

Gray matter, 2, 46, 51, 55
Great cerebral vein (of Galen), 12, 13,
　15
Gyral crests, 204
Gyri, 18
　of cerebral hemisphere, 38, 39
　of interior surface, 26, 27
　of lateral surface, 22, 23
　of medial surface, 24, 25
Gyrus rectus, 26

H
Habenula, 156
Habenulae, 36
Habenular nuclei, 174
Head, volitional control of, 140, 141
Hemianesthesia, 184, 186
Hemiplegia, 56
Hemorrhage, 214
Hemorrhagic infarction, 184
Hemorrhagic stroke, 184
Hindbrain, 4, 5
Hippocampal commissure, 32
Hippocampal formation, 170
Hippocampus, 166, 170
　exposure of, in dissection of right
　　hemisphere, 170, 171
Homonymous hemianopsia, 184, 186,
　190
Horizontal planes, 2, 3
Horizontal rami, 20
Huntington's disease, 154, 208
Hyperactive jaw reflex, 130
Hyperphagia, 174
Hypoglossal nerves, 110, 111
Hypothalamus, 2, 5, 36, 37, 62, 162,
　166
　medial view of, 163

I
Inferior cerebellar peduncle, 52, 126
Inferior colliculus, 37
　mesencephalon at level of, 82, 83
Inferior frontal gyrus, 35

Inferior frontal sulcus, 20, 39
Inferior horn, 170, 204
　of lateral ventricle, 166
Inferior occipitofrontal fasciculus, 40, 41
Inferior olivary nucleus, 62
　open medulla at level of, 70, 71
Inferior parietal lobules, 38, 39
Inferior petrosal sinus, 12, 13
Inferior sagittal sinus, 12, 13
Inferior temporal gyrus, 39
Inferior temporal sulcus, 39
Infratentorial, 2
Infundibulum, 174
Insula (island of Reil) lobe, 18, 20, 40, 41
Integrate sensory information, 166
Integrative cell column, 57
Intention tremor, 154
Intercavernous sinus, 13
Interhemispheric (longitudinal) fissure, 26,
　27, 34, 35
Intermediate septum, 46
Intermediate zone, 51, 57
Intermediolateral cell columns, 52, 53, 55
Intermediomedial cell columns, 52, 53, 55
Internal arcuate fibers, 132
Internal capsule, 2, 3, 170, 172, 188, 214
　blood supply of, 184, 185
　exposure of, in dissection of right hemi-
　　sphere, 172, 173
　horizontal section of brain through, 164,
　　165
Internal carotid, 190
Internal carotid aneurysm, angiography of,
　196, 197
Internal carotid system, 180
Internal cerebral vein, 12, 13
Internal genu, 98
Internal jugular vein, 12, 13, 15
Internal medullary lamina, 158
Internal obstructive hydrocephalus, 10
Interpeduncular fossa and cistern, 27
Interpeduncular nucleus, 62
Interstitial nucleus of Cajal, 62
Interthalamic adhesion, 36, 158

Interthalamic adhesion (anterior leader) and
　thalamus (lateral to third ventricle),
　37
Interventricular foramen (of Monro), 12, 156
Intracerebral bleeding, 90
Intracerebral hematomas, 214
Intracranial hemorrhage, 194
　computed tomography demonstration of,
　194, 195
Intracranial pressure, 214
Intraparietal sulcus, 20, 34, 35
Ipsilateral, 2
Ipsilateral paralysis, 130
Isthmus, 24, 36
　of cingulate gyrus, 37
　pons at level of, 80, 81

J
Jaw reflex, 96

K
Kinesthesia, 132
Klüver-Bucy syndrome, 174

L
Labyrinthine artery, 182
Lambda, 6, 7
Lambdoid suture, 7
Lateral cell column, 51, 53
Lateral corticospinal tract (LCST), 58, 126,
　136, 137, 142
Lateral funiculus, 51, 53, 55, 57
Lateral geniculate nucleus, 162, 190
Lateral horn, 46, 52
Lateral lemniscus, 126
Lateral occipital gyri, 38, 39
Lateral occipitotemporal, 172
Lateral stria of olfactory tract, 27
Lateral sulcus, 20, 38, 39, 172
Lateral surface, gyri of, 22, 23
Lateral ventricle, 154, 156, 170, 174, 188
　coronal T1 MRI through, 206, 207, 212,
　213
　midline sagittal T1 MRI through, 204, 205

Lateral ventricles, 154
Lateral wall, 14
Laterodorsal tegmental nuclei (acetyl-
    choline), 62
Left anterolateral fontanel, 7
Left cavernous sinus, 13
Left cerebral hemisphere, lateral surface
    of, 38, 39
Left hemisphere, dissection of, from lat-
    eral surface, 40, 41
Left posterolateral fontanel, 7
Lemniscal pathway, 64
Lemniscus, 50
Lenticular fasciculus, 158
Lenticular nucleus, 2, 2, 3, 170
Levator palpebrae muscle, 92
Limbic lobe, 166
Limbic system, 166
    connections, 168, 169
    output, 166
    structures, 166, 167
        exposure of, in dissection of right
            hemisphere, 174, 175
Limbs
    somatosensory pathways for, 136, 137
    volitional control of, 136, 137
Lingual gyrus, 24, 36, 37, 166, 190
Lissauer's tract, 128
Lissauer's zone, 51, 53, 55, 57
Locus ceruleus, 62
    rostral pons at level of, 78, 79
Longitudinal fasciculus, 32, 33
Loss
    of accommodation, 92
    of pupillary light reflex, 92
Lumbar cistern, 46
Lumbosacral enlargement, spinal cord at,
    50, 51

M
Macrocephaly, 10
Magnetic resonance angiography, 196
Magnetic resonance imaging (MRI)
    axial T1

through the diencephalon, 214, 215
through the midbrain, 216, 217
through the open medulla, 220, 221
through the pons, 218, 219
coronal T1
    through caudate nucleus, 208, 209
    through internal capsule, 210, 211
    through lateral ventricle, 206, 207
    through the lateral ventricle, 212,
        213
midline sagittal T1
    through cerebral aqueduct, 200, 201
    through cerebral peduncle, 202, 203
    through lateral ventricle, 204, 205
Mamillary body, 166, 174
    of hypothalamus, 27
Mamillothalamic fasciculus, 166, 174
Mamillothalamic tract, 158
Mammary glands, 162
Mandible, 7
Mass-occupying lesions, 16
Maxilla, 7
Maxillary division of trigeminal nerve, 14
Medial cell column, 51, 53, 55
Medial frontal gyrus, 37
Medial lemniscus, 54, 126, 132
    medulla at level of decussation, 68, 69
Medial longitudinal fasciculus (MLF), 64
Medial medullary syndrome, 122t
Medial occipitotemporal gyri, 172
Medial surface, gyri of, 24, 25
Median fissure, 46
Mediodorsal nucleus, 166
Medium septum, 46
Medulla
    axial T1 MRI through the open, 220,
        221
    characteristics of, at level of inferior
        olivary nucleus, 70, 71
    at level of decussation of medial lem-
        niscus, 68, 69
Medulla oblongata, 5, 14, 36, 37, 150
Meningeal artery, 214
Meninges, 14, 16

relation of spinal cord and spinal
    nerves to, 46, 47
Meningiomas, 36, 46
Meningocele, 4
Meningomyelocele, 4
Mesencephalic nucleus, 130
Mesencephalon, 4, 5
    at level of inferior colliculus, 82, 83
    at level of superior colliculus, 84, 85
Metencephalon, 4, 5
    fourth ventricle of, 8, 9, 11
Meyer's loop, interruption of, 90
Midbrain, 174
    axial T1 MRI through, 216, 217
Middle cerebellar peduncle (MCP), 126
Middle cerebral artery (MCA), 180
Middle frontal gyrus, 35, 38, 39
Middle temporal gyrus, 39
Midthalamus, forebrain at the level of,
    158, 159
Mitral cells, 88
Modalities, 48
Motor aphasia, 40
Motor cell column, 57
Motor disturbances, 50
Motor neurons, 48
    descending pathways convergence on,
        138, 139
Motor symptoms, 50
Motor unit, 48
Mydriasis, 92
Myelencephalon, 4, 5
    fourth ventricle of, 8, 9, 11
Myelin, 34

N
Neonate, sutures and fontanels in skull of,
    6, 7
Neoplasms, 218
Nerve, 46
Neural crest, 4
Neural folds, 4
Neural plate, 4
Neural tube, 4

Neurohypophysis, 174
Neuronal elements, 34
Neurulation, 4
Night vision, 90
Nissl staining method, 56
Noncommunicating hydrocephalus, 202
Nondiscriminative touch, 128, 129
Noradrenergic fibers, 170
Norepinephrine, 144
Nucleus accumbens, 154
    forebrain at the level of, 154, 155
Nucleus ambiguus, 68
Nucleus of Darkschewitsch, 62
Nucleus proprius, 50, 51, 53, 55, 57, 128

O
Obesity, 174
Oblique section, through caudal pons
    medullopontine junction, 74, 75
Occipital bone, 7
Occipital lobe, 18
Occipital sulcus, 20
Occipitofrontal fasciculus, 32, 33
Occipitotemporal gyrus, 24
Occipitotemporal sulcus, 20
Oculomotor, 14
Oculomotor nerves, 92, 93, 180
Oculomotor nucleus, 92
Olfactory bulb, 27, 88
Olfactory mucosa, 88
Olfactory nerves, 14, 88, 89
Olfactory tract, 27, 40, 41, 88
Olfactory trigone, 88
Olfactory tubercle, 27
Ophthalmic artery, 14, 190
Ophthalmic vein, 14
    superior, 14
Opthalmic division of trigeminal nerve,
    14
Optic canal, 14
Optic chiasm, 27, 40, 41
Optic disc, 90
Optic nerves, 14, 15, 27, 90, 91
Optic radiations, 164, 172, 214

Optic radiations—continued
    exposure of, in dissection of right
        hemisphere, 172, *173*
Optic tract, *27,* 158, 190
Orbital lesions, 26
Orbital plate, 14, *15*
Ossification centers, *7*

P
Pain, 128, *129,* 130, *131*
    perception of, 128
    transmission of, 62
Papilledema, 90
Paracentral lobule, 24
Parahippocampal gyrus, 24, 166, 172
Paramedian pontine reticular formation
        (PPRF), 98
Paraplegia, 56
Parasympathetic division of the automatic
        nervous system, 146, *147*
Paraventricular nuclei, 174
Paresis, 56
Parietal bone, *7*
Parietal cortice, 186
Parietal lobe, 18, 34
Parietal lobule, 22, *23*
Parieto-occipital sulcus, 18, 20, 36, *37,*
        166
Parkinson's disease, 82
Pars opercularis, 38, *39*
Pars orbitalis, 38, *39*
Pars triangularis, 38, *39*
Peduncle, 50
Pedunculopontine, 62
Perforated substance, 26, *27*
Periaqueductal gray (PAG), 62
Peripheral ganglion, 144
Peripheral lesion, 130
Petrosal sinus, *15, 17*
Phantom pain, 128
Phrenic nucleus, 56
Pia mater, 46
Picks' disease, 206
Pineal gland, 36, 150

Pituitary gland, *15*
    tumors of, 200
Planum sphenoidale, *14,* 15
Plexus, 14
Pons, *5*
    axial T1 MRI through the, 218, *219*
    at level of isthmus, 80, *81*
    at level of trapezoid body and facial
        colliculus, 76, *77*
Pontine nuclei, 62
Pontine reticulospinal tract, 58
Pontine tegmentum, 62
Position of pineal gland, *37*
Postcentral gyrus, 24, 34, *35,* 38, *39*
Postcentral sulcus, 20, 34, *35,* 38, *39*
Posterior cerebral arteries (PCAs), 180, 190
Posterior commissure, 92, 174
Posterior communicating arteries
        (PCoAs), 180
Posterior cranial fossa, 200
Posterior fontanel, *7*
Posterior horns, 10
Posterior hypothalamus, 174
Posterior limb, 170, 214
Posterior spinal arteries, *51, 53, 55, 57*
Posterolateral herniation, 50
Posteromarginal nucleus, 50, *51, 53, 55,*
        57, 128
Precentral gyrus, 24, 34, *35,* 38, *39*
Precentral sulcus, 20, 34, *35,* 38, *39*
Precommissural septal nuclei, 154
Precuneus, 24, 36, *37*
Prefrontal cortex, 154, 166
Preganglionic neuron, 144
Preoccipital notch, 18, 38, *39*
Pressure, 130, *131,* 132, *133*
Pretectal neurons, 92
Primary olfactory cortex, 88
Projectional fibers, *32,* 34
Proprioception, 130, *131, 132,* 132, *133*
Propriospinal fibers, *51, 53, 55, 57*
Prosencephalon, 4, *5*
Prosopagnosia, 172
Proximal, 2

Pterion, 6, *7*
Pulvinar of thalamus, *37*
Pupillary reflexes, 92
Putamen, *2,* 3, 154, 158, 164
    exposure of, in dissection of right
        hemisphere, putamen and
        hippocampus exposed, 170, *171*
Pyramidal decussation, 148
    caudal medulla at level of, 66, *67*
Pyramidal system, 142

Q
Quadriplegia, 56

R
Ramus, 20
Raphe nuclei (serotonin), 62
Recurrent artery of Heubner, 184
Red nucleus, *27,* 62, 150
Reflex
    consensual, 92
    direct pupillary light, 92
    loss of pupillary light, 92
Reticular formation, 62
Reticular pathways, 62
Reticulospinal tract, 58
Retinotopic, 48
Retrolenticular, 170
Rexed's laminae, 56
    of gray matter, *57*
Rhinal sulcus, 20
Rhombencephalon, 4, *5*
Right cavernous sinus, *13*
Right visual pathway, 90
Rods, 90
Rostral, 2
Rostral medulla at level of dorsal
        cochlear nucleus, 72, *73*
Rostral neuropores, 4
Rostral pons at level of locus ceruleus,
        78, *79*
Rostrum, 36
    of corpus callosum, *37*
Rubrospinal tract, 58

S
Sagittal plane, 2, *3*
Sagittal suture, *7*
Satiety center in medial hypothalamic
        area, 174
Schizophrenia, 204
Segmental pathology, 54
Sella turcica, 14
Senile brain, 34
Sensory aphasia, 40
Sensory decussation, 68, *69*
    characteristics of level of, 68
Sensory disturbances, 50
Sensory neurons, 48
Sensory symptoms, 50
Septal area, 36, *37*
Septal nuclei, 154
Septum pellucidum, 36, *37,* 154, 156
Serotonergic fibers, 170
Serotonin, 62
Sigmoid sinus, 12, *13, 15*
Skull
    base of, calvaria removed, internal as-
        pect, 116, *117*
    fractures of, 214
    median section through, internal aspect
        of the left basal portion, 118,
        119
    sutures and fontanels in neonate, 6, *7*
Somatic reflex arc, 48, *49*
Somatosensory cortex, 128
Somatosensory pathways, 134, *135*
Somatotopic, 48
Special somatic afferent (SSA) fibers, 48
Special visceral afferent (SVA) fibers, 48
Special visceral efferent (SVE) fibers, 48,
        130
Sphenoid bone, *7*
Sphenoparietal sinus, 12, *13,* 14, *15*
Sphincter pupillae, 92
Spina bifida cystica, 4
Spina bifida occulta, 4
Spinal accessory nucleus, 56
Spinal arteries, 46, 58, 182

Spinal cord, 54
  ascending pathways, 134, *135*
  blood supply for, 58, *59*
  at cervical enlargement, 56, *57*
  at high lumbar level, 52, *53*
  at high thoracic level, 54, *55*
  at lumbosacral enlargement, 50, *51*
  relation of, to meninges and vertebral column, 46, *47*
  transverse section of, showing somatic reflex arc, 48, *49*
Spinal nerves, 46, 50
  compression, 50
  relation of, to meninges and vertebral column, 46, *47*
Spinal taps, 46
Spinal trigeminal nucleus, 130
Spinoreticular, 128
Spinoreticular fibers, 128
Spinoreticulothalamic pathway, 134
Spinotectal fibers, 128
Spinothalamic tract, 52, 126, 128
Splenium, 36, 166, 212
  of corpus callosum, *27, 37*
Stenosis of the cerebral aqueduct, 10
Stoicism, 128
Straight sinus, 12, *13, 15, 17*
Stria medullaris thalami, 36, *37,* 156, 174
Striate arteries, 184
Stria terminalis, 156
Striatum, 154, 188
  forebrain at the level of, 154, *155*
Stroke, 184
Subacute combined degeneration, 52
Subarachnoid hemorrhage, 214
Subarachnoid space, 46, 216
Subcallosal area, 24
Subiculum, 170
Sublenticular, 170
Substantia gelatinosa, 50, *51, 53, 55, 57*
Substantia innominata, 154
Substantia nigra, *27,* 62, 150, 154, 158
Subthalamic nucleus, 154, 158
Subthalamus, 2, *5*

Sulcus, 18, 172
  of cerebral hemisphere, 20, *21,* 38, *39*
Superior cerebellar artery, 180
Superior cerebellar peduncle, 52, 126
Superior colliculus, *37*
  mesencephalon at level of, 84, *85*
Superior frontal gyrus, *35*
Superior frontal sulci, 20
Superior longitudinal fasciculus, 40, *41*
Superior medullary velum, 36, *37*
Superior occipitofrontal fasciculus, 156
Superior olivary nucleus, 62
Superior ophthalmic vein, 12, *13, 15*
Superior orbital fissure, 94, 98
Superior parietal lobules, 34, *35,* 38, *39*
Superior petrosal sinus, 12, *13, 15*
Superior sagittal sinus, 12, *13*
Superior temporal gyrus, *39*
Superior temporal sulcus, *39*
Suprachiasmatic nucleus, 162
Supratentorial, 2
Sutures in skull of neonate, 6, *7*
Sympathetic division, of the automatic nervous system, 144, *145*
Syringomyelia, 56

T
Tectum, *5,* 26, 188, 216
Tegmentum, 26, 64, 216, 218
  ascending pathways in, 126
Telencephalon, *2,* 3, 4, *5,* 154
  lateral ventricle of, *8, 9,* 10
Temperature, 128, *129,* 130, *131*
  impulses, 96
Temporal bone, *7*
Temporal cortex, 186
Temporal gyri, 38
Temporal lobe, 18, 172, 204
  epilepsy, 170
Temporal sulci, 20, 38
Tentorial incisure, 16, *17*
Tentorial notch, 16
Tentorium cerebelli, *3,* 14, *15,* 16, *17*
  descending herniation, 16, *17*

Thalamic fasciculus, 158
Thalamic nuclei, 160, *161*
Thalamic radiations, 166, *167*
Thalamic reticular nucleus, 158
Thalamic syndrome, 188
Thalamocortical fibers, *32*
Thalamogeniculate, 188
Thalamogeniculate arteries, 184
Thalamoperforating branches, 188
Thalamostriate vein, 12, *13*
Thalamus, 2, *2,* 3, *5,* 36, 88, 166, 188
  blood supply of, 184, *185*
  forebrain at the level of the anterior nucleus of, 156, *157*
  horizontal section of brain through, 164, *165*
Third ventricle, 4, *8, 9,* 11, 188
Tic douloureux, 96, 130
Tonotopic, 48
Tonsillar displacement, 202
Touch, 130, *131*
  discriminative, 132, *133*
  nondiscriminative, 128, *129*
Touch pressure, 132
Tract, 50
Transient ischemic attacks (TIAs), 184
Transient monocular blindness, 182
Transverse fissure, 16, 38, *39*
Transverse lesion, 52
Transverse sinuses, 12, *13, 15,* 16, *17*
Trapezoid body, pons at level of, 76, *77*
Trigeminal, 130
Trigeminal nerves, 14, 96, *97*
Trigeminal neuralgia, 96, 130
Trigeminal system, 130, *131*
Trigone, 164
Trochlear nerves, 14, 94, *95*
Trochlear nucleus, 94
Trunk (body), 36
  of corpus callosum, *37*
  somatosensory pathways for, 136, *137*
  volitional control of, 136, *137*
Tuber cinereum and infundibulum, *27*
Tumors, 172

U
Uncal herniation, 16
  syndrome, 6
Uncinate fasciculus, *32,* 40, *41*
Uncinate fits, 88
Unilateral, 2
Unilateral demyelination, 52

V
Vagus nerves, 106, *107*
Vascular accidents, 172
Velum interpositum, 164
Venous angle, 12, *13*
Venous sinuses
  dural, 14, *15*
  of dura mater, 12, *13*
Ventral area of dorsal horn, *51, 52, 53, 55, 57*
Ventral corticospinal tracts (VSCT), 126, 136, *137,* 142
Ventral funiculus, *51, 53, 55, 57*
Ventral median fissure, *51, 53, 55, 57*
Ventral pallidum, 154
Ventral posterolateral nucleus, 128, 132
Ventral root exit, *51, 53, 55, 57*
Ventral roots, 46, 50
Ventral spinocerebellar tract (VSCT), 52, 58, 120, *121,* 126
Ventral striatum, 154
Ventral tegmental area (dopamine), 62
Ventral thalamus, 162
Ventral trigeminothalamic tract, 130
Ventral white commissure, 50, *51, 53, 55, 57*
Ventricles
  lateral view of, 8, *9*
  superior view of, 10, *11*
Ventricular cavity, 64
Ventricular enlargement, 204
Ventricular system, 206
Ventrolateral funiculus, 128
Ventrolateral system, 54, 128, *129*
  fibers of, 58

Ventromedial nuclei, 162
Vermis, 36
   of cerebellum, *37*
Vertebral arteries, 14, 180, 182
Vertebral-basilar systems, 180, 190
Vertebral canal, 46
Vertebral column, relation of spinal cord
      and spinal nerves to, 46, *47*
Vestibulocochlear nerves, 102, *103*
Visual acuity, 90
Visual commissural fiber systems, 212
Visual field, 90
Visual system, blood supply of, 190, *191*

Vitamin B_{12} deficiency, 52
Volitional control
   of face and head, 140, *141*
   of limbs and trunk, 136, *137*

W
Watershed zones, 186
Wernicke's aphasia, 40
Wernicke's area, *32,* 38
White matter, 2, 34, 46, *51, 53, 55, 57*

Y
Yoke-like deficit, 128

ARAS	Ascending Reticular Activating System
ANS	Automatic Nervous System
BBB	Blood – Brain Barrier
CSF	Cerebrospinal Fluid
CVA	Cerebro vascular Accident
CVO	Circum ventricular Organ
CAT	Computerized Axial Tomography
CCT	Cuneo cerebellar Tract
DSCT	Dorsal Spino Cerebellar Tract
GSA	General Somatic Afferent
GSE	" " Efferent
GVA	" Visceral Afferent
GVE	" " Efferent
LCST	Lateral Cortico Spinal Tract
MRI	Magnetic Resonance Imaging
MCP	Middle Cerebellar Peduncle
MCA	Middle cerebral Artery
PPRF	Paramedian Pontine Reticular Formation
PAG	Peri aqueductal Gray
PCA	Posterior Cerebral Artery
PCoA	Posterior Communicating Artery
SSA	Special Somatic Afferent
SVA	" Visceral "
SVE	" " Efferent
TIA	Transient Ischemic Attack
VSCT	Ventral spino cerebellar Tract
VCST	Ventral cortico Spinal Tract